HEALTHCARE RECORDS MANAGEMENT, DISCLOSURE & RETENTION

HEALTHCARE RECORDS MANAGEMENT, DISCLOSURE & RETENTION

The Complete Legal Guide

Jonathan P. Tomes, J.D.

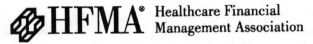HFMA® Healthcare Financial
Management Association

McGraw-Hill
New York San Francisco Washington D.C. Auckland Bogotá
Caracas Lisbon London Madrid Mexico City Milan
Montreal New Delhi San Juan Singapore
Sydney Tokyo Toronto

McGraw-Hill

A Division of The McGraw-Hill Companies

4 5 6 7 8 BRBBRB 98 1 0 9 8

ISBN:0-07-413117-6

This publication is designed to provide accurate and authoritative information in regard to the subject matter covered. It is sold with the understanding that neither the author nor the publisher is engaged in rendering legal, accounting, or other professional service. If legal advice or other expert assistance is required, the services of a competent professional person should be sought.

> *—From a declaration of Principles jointly adopted by a Committee of the American Bar Association and a Committee of Publishers.*

McGraw-Hill books are available at special quantity discounts to use as premiums and sales promotions, or for use in corporate training programs. For more information, please write to the Director of Sales, McGraw-Hill, 11 West 19th Street, New York, NY 10011. Or contact your local bookstore.

Contents

CHAPTER 2

Who Owns Medical Records?

PART II
How Do You Keep Your Medical Records?

CHAPTER 4
Which Media Can You Use to Maintain Medical Records?

CHAPTER 6

Correcting Medical Records

PART III
When Should You Refuse to Release Records and When Is Disclosure Permitted?

CHAPTER 7
Patients' Rights to Privacy

CHAPTER 8
Disclosure on Request

CHAPTER 9
Disclosure of Drug and Alcohol Abuse Records 345

CHAPTER 11
Disclosure When a Court Orders You To   394

CHAPTER 12
Disclosure for Medical Research   418

PART IV
How Do You Dispose of Your Medical Records?

CHAPTER 13
How Do You Destroy Your Medical Records?

CHAPTER 14

Disposing of Records During Acquisitions, Mergers, and Closings 451

PART V

Healthcare Business Records

CHAPTER 15

What Are Healthcare Business Records?

CHAPTER 16

Which Business Records Must You Keep and for How Long?

CHAPTER 17

What Media Can You Use for Business Records?   584

PART I

What Is a Record, Who Owns It, and What Do You Do with It?

In order to develop a good program for keeping healthcare records, we need to define our terms. What's a record? What's a medical record? Chapter 1 will provide these definitions and start you on your way to developing a good records retention program. Chapter 2 answers the question of who owns hospital and medical records, and Chapter 3 specifies which records you must keep and for how long.

What Is a Record?

Records Generally

A record is nothing more than an account of an event preserved in some medium so that it can be read at some later time. Rule 803 of the Uniform Rules of Evidence, which has been adopted by more than half of the states, focuses on business records, but its language is applicable to any record as being "a memorandum, report, record, or data compilation, in any form, of acts, events, conditions, opinions, or diagnoses, made at or near the time by, or from information transmitted by a person with knowledge."

The federal Privacy Act, 5 U.S.C. § 552a (1991), defines "record" as "any item, collection or grouping of information about an individual."

Medical Records

Some states define the term "medical record," while others merely specify what information such a record must contain. Colorado, for example, defines a medical record as

> the written or graphic documentation, sound recording, or computer record of services pertaining to medical and health care which are performed at the direction of a physician or other licensed health care provider on behalf of a patient by physicians, dentists, nurses, technicians, or other health care personnel. "Medical record" includes such diagnostic documentation as X rays, electrocardiograms, electroencephalograms, and other test results. (Colorado Revised Statutes § 18-4-412 [1991]).

Other states define related terms, such as medical information (Arizona), health records (Indiana), hospital records (Louisiana), or healthcare records (Nevada). Some states, such as North Dakota, do not define these terms as such, but require that medical records contain sufficient information to justify the diagnosis and warrant the treatment and end results.

Perhaps more important than what medical records are is what they must include. Some states provide detailed guidelines on what a medical record must contain; other states leave it up to the facility to define what a medical record comprises. In such an event, "sufficient information to justify the diagnosis and warrant the treatment and end results" probably is not sufficient both to provide proper health care and to minimize litigation losses.

Thus, to ensure that patients receive proper care and to avoid paying malpractice claims because the facility cannot document proper care, the facility must keep thorough medical records that document everything of significance. Each entry should be legible, accurate, complete, and objective, and cover all required aspects of patient care without assigning blame or covering up an adverse event. In a malpractice case, if the record does not reflect that a treatment or medication was given, it was not.

Use proper terminology for diseases and conditions such as that given in the *Terminology of the International Classification of Diseases*. Document patient behavior and other items factually, not emotionally. For example, rather than charting that a patient was extremely upset, record what he said and what his actions were.

Healthcare facilities should be cognizant of what their own states and other states require medical records to contain. Medical records managers may also wish to consult the *Accreditation Manual for Hospitals* of the Joint Commission on Accreditation of Healthcare Organizations. No jurisdiction prohibits healthcare providers from adding to a medical record information not required by a statute or regulation if the facility needs that information.

Federal Laws

Patient records of hospitals participating in Medicare must contain sufficient information to identify the patient and justify admission and hospitalization; support diagnoses; and describe the patient's progress and responses to treatment. Each record must also contain reports of physical examinations, patient's medical history, admitting diagnosis, results of consultative evaluations, documentation of infection or adverse reactions or complications, patient consent forms, patient monitoring information (i.e., medication schedules, lab reports, radiology reports), and a discharge summary that includes a final diagnosis, disposition of the case, and follow-up provisions.[1]

State Laws

ALABAMA

Alabama does not define the term "medical record," but sets forth the criteria various medical records must comprise:

The Alabama State Board of Health Division of Licensure and Certification Alabama Administrative Code r. 420-5-7.07 (1990) sets forth the criteria various *hospital medical records* must comprise

---

1. 42 C.F.R. Part 482 (1990).

- *Admission record,* either typewritten or legibly written with pen and ink, must be kept for each patient. It must include name, address, age, sex, nationality, marital status, name and address of closest relative, date of admission, date of discharge or death, and any other personal and statistical particulars required by the State Registrar of Vital Statistics on certificates of births, deaths, and stillbirths.

- *Medical and surgical record,* including the following data, when applicable:

    - Identification data (name, age, sex, referring and attending physician, etc.)

    - Complaint

    - Present illness

    - Past history

    - Family history

    - Review of systems

    - Physical examination

    - Provisional diagnosis

    - Clinical laboratory reports

    - X-ray reports

    - Consultations

    - Treatment (medical and surgical)

    - Operative report

    - Tissue report

    - Progress notes

    - Final diagnosis

    - Discharge summary on cases over 48 hours

    - Autopsy findings, if performed

- *Obstetrical record,* which must include the prenatal record (medical and obstetric history), labor record (observation and proceeding during labor), and postpartum record

- *Newborn record,* including the birth record and physical examination of the infant and the nurses' record (number and character of stools, bleeding from the umbilical cord, type and time of feeding, reaction of infant to feedings, and other such pertinent information)

- *Physician's orders,* which must be written on a specific form for each patient and signed or initialed by the attending physician. Verbal or telephone orders are considered to be in writing when dictated by the attending physician and later signed or initialed by him or her.

- *Nurses' record.* Personal services rendered and observations that may be of importance to the attending physician or to nursing personnel should be noted on the nurses' record.

The Alabama State Board of Health Division of Licensure and Certification Alabama Administrative Code r. 420-5-10-.16 (1988) also specifies requirements for nursing home medical records. The medical record should contain sufficient information to identify the patient clearly, to justify the diagnosis and treatment, and to document the results accurately. All medical records should contain the following general categories of data:

- *Admission record,* either typewritten or legibly written with pen and ink, for each patient, including the patient's name, address, date of birth, sex, nationality, marital status, religion, name and address and telephone number of sponsor and nearest relative, date of admission, date of discharge, and the name of the attending physician

- *Current medical evaluation* for each patient, including medical history, physical examination, mental status, diagnosis, and estimation of rehabilitation potential

- *Treatment records,* including

    - Physician orders for medications, treatments, diet, and other care and/or services to be rendered

    - Observations and progress notes

    - Reports of treatments and clinical findings

    - Medication administration record and treatment record

    - Documented evidence of an appropriate plan of treatment established within 30 days of admission by all disciplines involved in the care of the patient, with documentation of reviews and updates of the plan

    - Discharge summary completed by the physician to include final diagnosis, prognosis, and a summary of the course of prior treatment

    - Copies of transfer sheets received on admission and discharge

    - Signed and dated laboratory and x-ray reports

    - Signed and dated reports and evaluation of services and consultations from other health professionals, i.e., dental workers, social workers, activities workers, dietitians, mental health personnel, physical thera-pists, occupational therapists

- Medications given to the patient on discharge

- Copies of official death certificates when applicable

- *Care plans.* In coordination with other health professionals, a nursing home must develop a written patient care plan and maintain it in the medical record so as to reflect

  - Any changes in the patient's condition

  - Any accidents or injuries involving the patient

  - Care and/or services provided

  - Response to care provided

  - Changes in nutritional and hydration status, etc.

  - Administration of blood or blood products to include appropriate documentation of unification of blood type, patient condition (i.e., vital signs) prior to, during and after administration and any indica-tion of reactions

ALASKA

Alaska does not define a medical record, but regulations of the Department of Health and Social Services specify what information must be included in medical records.[2]

Inpatient medical records shall contain the following information, as appropriate:

- Identification sheet including

  - Patient's name

  - Medical record number

  - Patient's address on admission

  - Patient's date of birth

  - Patient's sex

  - Patient's marital status

  - Patient's religious preference

---

2. *See* Alaska Administrative Code tit. 7, § 12.425 (April 1988) (medical records for birth centers); *Id.* tit. 7, § 12.530 (medical records for home health agencies); and *Id.* tit. 7, § 12.770 (all other facilities except intermediate care facilities for the mentally retarded).

- Date of admission
- Name, address, and telephone number of a contact person
- Name of the patient's attending physician
- Initial diagnostic impression
- Date of discharge and final diagnosis
- Source of payment

- Medical and psychiatric history and examination
- Consultation reports, dental records, and reports of special studies
- Order sheet that includes medication, treatment, and diet orders signed by a physician
- Nurses' notes, which must include
  - Accurate record of care given
  - Record of pertinent observations and response to treatment, including psychosocial and physical manifestations
  - Assessment at the time of admission
  - Discharge plan
  - Name, dosage, and time of administration of medication or treatment; route of administration; site of injection, if other than by oral administration; patient's response; and signature of the person who administered the medication or treatment
  - Record of any restraint used, showing the duration of usage
- Court orders relevant to involuntary treatment
- Laboratory reports
- X-ray reports
- Consent forms
- Operative report on inpatient and outpatient surgery including preoperative and postoperative diagnosis, description of findings, techniques used, and tissue removed or altered, if appropriate[3]

The regulation adds that in *outpatient departments* that are organized by clinics, the following information must be available:

---

3. Alaska Administrative Code tit. 7, § 12.770 (c) (April 1988).

- Patient's identification sheet

- History and physical examination

- Physician's orders

- Any laboratory and other diagnostic tests, diagnosis, and treatment

- Disposition

- Outpatient records of other than organized outpatient clinics

If outpatient services are provided in other than an organized outpatient clinic, the following information shall be available:

- Patient's identification

- Information pertaining to the patient's chief complaint including, but not limited to, physician's orders, treatment or service provided, and disposition

The *emergency services* record must contain the following:

- Patient identification

- Record of any treatment patient received prior to arrival

- History of disease or injury

- Physical findings

- Laboratory and x-ray reports, if applicable

- Diagnosis

- Record of treatment

- Disposition

- Name of physician who saw patient in the emergency room

ARIZONA

Arizona's definition of "medical information" includes "all clinical records, medical reports, laboratory statements or reports, any file, film, record or report or oral statement relating to diagnostic findings and treatment of patients, as well as information relating to contacts, suspects and associates of communicable disease patients."[4]

---

4. Arizona Compilation Administrative Rules and Regulations 9-1-311 (1977).

ARKANSAS

According to the Arkansas Register, Part 6, § 1, *hospital* medical record content includes

- Identification data:
    - Patient's full name and maiden name, if applicable
    - Patient's address, telephone number, and occupation
    - Date of birth
    - Age
    - Sex
    - Race
    - Religion
    - Marital status
    - Dates and time of admission and of discharge
    - Full name of physician (and, if necessary, address and telephone number)
    - Name and address of nearest relative or person or agency responsible for patient, and occupation of responsible party
    - Name, address, and telephone number of person(s) to notify in case of emergency
    - Medical record number
    - General consent for medical treatment and care signed by the patient or legal guardian

    Clinical reports must record the following:

- History and physical examination (HPE) performed within 48 hours of the patient's admission to the facility and placed in the patient's record. The HPE must be documented by the attending physician and must contain
    - Family medical history and review of systems (respiratory, circulatory, etc.). If noncontributory, the record should reflect such.
    - Past (medical) history
    - Chief complaint(s)—brief statement of nature and duration of the symptoms that caused the patient to seek medical attention as stated in the patient's own words
    - Present illness with dates or approximate dates of onset

- Physical examination report

- Provisional or admitting diagnosis(es)

- If a patient is readmitted within 30 days with the same condition, an interval note may be used by the physician. The interval notes should include any changes that have taken place in the patient's HPE since the previous stay and the present reason for the patient's admission.

- *Short stay medical records* are acceptable in cases of a minor nature, which require less than 48 hours' hospitalization, with the exception of deaths and obstetrical cases. The short form should include identification data, pertinent physical findings, description of the patient's condition, summary of treatment given, and any other information necessary to justify the diagnosis(es) and treatment.

- *Progress notes* must be recorded, dated, and signed by the physician. The frequency of these notes is determined by the condition of the patient. Dictated progress notes are acceptable, if they are dictated by the attending physician, transcribed by the transcriptionist, and placed on the patient's medical record within 24 hours to 48 hours of dictation.

- *Treatment orders* must be recorded, dated, and signed by the attending physician. Verbal orders are acceptable, if they are recorded by the appropriate personnel (registered pharmacist or licensed nurses) and cosigned by the physician within 24 hours. Other professionals, such as physical therapists, may take verbal orders for patient treatments when nursing personnel are not available to coordinate services.

- *A discharge summary* recapitulating the significant findings and events of the patient's hospitalization and his/her condition on discharge must be documented by the attending physician within 20 days of the patient's discharge. The final diagnosis shall be stated in the discharge summary. If the patient dies, the date, time, and cause of the patient's death must be stated in the discharge summary and death note. A physician must pronounce the patient dead and document the required information.

- *Autopsy findings* must be documented in complete protocol within 60 days and the provisional anatomical diagnosis recorded within 72 hours. A signed authorization for autopsy must be obtained from the next of kin and documented in the medical record before an autopsy is performed.

- *Diagnostic and other reports.* Original, signed diagnostic reports (laboratory, x rays, electrocardiographs [EKGs], fetal monitoring, electroencephalograms [EEGs]) must be filed in the patient's medical record, and physicians' orders must accompany all treatment procedures. Reports of ancillary services (dietary, physical therapy, respiratory therapy, and social services) must be included in the patient's medical record if ordered by the physician. Reports of medical consultation, if ordered by the attending physician, must also be included in the patient's medical record within time frames established by the medical staff of the facility. The normal and customary time for consultant reports is 48 hours. An individualized nursing care plan must be developed for each patient and made a part of the permanent medical record. In addition, a medication administration record (MAR) must be maintained documenting the date, time, dosage, and manner of administration of all medications. The initials of the nurse administering the medication must also be recorded. If a MAR is not utilized by the facility, documentation must be reflected in the nurses' notes.

In addition to the general record content requirements, facilities are required to maintain *surgical, obstetric, and newborn records.*

A specific consent for *surgery* must be documented prior to the surgical procedure's being performed, except in cases of emergency. This consent must include the date, time, and signatures of the patient, physician, and witness. (Abbreviations are not acceptable.) A history and physical examination (HPE) on admission containing pertinent medical history and physical findings must be documented by the attending physician on the patient's medical record prior to surgery. In cases of emergency surgery, an abbreviated physical examination and a brief description of why the surgery is needed should be written by the physician.

A complete *anesthesia report,* including pre-evaluation and post–follow-up, must be documented by the anesthesiologist and/or certified registered nurse anesthetist (CRNA). The pre- and postanesthesia evaluations should be dated and timed and should include the following:

- Preoperative anesthesia evaluation (completed prior to the patient's surgery)

- Report of anesthesia (must be cosigned by a physician if completed by a CRNA)

- Postanesthesia evaluation (must be documented in the medical record within at least three to 48 hours of the patient's surgery)

- A postanesthesia care unit record or recovery room record, if applicable

- An individualized operative report must be written or dictated by the physician immediately following surgery and must describe in detail techniques, findings, pre- and postoperative diagnosis, and tissues removed. A signed pathology report of either macroscopic or microscopic examinations on all tissue surgically removed must also be recorded. A specific list of tissues that are exempt from pathological examination should be developed by the medical staff and included in the medical staff rules and regulations.

Outpatient surgery records are required to contain the same information, with the exception of a complete HPE if a local anesthesia is administered. A brief history and physical evaluation, pertinent to the surgical procedure that the patient is to have, will suffice. A discharge note is not required if discharge criteria have been developed and approved by the medical staff, and documented by the nursing staff on the individual patient records.

Obstetrical records must contain

- A pertinent prenatal record, updated on admission, or an HPE signed by the physician, available on the patient's admission and maintained in the patient's medical record

- A labor and delivery record for every obstetrical patient, and documentation of the patient's recovery from delivery. Nurses' postpartum record or graphics and nurses' notes also must be maintained.

A *newborn* HPE must be completed by the physician within 24 hours of birth and must include the following additional data:

- History of the newborn delivery (sex, date of birth, type of delivery, and anesthesia given the mother during labor and delivery)

- Physical examination (weight, date, time of birth, and condition of infant after birth)

- Consent for circumcision (if applicable)

- A discharge note or summary must be documented by the physician describing the condition of the newborn at discharge, and follow-up instructions given to the mother. A procedure note for circumcision describing technique, blood loss, complications, and anesthesia, if used, shall be documented by the physician prior to the newborn's discharge.

Outpatient records completed for each outpatient must include the following:

- HPE of the patient (not applicable if for diagnostic services and/or outpatient therapy services)

- Orders and reports of diagnostic services and outpatient therapy services

- Patient's diagnosis and summary of treatment received recorded by the attending physician

- Documentation of any medications administered

- Progress notes for subsequent clinic visits recorded by applicable disciplines (practitioner)

- Outpatient surgery record requirements

An *emergency room record* must be completed for each patient who seeks treatment at the emergency room. This record must contain the following:

- Patient identification

- Date and the following times

- Admission

- When physician was contacted by phone

- Physician's arrival

- Discharge

- History (when the injury or onset of symptoms occurred)

- Vital signs

- Nurses' assessment and physical findings

- Diagnosis (as stated by the physician)

- Record of treatment, including documentation of verbal orders and drug quantities administered, with initials of person(s) administering the drugs. Also, type and amount of local anesthetic, if administered.

- Diagnostic reports with specific orders noted

- Instructions to patient for follow-up care (e.g., do not drive after receiving sedatives, return to physician's office for removal of sutures in one week)

- Disposition of case (how the patient left, condition of the patient on discharge, and whether he/she was accompanied)

- Signature of patient or his/her representative

- Physician's signature and date

Emergency room records must be completed immediately, or if the physician treats a patient by telephone orders, they must be completed within 24 hours. When a patient is admitted as an inpatient on an emergency room visit, the medical record of the emergency room visit must be integrated with the patient's overall medical record.

A record of every patient admitted to an *observation* bed or unit must be maintained and must contain the following information:

- Identification data

- Nursing admission assessment by a registered nurse

- Nurses' observations

- Physician's assessment of the patient

- Physician's order for admission and discharge from the unit and any orders for treatment

- Record of any treatment received (diagnostic tests, medication)

The basic medical record requirements for *psychiatric patients* are the same as for other patient records. However, these records must also include:

- Identification data, which shall include the patient's legal status (e.g., legally incompetent) on the record's face sheet

- Proper consent or authority for admission

- Provisional diagnosis, specifying both the intercurrent disease and the psychiatric diagnosis

- Statements and reasons for admission given by family and by others, as well as the patient, preferably verbatim, with informant identified

- Psychiatric evaluation, completed by the attending psychiatrist, including the following:

  - Patient's chief complaints and/or reaction to hospitalization, recorded in patient's own words, if possible

  - History of present illness including onset, and reasons for current admission

  - History of any psychiatric problems and treatment, including a record of patient's activities (social, educational, vocational, interpersonal, and family relationships)

  - Mental status, including, at least, attitude and general behavior; affect; stream of mental activity; presence or absence of delusions and hallucinations; estimate of intellectual functions; judgment; and assessment of orientation and memory

  - Strengths, such as knowledge, interests, skills, aptitudes, experience, education, and employment status

  - Nonpsychiatric medical history and past treatment

  - Diagnostic impressions and recommendations

  - Physical examination documented by a physician and including a neurological examination

  - Social service records, including reports of interviews with patients, family members, and others, must be included for each admission, as well as reports of consultation, psychological evaluations, reports of electroencephalograms, dental records, and reports of special studies, when applicable

- *Individual comprehensive treatment plan* must be included in the medical record. The planning of this treatment plan should involve all staff who have contact with the patient and should include, as a minimum:

  - Problems and needs relevant to admission and discharge as identified in the various assessments, expressed in behavioral and descriptive terms

  - Strengths and assets including skills and interests

  - Problems, both physical and mental, that require therapeutic intervention by the facility staff

  - Goals and objectives describing action or behavior to be achieved. Such goals and objectives should be relevant, observable, and measurable.

  - Treatment modalities, individualized in relation to patient's needs

  - Evidence of patient involvement in the formulation of the plan

- *Master treatment plans* cross-referenced with other treatment plans, such as nursing and activity therapy, and multidisciplinary treatment plans should include realistic discharge and aftercare plans.

- *Treatment* received by the patient must be documented in such a manner and with such frequency as to assure that all active therapeutic efforts, such as individual and group psychotherapy, drug therapy, milieu therapy, occupational therapy, industrial or work therapy, nursing care and other therapeutic interventions, are included. Progress notes must be recorded by the physician, nurse, social worker, and others involved in active treatment modalities at least weekly for the first two months and at least once a month thereafter and must contain recommendations for revisions in the treatment plan, when indicated, as well as previous assessment of the patient's progress.

- *Discharge summary* including a recapitulation of the patient's hospitalization and recommendations from appropriate services concerning follow-up aftercare, as well as a brief summary of the patient's condition on discharge. In addition, the psychiatric diagnosis contained in the final diagnosis and included in the discharge summary must be written in the terminology of American Psychiatric Association's *Diagnostic and Statistical Manual of Mental Disorders (DSM-III)*.

CALIFORNIA

California defines "medical information" as any individually identifiable information in possession of or derived from a provider of health care regarding a patient's medical history, mental or physical condition, or treatment.[5] California defines "patient records" as records in any form or medium maintained by, or in the custody or control of, a healthcare provider and relating to the health history, diagnosis, or condition of a patient, or relating to treatment provided or proposed to be provided to the patient. Patient records include only records pertaining to the patient requesting the records or whose representative requests the records.[6] Patient records do not include information given in confidence to a healthcare provider by a person other than another healthcare provider or the patient.

California Code Regulations tit. 22, § 70749(c) (1991) specifies that a general *acute care hospital* inpatient medical record must contain

- Inpatient and outpatient hospital records:
  - Identification sheets including at least the following
    - Name
    - Address on admission
    - Identification number (if applicable), such as
      - Social Security number
      - Medicare number
      - Medi-Cal number
    - Age
    - Sex
    - Marital status
    - Religion
    - Date of admission
    - Date of discharge
    - Name, address, and telephone number of person or agency responsible for patient
    - Name of attending physician
    - Initial diagnostic impression
    - Discharge and final diagnosis
  - History and physical examination

---

5. California Civil Code § 56.05(b) (1991).
6. California Health & Safety Code § 1795.10(d) (1991).

- Consultation reports

- Order sheet including medication, treatment, and diet orders

- Progress notes, including current or working diagnosis

- Nurses' notes, which must include at least the following:

  - Concise and accurate record of nursing care administered

  - Record of pertinent observations, including psychosocial and physical manifestations as well as incidents and unusual occurrences, and relevant nursing interpretation of such observations

  - Name, dosage, and time of administration of medications and treatment. Route of administration and site of injection must be recorded if other than by oral administration.

  - Record of type of restraint and time of application and removal. The time of application and removal are not required for soft tie restraints used for support and protection of the patient.

- Vital sign sheet

- Reports of all laboratory tests performed

- Reports of all x-ray tests performed

- Consent forms, when applicable

- Anesthesia record, including preoperative diagnosis, if anesthesia has been administered

- Operative report including preoperative and postoperative diagnosis, description of findings, technique used, tissue removed or altered, if surgery was performed

- Pathology report if tissue or body fluid was removed

- Labor record, if applicable

- Delivery record, if applicable

- A discharge summary, which must briefly recapitulate the significant findings and events of the patient's hospitalization, condition on discharge and the recommendations and arrangements for future care

- In addition, the inpatient medical record must also contain the following information when applicable:

  - Surgical service records

  - Drug order records

  - Emergency service records

- Dental service records

- Psychiatric unit records, including legal authorization for admission

- Outpatient medical records must contain the same information as inpatient records, when applicable.

Acute psychiatric hospitals must maintain medical records containing the same general information as hospital inpatient medical records, when applicable, as well as the following additional items:

- Hospital admission number

- Name of patient's medical staff member responsible for care

- Disposition

- Psychiatric history

- Legal authorization for admission

- Treatment plan

Skilled nursing facilities must maintain patient health records that include the following items:

- Admission record, including

  - Name and social security number

  - Current address

  - Age and date of birth

  - Sex

  - Date of admission

  - Date of discharge

  - Name, address, and telephone number of guardian, authorized representative, person or agency responsible for patient, and the next of kin

  - Name, address, and telephone number of attending physician and the name, address, and telephone number of the podiatrist, dentist, or clinical psychologist, if such practitioner is primarily responsible for the treatment of the patient

  - Name, address, and telephone number of the designated alternate physician

  - Admission diagnoses, known allergies, and final diagnoses

  - Medicare and Medi-Cal numbers, when appropriate

- Inventory of jewelry, items of furniture, radios, televisions, other appliances, prosthetic and orthopedic devices, and any other valuable items identified by the patient, family, or authorized representative. The inventory list must be signed by a representative of the facility and the patient or the patient's authorized representative with one copy retained by each.

- Current report of physical examination, and evidence of tuberculosis screening

- Current diagnoses

- Correctly recapitulated physician orders, including drugs, treatment and diet orders, and progress notes, signed and dated on each visit

- Nurses' notes, signed and dated, including

  - Records made by nurse assistants, after proper instruction, including care and treatment of the patient as well as narrative notes of observation of the patient

  - Nurses' progress notes written by licensed nurses as often as the patient's condition warrants. Weekly nurses' progress notes must be written by licensed nurses on each patient and must be specific to the patient's needs, the patient care plan, and the patient's response to care and treatments.

- Name, dosage, and time of administration of drugs and the route of administration or site of injection, if other than oral. The person administering the dose must record both initials and the time of administration. Medication and treatment records must also contain the name and professional title of staff signing by initials.

- Justification for the results of the administration of all PRN medications and the withholding of scheduled medications

- Record of type of restraint and time of application and removal

- Medications and treatments administered and recorded as prescribed

- Documentation of oxygen administration

- Temperature, pulse, respiration, and blood pressure notations when indicated

- Laboratory reports of all tests prescribed and completed

- Reports of all x rays prescribed and completed

- Progress notes written and dated by the activity leader (at least quarterly)

- Discharge planning notes when applicable

- Observation and information pertinent to the patient's diet recorded in the patient's health record by the dietitian, nurse, or food service supervisor

- Records of each treatment given by the therapist, weekly progress notes, and a record of therapy reports to the physician

- Progress notes written by the social service worker if the patient is receiving social services

- Consent forms for prescribed treatment and medication not included in the admission consent for care

- Condition and diagnoses of the patient at time of discharge or final disposition

- Copy of the transfer form when the patient is transferred to another health facility

- Name, complete address, and telephone number where the patient was transferred on discharge from the facility

Intermediate care facilities must maintain patient health records containing the same general information as skilled nursing facility records, when applicable. In addition, intermediate care facilities must maintain patient health records for special rehabilitative program services.[7]

Special program health records must include

- List of the patient's problems or needs, as identified from the individual assessment

- Behavioral objectives for resolving problems or meeting needs of the patient. These objectives must be measurable, observable, within time frames, and subject to frequent review and updating.

- Statement of the plan for how the behavioral objectives will be met. The statement must include resources to be used, frequency of plan review and updating, and persons responsible for carrying out plans.

- Progress notes written by all members of the staff providing program services to the patient, specific to the needs or problems of the patient, and specific to the patient's program objectives and plans

- Summary of the progress of the patient in the program, appropriateness of program objectives, success or failure of the plan, and any other pertinent information regarding the patient's program

---

7. California Code Regulations tit. 22, § 73423 (1991). Special Subacute Psychiatric Program Services, *Id*. tit. 22, § 72431, and any other special program services. *Id*. tit. 22, § 73439.

Intermediate care facilities for the *developmentally disabled*—nursing must maintain unit client records,[8] including the following items:

- Admission record

- Client assessment as follows

    - Medical, social, and psychological evaluations.

    - Review and update of initial assessments

    - Interdisciplinary professional staff/team assessment

    - Nursing evaluation/assessment of health status

    - Assessment of bowel and bladder functions

    - Recreational interests

    - Assessment of behavior

    - Nutritional status, if food is refused

- Physical examination

- Dental examination

- Integrated and coordinated individual service plan developed by the interdisciplinary professional staff/team with input from direct-care staff

- Recreational activity plan

- Health care plan

- Measures to prevent decubitus ulcers, contractures, and deformities

- Bowel and bladder training plan, if applicable

- Behavior management plan, if applicable

- Discharge plan, when anticipated

- Review and update of individual service plan

- Progress notes as required

- Notification of medication errors and adverse reactions to the practitioner who ordered the drug

- Dental records

- Medication history

- All diagnostic and therapeutic prescriptions including diet and medications

---

8. *Id.* tit. 22, § 73928.

- Medication and treatment administration records

- Weight and height records

- Vital signs and other flow sheet records, if ordered

- Restraint records

- Developmental, medical, and psychiatric diagnoses comprising all admitting, concurrent, and discharge conditions, including allergies

- Discharge summary of treatment, including goals achieved and not achieved, and healthcare treatment prepared by the responsible practitioners

- Consent(s) to treatment

- An inventory, made upon admission and discharge, of all client's valuables, including items of jewelry, items of furniture, radios, televisions, other appliances, prosthetic and orthopedic devices, and any other valuable items identified by client, family, or authorized representative. The inventory list must be signed by a representative of the facility and the client or the client's authorized representative with one copy retained by each.

Intermediate care facilities for the *developmentally disabled—habilitative* must maintain similar unit client records,[9] including an admission record.

Referral services must maintain patient records containing patient's name and home address; age; client's name, if other than patient, and home address; diagnosis, disabilities, name of attending physician; amount of all fees, deposits, and remuneration received by the referral service from the client, and date of receipt; and facility chosen by the client.[10] The referral service must enter the name of each facility to which a client is referred in the referral service patient record.[11]

Home health agencies must maintain patient health records,[12] including the following items:

- Admission record including

  - Name and social security number

  - Current address

  - Age and date of birth

  - Sex

---

9. *Id.* § 76927.
10. *Id.* § 74211(a).
11. *Id.* § 74309.
12. *Id.* § 74735.

- Occupation or former occupation

- Date of admission and source of referral

- Date of discharge from referring facility, if applicable

- Name, address, and telephone number of person or agency responsible for patient and next of kin

- Name, address, and telephone number of attending physician

- Admission and subsequent diagnosis and known allergies

- Diagnosis and conditions with notation of those relevant to the plan of treatment

- Plan of treatment

- Statement of goals

- Allergies and known untoward reactions to drugs and food. This information must be given such prominence in the record that it cannot be missed by any agency personnel who have reasons to provide food or medication to the patient.

- Medication and treatment orders, diet orders, orders for other therapeutic services, including the frequency of visits for nursing, physical, occupational or speech therapy, social services, or other services

- Special side effects of certain medications and treatments requiring special precautions must be indicated.

- Degree of functional activity allowed

- Rehabilitation plan, if applicable

- Medical supplies and appliances or special devices needed

- Clinical notes dictated or written on the day of service by personnel rendering such service. Clinical notes must also be signed and incorporated into the patient's health record at least weekly, and must include

  - Concise and accurate record of care and treatment administered

  - Record of pertinent observations of the patient including psychosocial and physical manifestations as well as specific observations to be brought to the immediate attention of the physician. Observations must be recorded with sufficient frequency to indicate progress in achieving goals of the plan of treatment and changes in status that occur in the patient.

  - Evidence of coordination of services when patient is receiving more than one service

- Name, dosage, and time of administration of medications and treatments. Route of medication administration and site of injection must be recorded, except if by oral administration.

- Laboratory and x-ray reports, if applicable

- Treatment consent forms

- Discharge notes and summary by all professional personnel, including

  - Summary of patient's physical, mental, and emotional status at the time of discharge

  - Method of initiation of discharge (i.e., by physician, agency, or patient/family)

  - Date and reason for termination of service

  - Extent to which treatment goals were attained

  - Referrals made, if indicated

  - Documentation of notification of the termination of services to patient, family, and physician

Primary care clinics and *psychology clinics* also must maintain patient health records,[13] including an admission record for each patient.

Intermediate care facilities for the *developmentally disabled* must maintain a record for each client,[14] containing the following items:

- Individual program plan

- Report(s) of the preadmission evaluation(s)

- Reports of histories and previous evaluations

- Statement of the client's developmental potential and service needs that can be used as basis for programming and placement potential

- Drug and treatment orders

- Diet orders

- Comprehensive evaluation and individual program plan designed by an interdisciplinary team

- Reports of accidents, seizures, illnesses, and immunizations

- Records of all periods of restraint, with justification and authorization for each

---

13. *Id.* § 75055.
14. *Id.* § 76561.

- Progress notes written by members of the interdisciplinary team at least monthly, in addition to progress notes written by members of the other disciplines who are requested to assess the client

- Medications and treatments prescribed and recorded as given

- Annual physical examination

- Temperature, pulse, and respiration where indicated

- Reports of all laboratory tests and x rays ordered

- Discharge summary, including condition, diagnosis, and final disposition

- Summary of findings, progress, and plans recorded at time of permanent release or transfer

- Physicians' orders, including drug, treatment, and diet orders signed on each visit, with physicians' orders recapitulated as appropriate

- Consent forms for prescribed treatment and medication

- Inventory of all client's valuables made upon admission and discharge. The inventory list must be signed by a representative of the facility and the client or the client's authorized representative with one copy retained by each.

- Name, dosage, and time of administration of drugs, the route of administration, if other than oral, and site of injection

- Justification for the results of the administration of all PRN medications and withholding of scheduled medications

- Nursing progress notes for specific medical episodes

- Program staff documentation, including

    - List of the client's problems or needs, as identified from the individual assessment

    - Program objectives for resolving problems or meeting needs of the client. These objectives must be measurable, observable, within time frames, and subject to frequent review and updating.

    - Written plan for meeting the program objectives, noting resources to be used, frequency of plan review and updating, persons responsible for carrying out the plan, and evaluation criteria

    - Summary of the progress of the client, written at least monthly, evaluating the program objectives and the success or failure of the plan, as well as any other pertinent information

    - Temperature, intake of food and liquid, restraint observation, behavior counts, and other similar items must be recorded in a timely manner using a flow chart or other method that meets the approval of the Department.

- Height and weight, as required

- Client's admission record

Psychiatric health facilities must maintain patient health records containing the same general information as hospital inpatient medical records, when applicable,[15] as well as the following additional items:

- Disposition, including aftercare arrangements

- Mental status of patient

- Dated and signed observations and progress notes recorded as often as the patient's condition warrants by the person responsible for the care of the patient

- Any necessary legal authorization for admission

- Social service evaluation, if applicable

- Psychological evaluation, if applicable

- Rehabilitation evaluation, if applicable

- Interdisciplinary treatment plan

- Progress notes including the patient's response to medication and treatment rendered and observation(s) of patient by all members of treatment team providing services to the patient

- Medication records including name, dosage, and time of administration of medications and treatments given. The route of administration and site of injection must be recorded if other than by oral administration.

- Treatment records including group and individual psychotherapy, occupational therapy, recreational or other therapeutic activities provided

- All dental records, if applicable

- Reports of all cardiographic or encephalographic tests performed

- Reports of special studies ordered

- Acknowledgment in writing of patient's rights, signed by patient or person responsible for the patient; or denial of patient rights documentation

---

15. *Id.* § 77141.

Adult day health centers must maintain a standard health record for each participant, including the following items:

- Identifying information including name, address, telephone number, birth date, social security and Medi-Cal numbers; directions between home and adult day health center; name, address, and telephone number of personal physician; name, address, and telephone number of responsible person

- Admission data including referral source, reason for application as given by referral source, participant and family or others, number of days scheduled for attendance, method of transportation, and fee

- Daily records of participant's attendance and services utilized, including transportation

- Records of referrals to other providers, and dates and substance of communication with the participant's physician, family members, and other persons providing assistance

- Medication records

- Progress notes by providers of basic services

- Assessment of the participant by the multidisciplinary team

- Record of physician's health examination of participant

- Individual plan of care

- Written clearance by a physician for participants who have been absent for 30 days due to illness[16]

Chemical dependency recovery hospitals (CDRH) must maintain patient health records containing the same general information as hospital inpatient medical records, when applicable,[17] and including the following additional items:

- Progress notes, including at least pertinent observations of the patient by the staff responsible for the implementation of the recovery plan

- Records including pertinent observations of the patient by staff responsible for the patient's care

- Signed consent forms, including refusal of medication and treatment and authorization for release of information, if requested

- Discharge summary, including

---

16. *Id.* § 78431.
17. *Id.* § 79349(a).

- All final diagnoses, including complications of care, stated in standard medical terminology without abbreviations

- All procedures performed

- Brief recapitulation of significant findings and events of the patient's hospitalization

- Critical evaluation of patient's progress in attaining goals of the individual recovery plan

- Condition on discharge

- Instructions and arrangements for aftercare

- Discharge medications, if any

  - Copy of the transfer information and, upon discharge, the individual recovery plan

Under Title 8, Industrial Relations, California Code of Regulations section 3204(c)(6) (1991), all employers must maintain a medical record for each employee. This record concerns the health status of the employee and is made or maintained by a physician, nurse, or other healthcare personnel, or technician. An employee medical record includes

- Medical and employment questionnaires or histories (including job description and occupational exposures)

- Results of medical examinations (pre-employment, preassignment, periodic, or episodic) and laboratory tests (including chest and other x-ray examinations done for the purposes of establishing a baseline or detecting occupational illness, and all biological monitoring not defined as an "employee exposure record")

- Medical opinions, diagnoses, progress notes, and recommendations

- First-aid records

- Descriptions of treatments and prescriptions

- Employee medical complaints

An employee medical record does not include medical information in the form of physical specimens (e.g., blood or urine samples), records concerning health insurance claims, records created solely in preparation for litigation (which are protected from discovery under the applicable rules of procedure or evidence), or records concerning voluntary employee assistance programs (alcohol, drug abuse, or personal counseling programs).

COLORADO

Colorado defines "medical record" as

> the written or graphic documentation, sound recording, or computer record of services pertaining to medical and health care which are performed at the direction of a physician or other licensed health care provider on behalf of a patient by physicians, dentists, nurses, technicians, or other health care personnel. "Medical record" includes such diagnostic documentation as X rays, electrocardiograms, electroencephalograms, and other test results.[18]

6 Code of Colorado Regulations § 1011-1 for *general hospitals* states that a complete medical record must include

- Admission and discharge record
  - Date and time of admission and discharge
  - Adequate identification and sociological data
  - Admission diagnosis, final diagnosis, secondary diagnosis, and complications
  - Operative procedures
  - Condition on discharge
  - Signature of attending physician
- Medical-surgical data
  - Chief complaint and present illness
  - Past, family, and personal history
  - Physical examination reports
  - Provisional diagnosis
  - Reports of any special examinations
  - Reports of consultations
  - Treatment and progress notes
  - Complete surgical and dental reports
  - Condition on discharge
  - Final diagnosis
  - Autopsy protocol
  - Discharge summary

---

18. Colorado Revised Statutes § 18-4-412 (1990).

- Signed permissions for procedures
- Surgical records, which must include, in addition to the foregoing
  - History
  - Physical and special examinations
  - Diagnosis recorded prior to the operation
  - Anesthesia record, including postanesthetic condition
  - Complete description of operative procedures and findings including postoperative diagnosis
  - Pathologist's report on all tissues removed

Obstetric records must include

- Record of obstetric history and prenatal care, including blood serology and RH factor determination
- Admission obstetrical examination report describing condition of mother and fetus
- Complete description of progress of labor and delivery, including reason for induction and operative procedures
- Records of anesthesia, analgesia, and medications given in the course of labor and delivery
- Records of fetal heart rate and vital signs
- Signed report of consultants
- Names of assistants present during delivery
- Progress notes, including descriptions of involution of uterus, type of lochia, condition of breast and nipple
- Report of condition of infant following delivery
- Newborn records

Newborns' records must contain:

- Date and time of birth, weight and length, period of gestation, sex
- Parents' names and addresses
- Type of identification
- Description of complications of pregnancy or delivery
- Condition at birth

- Record of prophylactic instillation into each eye

- Results of PKU tests

- Report of initial physical examination

- Progress notes including temperature, weight, and feeding charts

- Condition of eyes and umbilical cord

- Number, consistency, and color of stools

- Condition and color of skin

- Motor behavior

CONNECTICUT

Connecticut Public Health Code § 19-13-D3 (d) (3) governs medical records.

All medical records must include proper identification data; the clinical records must include sufficient information including progress notes to justify the diagnosis and warrant the treatment; doctor's orders, nurses' notes, and all entries must be signed by the person responsible.

A complete *obstetrics record* will include such information as may be required by the commissioner of health services and include all items necessary to fill out a death certificate for the mother and all items necessary to fill out a birth certificate or a death certificate for the baby.

According to section 19-13-D8t (o) of the Public Health Code, January 30, 1990, chronic and *convalescent nursing homes* and rest homes with nursing supervision medical records must include

- Patient identification data including

  - Name

  - Date of admission

  - Most recent address prior to admission

  - Date of birth

  - Sex

  - Marital status

  - Religion

  - Referral source

  - Medicare/Medicaid number(s) or other insurance numbers

  - Next of kin or guardian

- Address and telephone number
- Name of patient's personal physician
- Signed and dated admission history and reports of physical examination
- Signed and dated hospital discharge summary, if applicable
- Signed and dated transfer form, if applicable
- Complete medical diagnosis
- All initial and subsequent orders by the physician
- Patient assessment, completed within seven days of admission, including
  - Health history
  - Physical, mental, and social status
  - Evaluation of problems
  - Rehabilitation potential
- Patient care plan
- Record of visits and progress notes by the physician
- Nurses' notes including:
  - Current condition
  - Changes in patient condition
  - Treatment
  - Responses to such treatments
- Record of medications administered, including
  - Name and strength of drug
  - Date, route, and time of administration
  - Dosage administered, and, with respect to PRN medications, reasons for administration and patient response/result observed
- Documentation of all care and ancillary services rendered
- Summaries of conferences and records of consultations
- Record of any treatment, medication, or service refused by the patient including physician's visits
- Discharge plans

DELAWARE

Delaware specifies the contents of medical records only for *nursing homes*. Other facilities follow the federal rules. Section 57.810 of the Nursing Home Regulations for Skilled Care (1986) states that nursing homes must maintain a separate clinical report on each patient, which will be a chronological history of the patient's stay in the nursing home. Every record must contain

- Admission record, including

  - Patient's name, birthdate, home address prior to entering the facility, identification numbers (social security, Medicaid, Medicare, etc.)

  - Date of admission

  - Physician's name, address, and phone number

  - Admitting diagnosis

  - Relationship, name, address, and phone number of the next of kin.

  - Facility's medical record number

- History and physical examination prepared by a physician within seven days of the patient's admission to the home. If the patient has been admitted immediately after discharge from a hospital, the patient's summary and history prepared at the hospital and the patient's physical examination performed at the hospital (if performed within seven days prior to admission to the home) may be substituted in lieu of the above records. Additionally, a record of an annual medical evaluation performed by a physician must be contained in each patient's file.

- Statement of complete diagnosis and prognosis

- Physician's orders, including

  - Complete list of medication names, dosage, frequency, and route of administration

  - Treatments

  - Diets

  - Level of permitted activity

  - Use of restraints (if the patient's condition requires them)

- Physician's progress notes

- Nursing notes

- Medication sheets, including

  - Medication name, dosage, frequency, and route of administration

- Space for recording initials of the nurse for dosage administered
- Signature identifying administering nurse's initials and professional status (R.N., L.P.N., etc.)

- Inventory of personal effects

- Accident reports

- Results of laboratory and special tests and x rays ordered by the physician

- Discharge record or notes, including
  - Condition on discharge
  - Place to which discharged
  - Prognosis, if appropriate

- Special service notes, including
  - Social services and activities
  - Results of specialty consultations requested by the physician
  - Physical therapy
  - Dental and podiatry consultations and treatments
  - Interagency transfer form, if patient was admitted from an acute care or another long-range care facility

DISTRICT OF COLUMBIA

The District defines "primary health record" as "the record of continuing care kept by a physician, psychologist, hospital, or extended care facility regarding a patient which reflects the diagnostic and therapeutic services rendered by the practitioner."[19]

Public health and medicine regulations provide that a facility must maintain a medical record on each inpatient.[20] A newborn's medical record must be maintained separately from that of its mother and assigned a separate record number.[21] The newborn's medical record must contain, in addition to the medical information required by the D.C. code, the name, address, race, age, and occupation of each parent, except that identifying data about the father need not be included when the infant is illegitimate.

The regulations stipulate that each medical record must conform to the requirements of the *Standards for Hospital Accreditation* (1960) by the Joint

19. District of Columbia Code Annotated § 32-501 (1990).
20. District of Columbia Municipal Regulations tit. 22, § 2216.3 (1986).
21. *Id.* § 2216.5. (1986).

Commission on Accreditation of Hospitals,[22] and specify that the nomenclature used in the medical records must conform to the *Standard Nomenclature of Diseases and Operations,* 5th edition.[23]

FLORIDA

Florida requires each *hospital* to maintain a current and complete medical record for every patient admitted for care. The medical record must contain at least the following information required for completion of birth, death, and stillbirth certificates[24] :

- Identification data

- Chief complaint

- Present illness

- Past history

- Family history

- Physical examination

- Provisional diagnosis

- Clinical laboratory reports

- X-ray reports

- Consultation reports

- Medical and surgical treatment notes and reports

- Evidence of appropriate informed consent

- Evidence of medication and dosage administered

- Copy of ambulance run reports given to the hospital as required, if patient was delivered to the hospital by ambulance

- Tissue reports

- Physician and nurse progress notes

- Final diagnosis

- Discharge summary

- Appropriate social work services, if provided

- Autopsy findings, when performed

---

22. *Id.* § 2216.4.
23. Published for the American Medical Association by McGraw-Hill Book Co., Inc. *Id.* § 2216.6.
24. Florida Administrative Code Annotated r. 10D-28.158(1) (1991).

Nursing home facilities must maintain similar medical records on all residents in accordance with accepted professional standards and practices and specific standards.[25]

Hospital clinical records must minimally conform to the following standards[26]:

- All clinical records must contain all pertinent clinical information, including, but not be limited to

    - Identification data and consent forms. When these are not obtainable, reason must be noted.

    - Source of referral

    - Reason for referral (e.g., chief complaint or presenting problem)

    - Record of complete assessment

    - Initial formulation and diagnosis based on assessment

    - Written treatment plan

    - Medication history and record of all medications prescribed

    - Record of all medication administered by facility staff, including type of medication, dosages, frequency of administration, persons who administered each dose, and route of administration

    - Documentation of course of treatment and all evaluations and examinations, including those from other facilities (e.g., emergency rooms or general hospitals)

    - Periodic treatment summaries, updated at least every 90 days

    - All consultation reports

    - All other appropriate information obtained from outside sources pertaining to patient

    - Discharge or termination summary report

    - Plans for follow-up and documentation of its implementation

- Identification data and consent form must include

    - Patient's name

    - Address

    - Home telephone number

---

25. *Id.* r. 10D-29.118(2)–(7).
26. *Id.* r. 10D-28.110(10).

- Date of birth

- Sex

- Next of kin

- School and grade

- Date of initial contact or admission to program

- Legal status and legal documents

- Other identifying data, as indicated

- Progress notes must include regular notations at least weekly by staff members, consultation reports, and signed entries by authorized identified staff. Progress notes by the clinical staff must

  - Document chronological picture of patient's clinical course

  - Document all treatment rendered to patient

  - Document implementation of treatment plans

  - Describe each change in each of the patient's conditions

  - Describe responses to and outcome of treatment

  - Describe responses of patient, family, or significant others to significant intercurrent events

- Discharge summaries must include

  - Initial formulation and diagnosis

  - Clinical resume

  - Final formulation, which must reflect the general observations and understanding of the patient's condition during appraisal of the fundamental needs of the patient. The relevant discharge diagnoses must be recorded and coded in the standard nomenclature of the current *Diagnostic and Statistical Manual of Mental Disorders,* published by the American Psychiatric Association, and the latest edition of the *International Classification of Diseases,* regardless of the use of other additional classification systems.

  - Final primary and secondary diagnoses

  - Psychiatric and physical categories

- Records of discharged patients must be completed following discharge, within a reasonable length of time (not to exceed 15 days). In the event of death, a summation statement must be added to the record, either as a final progress note or as a separate resume. This final note should take the form of a discharge summary and should include circumstances leading to death. All discharge summaries must be signed by a staff or consultant physician.

Nursing homes[27] and *home health agencies*[28] are required to maintain similar clinical records for every patient receiving healthcare services.

Primary care facilities are required to maintain a current and complete problem-oriented healthcare record for every client receiving primary care services.[29]

Each *hospital surgical department* is required to maintain current records that contain at least the following information:

- Patient's name

- Hospital number

- Preoperative diagnosis

- Postoperative diagnosis

- Procedure

- Names of surgeon, first assistant, and anesthetist

- Type of anesthetic

- Complications, if any[30]

- Ambulatory surgical center records

Ambulatory surgical centers must maintain medical records containing the original of the following (as appropriate to the service provided):

- Identification data

- Chief complaint

- Present illness

- Patient's history and family's history

- Physical examination

- Provisional diagnosis

- Clinical laboratory reports

- X-ray reports

---

27. *Id.* r. 10D-29.082(1).
28. *Id.* r. 10D-68.022.
29. *Id.* r. 10D-101.009.
30. *Id.* r. 10D-28.165(7).

- Consultation reports

- Medical and surgical treatment reports

- Surgical consent forms

- Tissue reports

- Physician orders

- Physician and nurse progress notes

- Final diagnosis

- Discharge summary

- Autopsy report, if appropriate[31]

Each *health maintenance organization* (HMO) must maintain a medical records system that includes a summary of significant surgical procedures, past and current diagnoses or problems, allergies, and untoward reactions to drugs and current medications.[32] This record also identifies the patient by providing the following:

- Name

- Member identification number

- Date of birth

- Sex

- Chief complaint or purpose of visit

- Objective findings of practitioner

- Diagnosis or medical impression

- Studies ordered (e.g., lab, x ray, EKG)

- Therapies administered and prescribed

- Name and professional status of practitioner rendering services (e.g., medical doctor [M.D.], registered nurse [R.N.], licensed practical nurse [L.P.N.]), including signature or initials of practitioner

- Disposition, recommendations, instructions to the patient, and evidence of whether there was follow-up

- Outcome of services

31. *Id.* r. 10D-30.012.
32. *Id.* r. 10D-100.005.

Chiropractors are required to maintain legible patient records including, at least

- History

- Symptomatology

- Examination, diagnosis, prognosis, and treatment.[33]

Dentists must maintain patient dental records under r. 21G-17.003 containing at least the following information:

- Appropriate medical history

- Results of clinical examinations and tests

- Treatment plan

- Treatment rendered

GEORGIA

Georgia defines a record as "a patient's health record, including, but not limited to, evaluations, diagnoses, prognoses, laboratory reports, X-rays, prescriptions, and other technical information used in assessing the patient's condition, or the pertinent portion of the record relating to a specific condition or a summary of the record."[34]

According to Georgia Compilation Code & Regulations r. 290-5-6-.11 (1977), *individual clinical records* must contain

- Admission and discharge data

  - Name, address, birth date, sex, and marital status

  - Date and time of admission

  - Date and time of discharge

  - Admitting diagnosis

  - Final diagnosis

  - Condition on discharge

  - Attending practitioner's signature

- History and physical examination

  - Personal history

  - Family history

---

33. *Id.* r. 21D-17.0065.
34. Georgia Code Annotated § 31-33-1.(3) (1991).

- Physical examination
- Psychiatric examination, if applicable
- Treatment
  - Practitioner's orders
  - Progress notes
  - Nurses' notes
  - Medication
  - Temperature, pulse, respiration (T.P.R.) (graphic chart)
  - Special examinations and reports
  - Operation record, if applicable
  - Anesthesia record, if applicable
  - Consultation record, if applicable
  - Autopsy findings, when performed
  - Discharge summary
  - If dental services are rendered, a complete dental chart with dental diagnosis, treatment, prescription and progress notes

HAWAII

Hawaii defines "medical records" as records of patients kept by a medical facility.[35]

The statute does not list the contents of all medical records but states that certain basic information must be retained by physicians and surgeons, even if the medical records are destroyed after the retention period or after microfilming. This information includes the patient's name and birthdate, a list of dated diagnoses and intrusive treatments, and a record of all drugs prescribed or given.[36]

Health care facilities must retain records including

- Patient's name and birth date
- Dates of admission and discharge
- Names of attending physicians
- Final diagnosis

---

35. Hawaii Revised Statutes § 622-51 (1990).
36. *Id.* § 622.58(d).

- Major procedures performed
- Operative reports
- Pathology reports
- Discharge summaries

IDAHO

While Idaho does not specify the contents of hospital medical records, it requires *health maintenance organizations* (HMOs) to maintain medical records that adequately and accurately document health maintenance care utilization by each enrollee.[37] Such records must

- Identify the patient by name, age, and sex
- Indicate the services provided, when, where, and by whom
- Indicate the diagnosis, treatment, and drug therapy employed

ILLINOIS

Illinois Administrative Code tit. 77, § 250.1510 (b) (2) (1985) specifies minimum requirements for medical record content:

- Patient identification and admission information
- Pertinent history of patient
- Chief complaints and present illness
- Family history
- Social history
- Physical examination report
- Provisional diagnosis
- Diagnostic and therapeutic reports on laboratory test results, x-ray findings, any surgical procedures performed, any pathological examinations, any consultations, and any other diagnostic or therapeutic procedures performed
- Orders and progress notes made by attending physician and, when applicable, by other members of the medical staff and allied health personnel
- Observation notes and vital sign charting made by nursing personnel

---

37. Idaho Code § 41-3909 (1990).

- Conclusions as to the primary diagnosis, any associated diagnoses, and brief clinical resume

- Disposition at discharge, including instructions and/or medications

- Any autopsy findings on a hospital death

Obstetrical records should include medical and obstetric history and findings during the prenatal period, which should be available in the maternity department prior to the patient's admission. Complete obstetrical records should also include observations and proceedings during labor, delivery, and postpartum period, and laboratory and x-ray findings that meet the criteria of the most current edition of the *Manual of Standards* of the American College of Obstetricians and Gynecologists. Such records must include

- Birth data, including time of birth, condition of infant at birth (including Apgar score at one and five minutes), age at which respiration becomes spontaneous and sustained, description of resuscitation, if required, and description of abnormalities and problems occurring from birth until transfer to the delivery room. Further, hospitals must keep records of births containing sufficient data to duplicate the birth certificate. (Facilities fulfill this requirement by retaining the yellow "hospital copy" of the birth certificate either properly bound in chronological order or with the individual medical record.)

- In addition to the items required in obstetric and birth records, infant records must include

  - History of maternal health and prenatal course

  - Description of labor, including drugs administered, method of delivery, complications of labor and delivery, and description of placenta and amniotic fluid

  - Report of complete and detailed physical examination of infant within 24 hours following birth

  - Report of a medical examination at least every three days during the hospital stay and within 24 hours of discharge

  - Physical measurements including length, weight, and head circumference at birth

  - Charting of weight every day and temperature twice daily

  - Documentation of infant feeding (intake, content, and amount, if by formula)

  - Clinical course during hospital stay including treatment rendered and patient response

- Clinical note of status at discharge

Medical records for *special care or special service units* must include

- Comprehensive treatment plan, based on strengths and liabilities, short-term and long-term goals, and the specific treatment modalities utilized as well as the responsibilities of each member of the treatment team in such a manner that provides adequate justification and documentation for the diagnoses and for the treatment and rehabilitation activities carried out

- Treatment received

- Progress notes

- Discharge summary

In addition, special care or service units must have written policies and procedures in place and maintained that detail how to maintain the confidentiality of patient information.[38]

Intermediate care facilities, and long-term care facilities are governed by Illinois Administrative Code tit. 77, § 300.1810 (1985) (Skilled Nursing Facilities and Intermediate Care Facilities); tit. 77, §§ 350.1610, 350.1620, and 350.1630 (1985) (Long-Term Care Facilities). Such records must contain

- *Identification sheet(s)* and/or admission forms with demographic information and name of dentist, admitting diagnosis, final diagnosis, and condition at time of discharge and disposition

- *Medical examination* containing medical history, physician findings, diagnosis, and restoration potential

- Initial medical evaluation and physical examination

- *Physician's order sheet* with orders for all medications, treatments, diet, activities, and special procedures or orders required for the safety and well-being of the resident

- *All physician's orders,* plans of treatment, Medicare/Medicaid certification and recertification statements and similar documents must have the original written signature of the physician. The use of physician's rubber stamp signature with or without initials is *not* acceptable.

- *Progress record* containing:

  - Changes in patient's condition noted

  - Actions, responses, attitude, appetite, etc.

  - Changes recorded by appropriate staff as they occur

---

38. *Id.* tit. 77, § 250.2860.

- Nursing personnel and other resident care staff must make notations at least monthly. Any significant observation should be recorded at the time it occurs. Physicians and consultants must make notations at the time of each visit. Notations by the person or persons directing the activity program and/or work program regarding resident response to these programs must be made at least monthly.

- *Medication sheet* or nurses' notes with date, time administered, name of drug, dosage, and by whom administered. The administration of each dose, and of any resident refusal, must be recorded on this sheet by the person administering medication. Persistent refusal of medication (other than PRN medications) must be communicated to the resident's physician promptly.

- *Treatment sheets* maintained specifying all nonregistered personnel and nursing care procedures ordered by each resident's attending physician. These procedures must include, but not be limited to, prevention and treatment of decubitus ulcers (bedsores) and weight monitoring to determine a weight loss or gain, if so ordered by physician.

- *Full written report of serious incident* or accident involving a resident placed in the patient's medical record, which includes the date and time of each incident or accident and the action taken concerning it. These incidents and accidents must include medication errors and drug reactions and all situations requiring the emergency services of a physician, a hospital, the police, the fire department, the coroner, etc. The department must be notified of all such serious incidents or accidents by a phone call to the regional office. Such notification must be within 24 hours of their occurrence. A written notification must be sent to the department within seven days of such incident or accident.

- *Nurses' notes,* descriptive of the nursing care provided, assessment and observations of symptoms, reactions to treatments and medications, and changes in the patient's physical or emotional condition

- Consultation reports with recommendations (dated and signed)

- Physician's visits

- Discharge record completed within 72 hours after the resident leaves facility, including date, time, condition of resident, to whom released, and planned destination

- All clinical records of discharged residents must be completed promptly.

- Facilities must also maintain reports of social service, dental, laboratory, x-ray, and special reports of consultations.

Illinois Administrative Code tit. 77, § 350.1610 (1985) specifies patient medical record requirement for *long-term health care facilities*.

- Residents admitted to the facility must have a summary discharge sheet (when admitted from a state-operated facility or a general hospital) that contains medical evaluation, physical examination, and psychological workup.

- Records maintained for each resident that are adequate for

  - Planning and continuous evaluating of the resident's habilitation program

  - Furnishing documentary evidence of the resident's progress and of his response to his habilitation program

  - Protecting legal rights

- *All entries* in the resident's record must be legible, dated, and authenticated by the written signature and identification of the individual making the entry. Symbols and abbreviations are used in record only if a legend is provided to explain them.

- *Social support personnel* and nursing personnel must make notations at least monthly. Any significant observation should be recorded at the time it occurs. Physicians and consultants should make notations at the time of each visit.

- *Consultants* must make written reports of their findings and recommendations at the time of each visit. Reports must be dated and indicate the specific time the consultant was in the facility. Recommendations must be included in the resident's progress record if concerned with an individual resident.

- *A full written report* of any serious incident or accident involving a resident must be placed in the resident's medical record. This report must include the date and time of each incident or accident and the action taken concerning it. These incidents and accidents must include medication errors and drug reactions and all situations requiring the emergency services of a physician, a hospital, the police, the fire department, the coroner, etc.

- Active current record dated, signed, complete, legible, and available at all times to the personnel of the facility and the department's representatives

INDIANA

Indiana defines "health records" as "written or printed information possessed by a provider concerning any diagnosis, treatment, or prognosis of the patient."[39]

---

39. Indiana Code Annotated § 16-4-8-1 (West 1991).

The Board of Health's licensure rules state that an *inpatient hospital record* should include[40]

- Identification data

- Chief complaint

- Present illness

- Past history

- Physical examination

- Progress notes

- Reports on consultations

- Copy of transfer form

- Reports on laboratory, x-ray, and operative procedures

- Special reports

- Physicians' orders (signed and dated)

- Notes and observations

- Treatment records of nurses, dietitian, therapists and other personnel

- Reports on vital signs

- Final discharge summary

- Summary sheet giving final diagnosis, complications, operative procedures, and signature of attending physician

Readmissions within a reasonable time (with the same diagnosis) require only a readmission note on the patient's condition and the reason for readmission. The facility may use a short form for patients hospitalized for less than 48 hours, which must include identification data, description of patient's condition, physical findings, treatments given, procedures carried out, operative procedures and anesthesia, medical orders, and other data to support the diagnosis and treatment, disposition, necessary signatures, and a dismissal diagnosis.

Emergency and outpatient records must include

- Identification data

- Description of the illness or injury

- Description of the treatment

- Signature of the physician

---

40. Indiana Administrative Code tit. 410, r. 15-1-9 (1988).

- Instructions given on release

- Condition on discharge

- Follow-up care

- Name of person giving instructions

- Copy of transfer form

If the facility does not provide care for the patient or transfers him elsewhere, the record should reflect the reason(s) therefor.

IOWA

Iowa public health regulations state that "Accurate and complete medical records must be written for all patients and signed by the attending physician."[41] The regulation governing *emergency services* provides that hospitals must have written policies and procedures that require a medical record on every patient given treatment in the emergency service and establish the medical record documentation. The documentation should include, at a minimum

- Appropriate information regarding the medical screening provided

- Notation of patient refusal to provide information

- Physician documentation of the presence or absence of an emergency medical condition or active labor

- Physician documentation of transfer or discharge, stating the basis for transfer or discharge and, where transfer occurs, identity of the facility of the transfer, acceptance of the patient by the facility of transfer, and means of transfer of the patient.[42]

Nursing facilities that transfer a resident to another facility must summarize the following information from the facility's records to accompany the resident:

- A transfer form or diagnosis

- Aid to daily living information

- Transfer orders

- Nursing care plan

- Physician's orders for care

- The resident's personal records

---

41. Iowa Administrative Code r. 481-51.6(135B) (1990).
42. *Id*. r. 481-51.28(1)(135B).

- When applicable, the personal needs fund record

- Resident care review team assessment[43]

Records of *skilled nursing facilities* must include:

- The licensee must keep a permanent resident admission record on all residents admitted to a skilled nursing facility with all entries current, dated, and signed. This must be a part of the resident clinical record. The admission record form must include

  - Name and previous address of resident

  - Birthdate, sex, and marital status of resident

  - Church affiliation

  - Physician's name, telephone number, and address

  - Dentist's name, telephone number, and address

  - Name, address, and telephone number of next of kin or legal representative

  - Name, address, and telephone number of person to be notified in case of emergency

  - Mortician's name, telephone number, and address

  - Pharmacist's name, telephone number and address[44]

As to resident clinical records, there must be a separate clinical record for each resident admitted to a skilled nursing facility with all entries current, dated, and signed. The resident clinical record must include

- Admission record

- Admission diagnosis

- Physical examination. The record of the admission physical examination and medical history must portray the current medical status of the resident and must include the resident's name, sex, age, medical history, tuberculosis status, physical examination, diagnosis, statement of chief complaints, estimation of restoration potential and results of any diagnostic procedures. The report of the physical examination must be signed by the physician.

- Physician's certification that the resident requires no greater degree of nursing care than the facility is licensed to provide

---

43. *Id*. r. 441-81.5(249A).
44. *Id*. r. 481-59.19(1).

- Physician's orders for medication, treatment, and diet in writing and signed by the physician every 30 days

- Progress notes

  - Physician must enter a progress note at the time of each visit.

  - Other professionals, i.e., dentists, social workers, physical therapists, pharmacists, and others must enter a progress note at the time of each visit.

- All laboratory, x-ray, and other diagnostic reports

- Nurses' notes, signed at the time of entry, to include

  - Admitting notes including time and mode of transportation, room assignment, disposition of valuables, symptoms and complaints, general condition, vital signs, and weight

  - Routine notes, including

    - Physician's visits

    - Telephone calls to and from the physician

    - Unusual incidents and accidents

    - Change of condition

    - Social interaction

    - PRN medications administered including time and reason administered and resident's reaction

  - Organized nursing history and assessment of observed symptoms

  - Reaction to all treatments and medications

  - Changes in the resident's physical and emotional condition

  - Description of the nursing care provided

  - Discharge or transfer notes including time and mode of transportation

  - Resident's general condition

  - Instructions given to resident or legal representative

  - List of medications and disposition

  - Completion of transfer form for continuity of care

  - Death notes, including notifications of physician and family to include time, disposition of body, resident's personal possessions, and medications

- Complete and accurate notes of resident's vital signs and symptoms preceding death

- Medication record. Medication and treatment record, including all medications, treatments, and special procedures for each resident.

- Death record

  - The death record must include name, age, sex, and race of deceased; date and time of death; physician's name, address, and signature; immediate cause of death; name and address of relative or legal representative notified of death; name, address, and signature of mortician receiving the body.

  - If the physician does not sign the death record, a copy of the death certificate must be obtained by the facility as soon as it becomes available and made a part of the resident's medical record retained by the facility.

- Transfer form

  - The transfer form must include identification data from the admission record, name of transferring institution, and date of transfer.

  - The nurse's report must include resident attitudes, behavior, interests, functional abilities (activities of daily living), unusual treatments, nursing care, problems, likes and dislikes, nutrition, current medications (when last given), and condition on transfer.

  - The physician's report must include reason for transfer, medications, treatment, diet, activities, significant laboratory and x-ray findings, and diagnosis and prognosis.

- Consultation reports must indicate services rendered by allied health professionals in the facility or in health-centered agencies such as dentists, physical therapists, podiatrists, oculists, and others.[45]

Resident personal records may be kept as a separate file by the facility.[46]

- Personal records may include factual information regarding personal statistics, family and responsible relative resources, financial status, and other confidential information.

- Personal records must be accessible to professional staff involved in planning for services to meet the needs of the resident.

- On discharge of the resident, all statistical and financial information pertaining to the resident's stay must be centralized in the resident's medical record.

---

45. *Id.* r. 481-59.19(2).
46. *Id.* r. 481-59.19(3).

- Personal records must include a duplicate copy of the contract.

Each skilled nursing facility must maintain an incident record report and must have available incident report forms.

- Report of incidents must be in detail on a printed incident report form.

- The report must cover all accidents where there is apparent injury or where hidden injury may have occurred.

- The report must cover all accidents or unusual occurrences within the facility or on the premises affecting residents, visitors, or employees.

- A copy of the incident report must be kept on file in the facility.[47]

Intermediate care facility patient records must contain

- A permanent resident admission record on all residents admitted to an intermediate care facility with all entries current, dated, and signed. This must be a part of the resident clinical record. The admission record form must include

  - Name and previous address of resident

  - Birthdate, sex, and marital status of resident

  - Church affiliation

  - Physician's name, address, and telephone number

  - Dentist's name, address, and telephone number

  - Name, address, and telephone number of next of kin or legal representative

  - Name, address, and telephone number of person to be notified in case of emergency

  - Mortician's name, telephone number, and address

  - Pharmacist's name, telephone number, and address[48]

Each intermediate care facility must maintain a separate clinical record for each resident admitted to the facility with all entries current, dated, and signed.[49] The resident clinical record must include

- Admission record, including

  - Resident's name, sex, age, medical history, and tuberculosis status

---

47. *Id.* r. 481-59.19(4).
48. *Id.* r. 481-58.15(135C).
49. *Id.* r. 481-58.15(2).

- Physical examination, signed by the physician

- Diagnosis

- Statement of chief complaints

- Estimation of restoration potential

- Results of any diagnostic procedures

- Physician's certification that the resident requires no greater degree of nursing care than the facility is licensed to provide

- Physician's orders for medication, treatment, and diet in writing and signed by the physician quarterly

- Progress notes

- All laboratory, x-ray, and other diagnostic reports

- Nurses' record, including

  - Admitting notes including time and mode of transportation

  - Room assignment

  - Disposition of valuables

  - Symptoms and complaints

  - General condition

  - Vital signs

  - Weight

  - Routine notes, including

    - Physician's visits

    - Telephone calls to and from the physician

    - Unusual incidents and accidents

    - Change of condition

    - Social interaction

    - PRN medications administered, including time and reason administered and resident's reaction

- Discharge or transfer notes, which should include

  - Time and mode of transportation

  - Resident's general condition

  - Instructions given to resident or legal representative

- List of medications and disposition
- Completion of transfer form for continuity of care
- Death notes, which must include notification of physician and family, to include
  - Time
  - Disposition of body
  - Resident's personal possessions and medications
  - Complete and accurate notes of resident's vital signs and symptoms preceding death
- Medication record
  - An accurate record of all medications administered
  - Schedule II drug records kept in accordance with state and federal laws
- Death record, which must include
  - Name, age, sex, and race of deceased
  - Date and time of the death
  - Physician's name, address, and signature of mortician receiving the body
  - If the physician does not sign the death record, a copy of the death certificate must be obtained by the facility as soon as it becomes available and made a part of the resident's medical record retained by the facility.
- Transfer form
  - The transfer form must include
    - Identification data from the admission record
    - Name of transferring institution
    - Name of receiving institution
    - Date of transfer
  - The nurses' report must include
    - Resident attitudes, behavior, interests
    - Functional abilities (activities of daily living)
    - Unusual treatments

- Nursing care

- Problems

- Likes and dislikes

- Nutrition

- Current medications (when last given)

- Condition on transfer

- The physician's report must include

  - Reason for transfer

  - Medications

  - Treatment

  - Diet

  - Activities

  - Significant laboratory and x-ray findings

  - Diagnosis and prognosis

- Consultation reports must indicate services rendered by allied health professionals in the facility or in health-centered agencies, such as dentists, physical therapists, podiatrists, oculists, and others.

- Resident personal records may be kept as a separate file by the facility.[50]

  - Personal records may include factual information regarding personal statistics, family and responsible relative resources, financial status, and other confidential information.

  - Personal records must be accessible to professional staff involved in planning services to meet the needs of the resident.

  - When the resident's records are closed, the information must become a part of the final record.

  - Personal records must include a duplicate copy of the contract(s).

- Incident record. Each intermediate care facility must maintain an incident record report and must have available incident report forms.[51]

  - Report of incidents must be in detail on a printed incident report form.

  - The person in charge at the time of the incident must prepare and sign the report.

---

50. *Id*. r. 481-58.15(3).
51. *Id*. r. 481-58.15(4).

- The report must cover all accidents where there is apparent injury or where hidden injury may have occurred.

- The facility must keep a copy of the incident report on file in the facility.

The licensee must keep a permanent record on all residents admitted to a *residential care facility* with all entries current, dated, and signed.[52] The record must include

- Name and previous address of resident

- Birthdate, sex, and marital status of resident

- Church affiliation

- Physician's name, telephone number, and address

- Dentist's name, telephone number, and address

- Name, address, and telephone number of next of kin or legal representative

- Name, address, and telephone number of person to be notified in case of emergency

- Mortician's name, telephone number, and address

- Pharmacist's name, telephone number, and address

- Physical examination and medical history

- Certification by the physician that the resident requires no more than personal care and supervision, but does not require nursing care

- Physician's orders for medication, treatments, and diet in writing and signed by the physician quarterly

- A notation of yearly or other visits to physician or other professional services

- Any change in the resident's condition

- If the physician has certified that the resident is capable of taking his or her prescribed medications, the administrator must require residents to keep him or her advised of current medications, treatments, and diet. The administrator must keep a listing of medications, treatments, and diet prescribed by the physician for each resident.

- If the physician has certified that the resident is not capable of taking his or her prescribed medication, it must be administered by a qualified

---

52. *Id.* r. 481-57.16(10).

person of the facility. A qualified person must be defined as either a registered or licensed practical nurse or an individual who has completed the state-approved training course in medication administration.

- Medications administered by an employee of the facility must be recorded on a medication record by the individual who administers the medication.

- A notation describing condition on admission, transfer, and discharge

- In the event of the death of a resident, a death record must be completed, including the physician's signature and disposition of the body. A notation must be made on the resident record of the notification of the family.

- A copy of instructions given to the resident, legal representative, or facility in the event of discharge or transfer

- Disposition of valuables

  Records of residential care *facilities for the mentally retarded* must contain

- Name and previous address of resident

- Birthdate, sex, and marital status of resident

- Church affiliation

- Physician's name, telephone number, and address

- Dentist's name, telephone number, and address

- Name, address, and telephone number of next of kin or legal representative

- Name, address, and telephone number of person to be notified in case of emergency

- Mortician's name, telephone number, and address

- Pharmacist's name, telephone number, and address

- Physical examination and medical history

- Certification by the physician that the resident requires no more than personal care and supervision, but does not require nursing care

- Physician's orders for medication, treatment, and diet in writing and signed by the physician

- Notation of yearly or other visits to physician or other professional services

- Any change in the resident's condition

- If the physician has certified that the resident is capable of taking his or her prescribed medications, the resident must be required to keep the administrator advised of current medications, treatments, and diet prescribed by the physician for each resident.

- If the physician has certified that the resident is not capable of taking his or her prescribed medication, it must be administered by a qualified person of the facility. A qualified person must be defined as either a registered or licensed practical nurse or an individual who has completed the state-approved training course in medication administration.

- Medications administered by an employee of the facility must be recorded on a medication record by the individual who administers the medication.

- Notation describing condition on admission, transfer, and discharge

- In the event of the death of a resident, a death record must be completed, including the physician's signature and disposition of the body. A notation must be made on the resident record of the notification of the family and, as appropriate, the agency of financial responsibility.

- A copy of instructions given to the resident, legal representative, or facility in the event of discharge or transfer

- Disposition of valuables[53]

Each residential care facility for the mentally retarded must maintain an incident record report and must have available incident report forms.[54] Reports of incidents must be in detail on a printed incident report form. The person in charge at the time of the incident must oversee the preparation and sign the incident report. The report must cover all accidents where there is apparent injury or where hidden injury may have occurred, and cover all accidents or unusual occurrences within the facility or on the premises affecting residents, visitors, or employees. A copy of the incident report must be kept on file in the facility.

Concerning intermediate care facilities for the mentally retarded, the structure and content of the individual's record must be an accurate, functional representation of the actual experience of the individual in the facility. It must contain enough information to indicate that the facility knows the status of the individual, has adequate plans to intervene, and provides sufficient evidence of the effects of the intervention. The department must be able to identify this through interviews with staff, and when possible with individuals being served, as well as through observations.[55]

The regulations[56] specify that the licensee must keep a permanent record about each resident with all entries current, dated, and signed, including

- Name and previous address of resident

- Birthdate, sex, and marital status of resident

---

53. *Id.* r. 481-63.1(1).
54. *Id.* r. 481-63.17(2).
55. *Id.* r. 483.410(c)(1).
56. *Id.* r. 481-62.18(1).

- Church affiliation

- Physician's name, telephone number, and address

- Dentist's name, telephone number, and address

- Name, address, and telephone number of next of kin or legal representative

- Name, address, and telephone number of the person to be notified in case of emergency

- Funeral director, telephone number, and address

- Pharmacy name, telephone number, and address

- Results of annual evaluation of the patient

- Certification by the physician that the resident requires no more than personal care and supervision, but does not require nursing care

- Physician's orders for medication and treatments must be in writing and signed by the physician quarterly; diet orders must be renewed yearly.

- A notation of yearly or other visits to physician or other professionals, all consultation reports and progress notes

- Any change in the resident's condition

- A notation describing the resident's condition on admission, transfer, and discharge

- In the event of the death of a resident, a death record must be completed, including the physician's signature and disposition of the body. A notation must be made on the resident's record of the notification of the family.

- Copy of instructions given to the resident, legal representative, or facility in the event of discharge or transfer

- Disposition of personal property

- Copy of individual program plan (IPP)

- Progress notes

KANSAS

Kansas Administrative Regulations § 28-34-9a (e)(1)–(3) (1990) specify that medical records must contain sufficient information to identify the patient clearly, to justify the diagnosis and treatment, and to document the results accurately. At a minimum, the record should include

- Notes by authorized house staff members and individuals who have been granted clinical privileges, consultation reports, nurse's notes, and entries by specified professional personnel

- Findings and results of any pathological or clinical laboratory examinations, radiology examinations, medical and surgical treatment, and other diagnostic or therapeutic procedures

- Provisional diagnosis, primary and secondary final diagnosis, a clinical resume, and where appropriate, necropsy reports

The *emergency record,* when appropriate, must contain

- Patient identification

- History of disease or injury

- Physical findings

- Laboratory and radiological reports, if any

- Diagnosis

- Record of treatment

- Disposition of the case

- Signature of physician rendering the service.[57]

KENTUCKY

902 Kentucky Administration Regulations 20:016 § 3 (11) (d) (1991) specifies that medical records must include

- Identification data and signed consent forms, including name and address of next of kin, and of person or agency responsible for patient

- Date of admission and name of attending medical staff member

- Chief complaint

- Medical history including present illness, past history, family history, and physical examination

- Report of special examinations or procedures such as consultations, clinical laboratory tests, x-ray interpretations, EKG interpretations

- Provisional diagnosis or reason for admission

- Orders for diet, diagnostic tests, therapeutic procedures, and medications,

---

57. *Id.* § 28-34-16(f).

including patient limitations, signed and dated by the medical staff member; and, if given verbally, undersigned by the medical staff member on his next visit to hospital

- Medical, surgical, and dental treatment notes and reports, signed and dated by a physician, or dentist when applicable, including records of all medication administered to the patient

- Complete surgical record signed by the attending surgeon, or oral surgeon, to include anesthesia record signed by anesthesiologist or anesthetist, preoperative physical examination and diagnosis, description of operative procedures and findings, postoperative diagnosis, and tissue diagnosis by qualified pathologist on tissue surgically removed

- Physician's, or dentist's when applicable, progress notes and nurses' observations

- Record of temperature, blood pressure, pulse, and respiration

- Final diagnosis using terminology in the current version of the *International Classification of Diseases* or the American Psychiatric Association's *Diagnostic and Statistical Manual of Mental Disorders*, as applicable.

- Discharge summary, including condition of patient on discharge and date of discharge

- In case of death, autopsy findings, if performed

- In the case of death, an indication that the patient has been evaluated for organ donation in accordance with hospital protocol

The Kentucky Living Will Act, Kentucky Revised Statutes Annotated § 311.622-.634 (Michie/Bobbs-Merrill 1991) requires the written declaration and subsequent revocation of a declaration by a patient diagnosed with a terminal condition (instructing his/her physician to withhold or withdraw life-prolonging treatment) to be included in the patient's medical record.

LOUISIANA

Louisiana law defines "hospital record" as "a compilation of the reports of the various clinical departments within a hospital, as well as reports from health care providers, as are customarily catalogued and maintained by the hospital medical records department."

Louisiana Revised Statutes Annotated § 40:2144 A.(5) (West 1990) notes that hospital records include reports of procedures such as x rays and electrocardiograms, but they do not include the image or graphic matter produced by such procedures.

MAINE

Medical records in Maine must contain sufficient information to justify the diagnosis and warrant the treatment and results. Medical records should contain the following information according to Code Maine Rules & Regulations Governing the Licensing and Functioning of General and Specialty Hospitals, ch. XII:

- Identification data

- Chief complaint

- Present illness

- Past history

- Family history

- Physical examination

- Provisional diagnosis

- Clinical laboratory reports

- X-ray reports

- Consultations

- Treatment, medical and surgical

- Tissue report

- Progress notes

- Final diagnosis

- Discharge summary

- Autopsy findings

MARYLAND

Maryland defines "medical record" as "each record of medical care that a facility keeps on an individual and includes records kept in manual or automated form."[58]

The Code of Maryland Regulations, covering Comprehensive Care Facilities and Extended Care Facilities, Maryland Annotated Code art. 10, § .07.02.20 (1988) discusses maintenance of clinical records and specifies their contents.

- Identification and summary sheet or sheets, including

  - Patient's name

---

58. Maryland Health-General Code Annotated § 4-302 (1990).

- Social security number
- Armed forces status
- Citizenship
- Marital status
- Age
- Sex
- Home address
- Religion
- Names, addresses, and telephone numbers of referral agencies (including hospital from which admitted), personal physician, dentist, parents' names or next of kin, or authorized representative
- Documented evidence of assessment of the needs of the patient, of establishment of an appropriate plan of initial and ongoing treatment, and of the care and services provided
- Authentication of hospital diagnoses (discharge summary, report from patient's attending physician, or transfer form)
- Consent forms when required
- Medical and social history of patient
- Report of physical examination
- Diagnostic and therapeutic orders
- Consultation reports
- Observations and progress notes
- Reports of medication administration, treatments, and clinical findings
- Discharge summary including final diagnosis and prognosis
- Discipline assessment
- Interdisciplinary care plan

Home health agencies' clinical records must include, at a minimum

- All pertinent diagnoses
- Name, address, and telephone number of physician
- Physician's orders, including specific instructions for services to be rendered, activities and limitations, and medically necessary supplies and equipment

- Drug information, including type, dosage, route of administration, frequency, and history of sensitivities or allergic reactions

- Nutritional requirements, including specific dietary plans

- Prognosis, including rehabilitation potential

- Patient care plans, which should include

  - Long and short-range goals

  - Physical needs, including safety measures to protect against injury

  - Psychosocial needs

  - Actions taken by individual disciplines

  - Evidence of periodic reappraisal of the needs of the patient

- Progress notes and modifications to the treatment plan

- Discharge summary[59]

Maryland requires the following contents for medical records of health maintenance organizations (HMOs):

- Identification and summary sheets

- Prior medical findings and referral information

- Information necessary to support the diagnosis and justify the treatment given as shown in the individual written plan of treatment

- Progress notes by a medical staff member, as appropriate; a physician must review and approve the progress notes within 24 hours of entry.

- Dated record of all treatments, medications, laboratory tests, x rays, operative reports, anesthesia records, and measurements

- Consultation report, if appropriate

- Record of any emergency care rendered to patient

- Discharge summary of inpatient hospitalization to include condition at time of discharge and postoperative instructions given to the patient[60]

Hospice care programs' patient records must include

- Age

- Sex

---

59. *Id*. art. 10, § .07.10.11.
60. *Id*. art. 10, § .07.11.05.

- Diagnoses
- Days of inpatient care
- Days of home-based care
- Patient assessments
- Plans of care
- Results of any physical examinations or laboratory studies
- Actual services provided by program employees and volunteers[61]

MASSACHUSETTS

The Department of Public Health, by regulation, has defined the contents of medical records:

- Identification data
- Complaint
- Present illness
- Past history
- Social and occupational history
- Family history
- Dietary history
- Contact with tuberculosis history
- Physical examination
- Provisional diagnoses
- Consultation requests and replies
- Clinical laboratory reports, roentgenologic reports, tissue reports
- Treatment, medical and surgical
- Operation reports
- Progress notes
- Nurses' notes
- Final diagnosis
- Complete summary
- Autopsy findings

---

61. *Id.* art. 10, § .07.21.

- The facility must use the *Standard Nomenclature of Disease and Operations* and the current *Diagnostic Standards* of the National Tuberculosis Association for nomenclature.[62]

The regulations require healthcare facilities that give patients *transfusions* to include the following in their medical records:

- Recipient's name, health facility identification number, location, ABO group and Rh type, and informed consent form

- Donor identification number, ABO group and Rh type

- Results of compatibility tests, dated and signed or initialed by the person performing the test

- Identification of blood product transfused

- Date, time transfusion started, time terminated, and amount administered. Time terminated and amount transfused is required only if the whole unit is not transfused.

- Signature of transfusionist

- Type of reaction, if any

- The original completed copy of the results of the investigation must be included in the patient's medical record, in the case of any adverse reaction.[63]

In addition to the above requirements for all hospital patient records, *obstetric maternal records* must include

- Mother's medical and obstetric history including prenatal course

- Antenatal blood serology, Rh factor, and blood type

- Admission obstetrical examination including the condition of both mother and fetus

- Complete description of progress of labor and delivery, signed by the attending physician, or certified nurse midwife, including reasons for induction and operative procedures

- Type of medications, analgesia, and anesthesia administered to the patient during labor and delivery

- Signed report of qualified obstetric or other consultant when such service has been obtained

- Names and credentials of all those present during delivery

---

62. Massachusetts Regulations Code tit. 105, § 134.330 (1990).
63. *Id.* tit. 105, § 135.903.

- Description of postpartal course, including complications and treatments, signed by the attending physician or certified nurse midwife

- Medications, including contraceptives, prescribed at discharge

- Infant's condition at birth including gestational age, weight, Apgar score, blood type, and results of initial physical assessment

- Nursing assessment, diagnosis, interventions, and teaching

- Method of infant feeding: progress and plans for further support of lactation or suppression of lactation

- If neonatal death occurs, cause of death, assessment of the family's coping mechanisms and plans for follow-up and/or referrals of the family

    Newborn records under this regulation must contain

- Significant maternal diseases

- Mother's obstetrical history including estimated date of confinement and prenatal care course

- Maternal antenatal blood serology, blood typing, Rh factors, rubella antibody titer, and Coombs test for maternal antibodies if indicated

- Results of any significant prenatal diagnostic procedures including genetic testing and/or chromosomal analysis

- Complications of pregnancy or delivery

- Duration of ruptured membranes

- Medications, analgesic and/or anesthesia administered to the mother

- Complete description of progress of labor including diagnostic tests, treatment rendered, and reasons for induction and operative procedures

- Date and time of birth

- Cause of death if it occurs

- Condition of infant at birth to include

    - Apgar score

    - Resuscitation

    - Time of sustained respirations

    - Description of congenital abnormalities

    - Gestational age

    - Head circumference

- Length

- Weight

- Pathological conditions

- Treatments

- Number of cord vessels

- Description of any placental abnormalities

- Written verification of eye prophylaxis and mandated screening tests, including time and date

- Method of feeding

- Report of infant's initial medical examination within 24 hours of birth, signed by the infant's attending physician or his/her physician designee

- Informed consent for circumcision or any other surgical procedures

- Physician progress notes written in accordance with hospital policy

- A report of discharge examination signed by attending physician, certified nurse midwife, or pediatric nurse practitioner within 24 hours of discharge

- Nursing assessment, diagnosis, interventions, and teaching[64]

Each *birth center* must keep the following information in client records:

- Client's name, date of birth, home address and telephone number, and spouse or other person to contact in an emergency

- Date of each client visit with birth center staff, at the birth center or elsewhere

- Obstetrical and medical history

- Diagnosis observations, evaluations, and therapeutic plans

- Orders for any medication, test, or treatment

- Records of any administration of medications, treatment, or therapy

- Laboratory, radiology, and other diagnostic reports

- Progress notes

- Reports of any consultations, special examinations, or procedures

---

64. *Id.* tit. 105, § 130.627.

- Referrals to other agencies
- Discharge summary where appropriate

Each birth center must record the following information with respect to each newborn:

- Condition of infant at birth to include Apgar score (or its equivalent) at one minute and repeat ratings in five minutes, resuscitation, time of sustained respirations, and details of physical abnormalities and pathological states
- Date and hour of birth, birth weight, and period of gestation
- Number of cord vessels and any abnormalities of the placenta
- Verification of eye prophylaxis
- Metabolic screening
- Treatments, medications, and special procedures
- Condition at discharge or transfer[65]

Hospice records must include

- Initial and subsequent assessments
- Plan of care
- Identification data
- Consent forms
- Pertinent medical history
- Complete documentation of all services and events (including evaluations, treatments, progress notes, etc.)
- Physician's orders
- Medication records
- Discharge/transfer records
- All pertinent diagnoses
- The patient's prognosis
- Designation of the attending physician
- A bereavement assessment and plan for intervention, if any

---

65. *Id.* tit. 105, § 142.504.

- Instructions to the family concerning care if patient is discharged[66]

Clinical records of *long-term care facilities* must contain

- Identification and summary sheet
- A healthcare referral form, hospital summary discharge sheets, and other such information transferred from the agency or the institution to the receiving facility
- Admission data
- Initial medical evaluation
- Physician's or physician-physician assistant team's or physician-nurse practitioner team's progress notes
- Consultation reports
- Medication treatment record
- A record of all fires and all incidents involving patients or residents and personnel while on duty
- A nursing care plan
- Nurses' notes
- Initial plans and written evidence of periodic review and revision of dietary, social service, restorative therapy services, activity, and all other patient or resident care plans
- Laboratory and x-ray reports
- A list of each patient's or resident's clothing, personal effects, valuables, fund or other property
- Discharge or transfer data
- Utilization review plan, minutes, reports, and special studies
- Individual service plan[67]

MICHIGAN

As to medical records in general, the Department of Public Health Administrative Rules and Procedures lists the requirements for *medical records:*

- Admission date
- Admitting diagnosis

---

66. *Id.* tit. 105, § 141.209 (1990).
67. *Id.* tit. 105, § 150.013.

- History and physical examination
- Physician's progress notes
- Operation and treatment notes and consultations
- The physician's orders
- Nurses' notes including temperature, pulse, respiration, conditions observed, and medication given
- Record of discharge or death
- Final diagnosis[68]

Surgical records should include the following:

- Details of the preoperative study and diagnosis
- Preoperative medication
- Name of the surgeon and his assistants
- Method of anesthesia
- Amount of anesthetic when measurable
- Name of the anesthetist
- Postoperative diagnosis, including pathological findings
- Reports of special examinations, such as laboratory, x-ray and pathology, must also be part of the record

Nursing home clinical records must include

- The identification and summary sheet, which must include all of the following patient information:
  - Name
  - Social security number
  - Veteran status and number
  - Marital status
  - Age, sex, and home address
- Name, address, and telephone number of next of kin, legal guardian, or designated representative
- Name, address, and telephone number of person or agency responsible for patient's maintenance and care in the home

---

68. Michigan Administrative Code r. 325.1028 (1987).

- Date of admission

- Clinical history and physical examination performed by the physician within five days before or on admission, including a report of chest x rays performed within 90 days of admission and a physician's treatment plan

- Admission diagnosis and amendments thereto during the course of the patient's stay at the home

- Consent forms as required and appropriate

- Physician's orders for medications, diet, rehabilitative procedures, and other treatment or procedures to be provided to the patient

- Physician's progress notes written at the time of each visit describing the patient's condition and other pertinent clinical observations

- Nurses' notes and observations by other personnel providing care

- Medication and treatment records

- Laboratory and x-ray reports

- Consultation reports

- Time and date of discharge, final diagnosis and place to which patient was discharged, condition on discharge, and name of person, if any, accompanying patient[69]

Resident records in *homes for the aged* must include

- Identifying information including name, social security number, veteran status and number, marital status, age, sex, and home address

- Name, address, and telephone number of next of kin or legal guardian

- Name, address, and telephone number of person or agency responsible for resident's maintenance and care in the home

- Date of admission

- Date of discharge and place to which resident was discharged

- Health information including physician reports and reports of diagnostic procedures

- Name, address, and telephone number of resident's attending physician[70]

---

69. *Id.* r. 325.21102 (1987).
70. *Id.* r. 325.1851.

MINNESOTA

Minnesota requires keeping of accurate and complete medical records on all patients from the time of admission to the time of discharge.[71] A complete record should include:

- Adequate identification data

- Admitting diagnosis, to be completed within 24 to 48 hours

- History and physical examination, including history of pregnancy on maternity cases, to be completed within 24 to 48 hours

- Progress notes

- Signed physicians' orders

- Operative notes, where applicable, to include course of delivery on maternity cases

- Special reports and examinations, including clinical and laboratory findings, x-ray findings, records of consultations, anesthesia reports, etc.

- Nurses' notes

- Discharge diagnosis

- Autopsy report, where applicable

Hospitals must maintain the following additional information on all *maternity patients*

- Full and true name of patient and her husband

- Place of residence of the patient prior to hospitalization

- Place of residence following discharge

Medical records on *newborn infants* must include a physical examination and a statement of the physical condition of the infant at discharge. If the child leaves the hospital with any person other than a parent, the hospital must record the true name of the person or persons with whom the child leaves and the residence where the child is to be taken.

An *individual permanent medical record* (which the hospital must retain permanently under Minnesota Statutes § 145.32) must consist of the following parts of the hospital record that are applicable to that patient:

- Identification data, which includes the patient's name, address, date of birth, sex, and if available, the patient's social security number

---

71. Minnesota Rules 4640.1000 (3) (1991).

- Medical history, which includes details of the present illness, the chief complaint, relevant social and family history, and provisional diagnosis

  - For obstetrical patients, the medical history must include prenatal information when available.

  - For newborns, a birth history consisting of a physical examination report and delivery record as it pertains to the newborn must be included.

- A physical examination report

- A report of all operations, which includes

  - Preoperative diagnosis

  - Names of all surgeons and assistants

  - Anesthetic agent

  - Description of the specimens removed with pathological findings

  - Description of the surgical findings

  - Technical procedures used

  - Postoperative diagnosis

- Discharge summary, which includes

  - Reason for hospitalization

  - Summary of clinical observations

  - Procedures performed

  - Treatment rendered

  - Significant findings (for example, pertinent laboratory, x-ray, and test results)

    - Condition at discharge

    - For newborns or others for whom no discharge summary is available, a final progress note must be included.

- Autopsy findings[72]

Medical records on *tuberculosis patients* must include, in addition to that required of records generally, above

- Tuberculosis classification at the time of discharge

- Reason for discharge

---

72. Minnesota Rules 4642.1000 (1991).

- Number of days of hospitalization[73]

Personal records of *adult foster care homes* must include the following medical information:

- Name, address, and phone number of the resident's physician, dentist, clinic, and other sources of medical care

- Health history and information on any health risks, allergies, currently prescribed medication, and documentation of the physical examination or transfer record

- Any emergency treatment needed or provided while the resident resides in the adult foster care home

- Medication record[74]

As a condition for *reimbursement* under the Surveillance and Utilization Review Program, medical and health care records must contain the following:

- Each page of the record must name or otherwise identify the patient.

- Each entry must be signed and dated by the individual providing health care. Record entries for health care provided by an individual under the supervision of an individual licensed provider must be countersigned by the provider. Institutional providers must not be required to countersign record entries for health care provided in the facility by an individual provider; however, the institutional providers must be responsible for monitoring the provision of such health care.

- Diagnoses, assessments, or evaluations

- Patient case history and results of oral or physical examination

- Plan of treatment or patient care plan must be entered in the physical record or otherwise available on site.

- Quantities and dosages of any prescribed drugs ordered and/or administered must be entered in the record.

- Results of all diagnostic tests and examinations

- Records must indicate the patient's progress, response to treatment, any change in treatment, and any change in diagnosis.

- Copies of consultation reports relating to a particular recipient

---

73. *Id.* R. 4640.4700.
74. *Id.* R. 9555.6245.

- Dates of hospitalization relating to service provided by a particular provider

- A copy of the summary of surgical procedures billed to the programs by the provider

MISSISSIPPI

Mississippi Code Annotated § 41-9-61 (b) (1990) defines "hospital records" as

> those medical histories, records, reports, summaries, diagnoses, and prognoses, records of treatment and medication ordered and given, notes, entries, X-rays, and other written or graphic data prepared, kept, made or maintained in hospitals that pertain to hospital confinements or hospital services rendered to patients admitted to hospitals or receiving emergency room or outpatient care. Such records must also include abstracts of the foregoing data customarily made or provided. . . . Such records must not, however, include ordinary business records pertaining to patient's accounts or the administration of the institution nor must "hospital records" include any records consisting of nursing audits, physician audits, departmental evaluations or other evaluations or reviews which are used only for inservice education programs, or which are required only for accreditation or for participation in federal health programs.

MISSOURI

Patient's medical records should include

- A unique identifying record number

- Pertinent identifying and personal data

- History of present illness or complaint

- Past and family history

- Physical examination results

- Provisional admitting diagnosis

- Medical staff orders

- Progress notes

- Nurses' notes

- Discharge summary

- Final diagnosis

- Evidence of appropriate informed consent

Where applicable, medical records must also contain reports such as clinical laboratory, x ray, consultation, electrocardiogram, surgical procedures, therapy, anesthesia, pathology, autopsy, and any other reports pertinent to the patient's care[75]

Medical records of *deceased patients* must contain

- Date and time of death

- Autopsy permit, if granted

- Disposition of the body

Nursing home admission records must include the following general information:

- Resident name and prior address

- Age (birthdate)

- Sex

- Marital status

- Social security number

- Medicare and Medicaid numbers

- Date of admission

- Name, address, and telephone number of responsible party

- Name, address, and telephone number of attending physician

- Height and weight on admission

- Inventory of resident's personal possessions on admission

- Names of preferred dentist, pharmacist, and mortician[76]

Nursing home medical records must include

- Admission diagnosis

- Admission physical and findings of subsequent examinations

- Progress notes

- Orders for all medications and treatments

- Orders for extent of activity

- Orders for restraints including type and reason for such restraint

- Orders for diet

75. Missouri Code Regulations tit. 19, § 30-20.021(D)(3) & (9) (1990).
76. *Id.* tit. 13, § 15-14.042 (104)–(110).

- Discharge diagnosis, or cause of death[77]

  Nursing progress notes must include

- Observations concerning the general condition of the resident

- Any change in the resident's physical or mental condition

- Any change in appetite

- Any injury, incident, or accident

- Observation of any resident being restrained

- Any significant item of care rendered to the resident

- Monthly weights

- Physician's visits[78]

- Discharge records

  Discharge records must include

- Date, condition, and reason for transfer or discharge

- Name of person to whom resident is discharged

- Forwarding address of discharged patient

- Date and time of death

- Disposition of the body[79]

MONTANA

Montana law does not define medical records or enumerate what all records should contain. Its Administrative Rules, however, list what must compose certain specialized records.

A *delivery record* must contain

- Starting time of patient's labor

- Time of birth of patient's newborn

- Anesthesia used on patient

- Whether an episiotomy was performed on patient

- Whether forceps were used in delivery

- Names of attending physicians

---

77. *Id.*
78. *Id.*
79. *Id.*

- Names of attending nurses

- Names of all other persons attending delivery

- Sex of the newborn

- Time of eye prophylactic treatment and name of drug used[80]

Obstetrical records must include the prenatal record, labor notes, obstetrical anesthesia notes, and delivery record.[81]

Records for newborns must include

- Observations of newborn after birth

- Delivery room care of newborn

- Physical examinations performed on newborn

- Temperature of newborn

- Weight of newborn

- Time of newborn's first urination

- Number, character, and consistency of newborn's stool

- Type of feeding administered to newborn

- Phenylketonuria report for newborn

- Name of person to whom newborn is released[82]

Medical records of hospices must contain

- Patient identification, diagnosis, prognosis

- Patient's medical history

- Patient/family plan of care

- A record of all physician's orders, verified at appropriate intervals

- Progress notes, dated and signed

- Evidence of timely action by the patient care team

Chapter 23 of the Montana Hospital Association Consent Manual does suggest that patient's records contain

- The patient's name, address, age, sex, and marital status

- Date of admission and date of discharge

---

80. Montana Administrative Rules 16.32.323 (1986).
81. *Id*. R. 16.32.328.
82. *Id*. R. 16.32.328 (1986).

- Name, address, and telephone number of person or agency responsible for patient

- Name, address, and telephone number of attending physician

- Diagnosis on admission

- Progress notes by physician

- Nurses' notes

- Medication and treatment orders

- Temperature chart, including pulse and respiration

- Condition and diagnosis of patient at time of discharge

- Complete surgical record, including anesthesia record, preoperative diagnosis, operative procedure and findings, postoperative diagnosis, and tissue diagnosis on all specimens surgically removed

- Complete obstetrical record, including prenatal record (if available), labor record, delivery record, and complete newborn record

Montana law does provide that a person's medical record may be abridged following the ten year retention date to a "core" record, which gives some guidance as to what a complete record must contain.[83] A *core record* must contain, at a minimum, the following:

- Identification of patient data, which includes

  - Name

  - Maiden name if relevant

  - Address

  - Date of birth

  - Sex

  - Social security number

- Medical history

- Physical examination report

- Consultation reports

- Report of operation

- Pathology report

---

83. Montana Administrative Rules 16.32.328(4) (1986).

- Discharge summary, except that for newborns and others for whom no discharge summary is available, the final progress note must be retained.

- Autopsy findings

- For each maternity patient, the information listed above

- For each newborn, the information listed above

Infirmaries must keep medical records for each patient, which include

- Identification data

- Chief complaint

- Present illness

- Medical history

- Physical examination

- Laboratory and x-ray reports

- Treatment administered

- Tissue report

- Progress reports

- Discharge summary[84]

Outpatient facility medical records must include the same information as infirmaries, immediately above.[85]

Personal care facility resident records must be composed of the following information:

- Admission record, including date of admission and discharge

- Name and address of resident

- Birthdate

- Marital status

- Financial responsibility

- Religious affiliation

- Telephone number of physician and of person to be notified in an emergency

- Discharge information concerning disposition of a resident's personal belongings

84. Montana Administrative Rules 16.32.340(4) (1987).
85. *Id.* R. 16.32.355(3).

- A care record, including date and dosage of each medication

- Date and time of visit to or by his physician[86]

NEBRASKA

Hospital medical records in Nebraska should contain sufficient information to justify the diagnosis and warrant the treatment and results.
  Hospital medical records must contain

- Identification data

- Chief complaint

- Present illness, history, and physical examination

- Provisional diagnosis

- Clinical pathology laboratory reports

- Radiology reports

- Consultations

- Treatment, medical and surgical

- Tissue report

- Progress notes (all disciplines)

- Discharge summary and autopsy findings

For purposes of retention and inclusion, Nebraska does not include original x-ray film or laboratory samples, slides, or tissues in medical records.[87]
Medical records for *intermediate care facilities* must include

- Documented evidence of initial and periodic assessment of the needs of the resident, of establishment of an overall plan of care and specific plans of care to meet the needs of the residents, including any changes, and of the care and services provided

- Admission information, including the medical and social history of the resident

- Identification data and consent forms

- Medical and nursing history of resident

- Reports of physical examination(s)

---

86. *Id.* R. 16.32.381(1).
87. Nebraska Administrative Rules & Regulations 175-9-003.04A (1979).

- Diagnostic and therapeutic orders signed by the physician

- Medical and nursing observations and progress notes

- Dental observations, orders, and progress notes

- Reports of treatments and clinical findings

- Medication administration records

- Rehabilitative services plans of care, evaluations, treatment notations, progress notes, and discharge summary and recommendations to the physician

- Social services records, resident activities assessment, and progress notes

- Nutritional assessments, plans, and care

- Transfer records and medical and other information necessary or useful in care and treatment of residents transferred between the facility and hospitals or other institutions[88]

Clinical (medical) records for each resident of a skilled nursing facility must include

- Documented evidence of assessment of the needs of the resident, of establishment of an overall plan of care and specific plans of care to meet the needs of residents, including any changes, and of the care and services provided

- Authentication of hospital diagnosis (discharge summary, report from patient's attending physician, transfer form)

- Identification data and consent forms

- Medical and nursing history of resident

- Reports of physical examination(s)

- Diagnostic and therapeutic orders signed by the physician

- Medical and nursing observations and progress notes

- Dental observations, orders, and progress notes

- Reports of treatments and clinical findings

- Medication administration records

- Rehabilitative services plans of care, evaluations, treatment notations, progress notes, and discharge summary and recommendations

- Social services records, resident activities assessment, progress notes[89]

88. *Id*. R. 175-8-003.04.
89. *Id*. R. 175-12-003.04.

Regulations and standards governing *health clinics* require that records of clients must include any medical examination, medical history, progress notes, and any other entries of pertinent observations and events.[90]

Records of *mental health clinics* must include identifying data, evaluation and admission data, client history, treatment plan, treatment course, and termination and disposition information.[91]

Outpatient records of *drug treatment centers* must include

- Presenting problem

- Health—basic physical status and significant medical history

- Substance use and history, including type and amount of substance

- Educational and occupational activities

- Criminality—to include past and current records of arrest, convictions, probation, sentence, parole, and pardon

- Psychological or psychiatric evaluation, or both, when indicated, and level of social functioning against which progress may be measured[92]

Resident records must contain the intake, medical examination, progress notes, and other entries of pertinent observations and events.[93]

Resident records of *domiciliary facilities* must contain

- Admission number

- Date of admission

- Full name, age, and sex

- Social security number

- Date of discharge

- Next of kin or person to be notified

- Name of attending physician

- Weight recorded at least quarterly[94]

Records of residents of *residential care facilities* must contain

- Certification by a physician that the resident does not require nursing care and requires only residential care services, if any services are required

- Admission number

90. *Id*. R. 175-7-004.04 (1975).
91. *Id*. R. 175-6-004.05 (1974).
92. *Id*. R. 175-6-004.04.
93. *Id*. R. 175-6-004.09 (1974).
94. *Id*. R. 175-4-007.06.

- Date of admission

- Full name of resident

- Age, sex, and date of birth

- The room assignment of the resident

- Signed written physician's orders for all medication, special diets, and any limitation of activities or conditions

- Social security number

- Date of discharge

- Next of kin or person to be notified

- Name of attending physician[95]

  Clinical records of *home health agencies* must contain

- Identification data and consent forms

- Name and address of the patient's physician(s)

- Physician's signed order for home health care and the approved plan of care must include, when appropriate to the services being provided

  - Medical diagnosis

  - Medication orders

  - Dietary orders

  - Treatment orders

  - Activity orders

  - Safety orders

- Initial and periodic assessments and care plans by disciplines providing services

- Signed and dated admission, observation, progress, and supervisory notes

- Copies of summary reports sent to the physician

- Diagnostic and therapeutic orders signed by the physician

- Reports of treatment and clinical findings

- Discharge summary[96]

---

95. *Id.* R. 175-11-007.07.
96. *Id.* R. 175-14-006.01A (1988).

NEVADA

Nevada defines "health care records" as "any written reports, notes, orders, photographs, X-rays or other written record received or produced by a provider of health care, or any person employed by him, which contains information relating to the medical history, examination, diagnosis or treatment of the patient."[97]

In addition, Nevada defines "medical records" to include bills, ledgers, statements, and other accounts showing the cost of medical services or care provided to a patient.[98]

The Nevada Administrative Code lists requirements for medical records. A medical record must be maintained for every patient admitted to a hospital,[99] extended care facility, or nursing home.[100] Records must contain sufficient information to justify the diagnosis, warrant treatment, and vindicate the end results. Records must be authenticated and signed by a licensed physician.

Under Nevada Administrative Code ch. 449 § 379(2) (1986), hospital records must contain

- Patient's name, address at time of admission, date of birth, sex, social security number, and marital status

- Date of admission

- Name, address, and telephone number of person or agency responsible for patient

- Name of attending physician

- Name and address of parents or guardians for minor patients

- Diagnosis on admission

- Race, religion, citizenship, state and county of birth

- Progress notes by physician

- Chief complaint

- Consultations

- Nurses' notes, which must conform to statute of limitation[101]

- Orders for medication and treatment

- Orders for diet[102]

---

97. Nevada Revised Statutes Annotated § 629.021 (Michie 1986).
98. *Id.* § 52.320.
99. Nevada Administrative Code ch. 449 § 379 (1986).
100. *Id.* § 403 (1986).
101. Nevada Revised Statutes Annotated § 629.051 (Michie 1986); *Id.* § 629.061 (Michie Supp. 1988).
102. Nevada Administrative Code ch. 449 § 337(3) (1986).

- History and physical examination

- Condition and diagnosis of patient at time of discharge

- Place where discharged

- Laboratory reports of all tests completed[103]

- Reports of all x rays completed[104]

- Complete surgical record, including anesthesia record, preoperative diagnosis, operative procedure and findings, postoperative diagnosis, and tissue diagnosis on all specimens surgically removed

- Complete obstetrical record, including prenatal, labor, delivery, and complete newborn record including birth certificate, test results, and the general condition of baby on discharge

- Copy of death certificate

  Extended care facilities and nursing homes must contain the following:

- Identification of patient, his address, and next of kin

- Medical notations

- Physician's orders

- Physical examination

- History and progressive notes signed by the attending physician

- Nursing notations

- Incident reports

- Laboratory and x-ray reports

- Consultation reports

- Reports of all tests, examinations, medical procedures, and services rendered to the patient in the facility by allied health professionals[105]

NEW HAMPSHIRE

New Hampshire Code of Administrative Rules, Department of Health & Human Services Regulation He-P 802.11 (1986), lists the contents of complete *hospital* medical records as including

- Identification data

---

103. *Id.* § 373(5)(b) (1986).
104. *Id.* § 376(3) (1986).
105. *Id.* § 403.

- Complaint
- Personal and family history
- History of present illness
- Physical examination
- Special examinations, such as consultants
- Clinical laboratory
- X-ray and other examinations
- Provisional or working diagnosis
- Medical or surgical treatment
- Gross and microscopic pathology findings
- Progress notes
- Final diagnosis
- Condition on discharge
- Follow-up and autopsy findings

  Nursing home records must contain

- Admission data including
  - Date of admission
  - Admitted from
  - Name, address, date of birth, marital status, sex
  - Name, address, and telephone number of nearest relative or other person responsible for the resident
  - Name and telephone number of the resident's physician
- Initial physician examination and periodic medical evaluation findings
- Medical history, diagnoses, and orders for medications, treatments, diet, and activities
- Physician's visits and progress notes
- Nurses' notes to include
  - Condition of resident on admission
  - Pertinent observations
  - Changes in the resident's physical or emotional condition

- Medications and treatments including reactions (if any)
- Vital signs
- Record of restraint monitoring

- Reports of accidents, injuries, or unusual incidents
- Consultation reports, laboratory reports, and other medical data
- Discharge or transfer information including date, time, health status, and future address. In the case of a deceased resident, the record must contain a licensed funeral director's receipt for removal of the body.[106]

Sheltered care facilities medical records must include

- Admission data, name and telephone number of next of kin or person responsible for the resident, and the telephone number of the resident's physician
- Admission health assessment
- Personal care and services needed by the resident
- Accounting of the patient's funds if managed by the facility
- Record of any accidents or injuries while in the facility
- In the case of a deceased resident, a receipt from a licensed funeral director[107]

Sheltered care facilities with nursing unit must keep more detailed records, including

- On admission, the resident's date of admission, name, address, date of birth, sex, and telephone number of the resident's physician
- Periodic medical evaluation findings, diagnoses, orders for medications, treatments, diet, and activities
- Physicians' visits and progress notes
- Nurses' notes, to include
  - Condition of resident on admission
  - Pertinent observations
  - Changes in the resident's physical or emotional condition
  - All medications and treatments including reactions (if any)
  - Vital signs

---

106. *Id.* R. 803.06.
107. *Id.* R. 804.04.

- Record of restraint monitoring

- Reports of accidents, injuries, or unusual incidents

- Consultation reports, laboratory reports, and the medical data, when applicable

- Discharge or transfer information including time, date, health status, and future address of the resident. In the case of a deceased resident, there must be a licensed funeral director's receipt for removal of the body.[108]

Outpatient clinic medical records must include

- Patient/client identification data

- Health assessment

- Medical evaluation and physical examination or other appropriate evaluation and diagnosis

- Physician orders for medications, treatments, diets, laboratory tests

- Progress notes by physician, health professional, and health worker

- Documentation of all services provided.

- Laboratory, x-ray, and other diagnostic tests and consultation reports

- Discharge summary

- Instructions given to patient/client[109]

Residential treatment and rehabilitation facilities' records must include

- Identification data, to include

  - Name

  - Address

  - Source of referral

  - Date of admission

  - Home telephone number

  - Age

- Pertinent history, assessment, diagnosis, rehabilitation problems, goals, prognosis

- Physician orders for medications, special diets, treatments, diagnostic services

---

108. *Id.* R. 805.05.
109. *Id.* R. 806.10.

- Individual treatment plan

- Progress notes

- Reports from consultation, laboratory, and all other diagnostic services

- Unusual events or occurrences and incident reports

- Discharge summary[110]

   Clinical laboratories must maintain accession logs containing

- The laboratory number identifying the specimen

- The identification of the person from whom the specimen was taken

- The name of other identification of the licensed physician, other authorized person, clinical laboratory, or collecting depot that submitted the specimen

- The date and time (if timing is critical) the specimen was collected

- The date and hour the specimen was received, if collected outside the laboratory doing the test

- The condition of the specimen when received if unsatisfactory

- The analysis performed

- The results of the laboratory test

- The date any required report was sent to the division of public health services or to other agencies[111]

   Home health care providers care records must include a plan of care containing

- Client identification data to include at least name, address, age, pertinent history, diagnosis, and goals

- Documentation of service provided

- Discharge summary[112]

NEW JERSEY

New Jersey defines medical records as "all records in a licensed hospital which pertain to the patient including X-ray films."[113]

---

110. *Id.* R. 807.07 (1986).
111. *Id.* R. 808.12.
112. *Id.* R. 809.07.
113. New Jersey Administrative Code tit. 8 § 43B-7.4 (c) 3.i (1985).

Patient's *individual medical records* should contain enough information to justify the diagnosis and treatment and to document the results accurately. Such records must contain

- Identification data and consent forms

- Admission and provisional diagnosis

- History

- Physical examination

- Physicians' progress notes

- Operative record

- Radiological diagnostic and treatment reports

- Laboratory reports

- Nursing notes

- Physicians' orders

- Medication and treatment record

- Consultations

- Record of discharge or death

- Autopsy findings

- Final diagnosis

- Discharge summary[114]

Obstetric medical records must contain

- Patient identification data

- Name of the patient's physician

- Physician's signed and dated admission note, medical and surgical history, and report of physical examination, completed within 24 hours of admission. Updating of the prenatal record fulfills this standard.

- Completed prenatal record

- Documentation of complete blood count and dipstick urinalysis including protein and sugar on admission

- Reports of laboratory, radiological, and other tests done prior to admission

---

114. *Id.* § 43B-7.2 (b) & (c).

- Documentation of the course of labor, delivery, and the immediate post-partum period

- All orders for the patient, written, signed, and dated

- Documentation of the patient's vital signs, condition of the uterus, blood loss, and any complications, prior to transfer to the postpartum unit

- A nursing care plan

- Signed informed consents

- An operative report, if surgery has been performed, recorded by the physician who performed the surgery, including a description of the technique used, surgical procedures, tissue removed or altered, sponge count, condition of the patient on leaving the operating or delivery room, estimated blood loss, postoperative diagnosis, and the names of the physician-in-charge and assistants

- For patients receiving anesthesia

  - Preanesthesia record, including at least drug history, anesthesia history, and potential anesthetic problems

  - Anesthesia record, describing at least induction and maintenance of anesthesia, including volume, route of admission, patient's vital signs, duration of anesthesia, any complications of anesthesia or analgesia management, and drugs, intravenous fluids, blood, and/or blood components administered

  - Postanesthesia note by the anesthetist describing the presence or absence of anesthesia-related complications, recorded after the patient's recovery from anesthesia

- Documentation of accidents and incidents, if any

- A record of any treatment, medication, or service refused by the patient, including a physician's visit

- Documentation of any medication released to the patient on discharge

- Progress notes by the physician

- Clinical notes

- A record of medications administered, including the name and strength of the drug, date and time of administration, dosage administered, method of administration, and signature and title of the person administering the drug

- Any referrals to outside resources

- A discharge summary

- Page 4 of the Prenatal Record, Form MCH-13 of the Maternal and Child Health Program of the department, or other form that includes the same information, included at the time of discharge[115]

Newborn records must include

- Summary of the mother's obstetric history

- Summary of labor and delivery, including

  - Anesthesia, analgesia, and medications given to the mother

  - Reasons for induction of labor and operative procedures (if performed)

  - Condition of the newborn at birth, including the one- and five-minute Apgar scores or the equivalent, time of sustained respirations, details of any physical abnormalities, and any pathological states observed and treatment given before transfer to the nursery

  - Any abnormalities of the placenta and cord vessels

  - Date and time of birth

  - Birth weight and length

  - Length of gestation

  - Procedures performed in the delivery room

  - Verification of eye prophylaxis

- The newborn's identification

- Record of newborn assessment, performed by a physician or registered professional nurse on the newborn's admission to the newborn nursery

- Nursing care plan

- Record of the initial physical examination

- Physical examination on discharge or transfer to another facility, including head circumference and body length (unless previously measured), signed by a physician[116]

Renal dialysis records must include

- Signed, dated admission and medical history

- Report of physical examination

---

115. *Id.* tit. 8 § 43B-8.17.
116. *Id.* tit. 8 § 43B-8.25.

- Medical, nursing, social service, and dietary portions of the patient care plan
- Clinical notes

Cardiac diagnostic and surgical services medical records must include

- Signed, dated admission, medical and surgical history, and a report of physical examination, completed within 24 hours of admission. The examination report must include results of all tests and procedures performed, diagnoses, prognosis, and rehabilitation potential.
- All orders for the patient, written, signed, and dated by the physician
- Physician's care plan, initiated on admission and kept current
- Nursing care plan, and a care plan for each of the services providing care to the patient, initiated on admission and kept current
- Signed informed consent prior to catheterization or surgery
- Cardiac catheterization summary sheet if cardiac catheterization is performed, including pre- and postcatheterization diagnoses and complications of the procedure, if any
- Operative report, if surgery has been performed, recorded immediately after surgery by the cardiovascular surgeon who performed the surgery, and including
  - Description of findings
  - Technique used
  - Surgical procedures
  - Tissue removed or altered
  - Sponge count
  - Estimated blood loss
  - Postoperative diagnosis
  - Names of the surgeon and assistants
- Preanesthesia record, including at least drug history, anesthesia history, and potential anesthetic problems
- Anesthesia record, describing at least the following: induction and maintenance of anesthesia, including volume, route of administration, patient's vital signs, duration of anesthesia; any complications of anesthesia or analgesia management; and other drugs, intravenous fluids, blood and/or blood components administered

- Postanesthetic note by the anesthesiologist describing any postoperative abnormalities or complications and stating the blood pressure, pulse, presence or absence of swallowing reflexes, cyanosis, and ability to move extremities

- Clinical notes

- Progress notes by physicians

- A record of medications administered, including the name and strength of the drug, date and time of administration, dosage administered, route of administration, and signature of the licensed nurse who administered the drug

- Summaries of conferences and consultations

- Any referrals to outside resources and documentation of follow-up

- A clinical resume

- Discharge plan for each of the services providing care to the patient[117]

The State Board of Medical Examiners of New Jersey[118] requires that *professional treatment records* must reflect

- Dates of all treatments

- Patient's complaint

- History

- Findings on appropriate examination

- Progress notes

- Any orders for tests or consultations and the results thereof

- Diagnosis or medical impression

- Treatment ordered, including specific dosages, quantities, and strengths of medications if prescribed, administered, or dispensed

- Identity of the treatment provider if the service is rendered in a setting in which more than one provider practices

NEW MEXICO

Regulations of the New Mexico Health and Social Services Department require that medical records include

---

117. *Id.* tit. 8 § 43B-17.10.
118. *Id.* tit. 8 § 35-6.5 (b).

- Identification data

- Complaint

- Personal and family history

- History of present illness

- Physical examination

- Nursing notes

- Temperature chart

- Special examinations and consultations

- Clinical laboratory examinations

- X-ray examinations

- Other examinations

- Provisional and final diagnosis

- Medical, surgical, and dental treatment

- Gross and microscopic pathology findings on tissues removed

- Progress notes

- Condition on discharge

- Follow-up and autopsy findings[119]

NEW YORK

New York's Department of Health requires an accurate, clear, and comprehensive medical record for every person evaluated or treated as an inpatient, ambulatory patient, emergency patient, or outpatient of the hospital. The record must contain information to justify admission and continued hospitalization, support the diagnosis, and describe the patient's progress and response to medications and services.[120]

All records must document

- Evidence of a physical examination, including a health history, performed no more than seven days prior to admission or within 24 hours after admission and a statement of the conclusion or impressions drawn

- Admitting diagnosis

---

119. Health Care Financial Management Association, New Mexico Hospital Association Legal Handbook, ch. 5, ¶ 5(2) (rev. ed. 1981).

120. New York Compilation Codes Rules & Regulations tit. 405 (1988–89).

- Results of all consultative evaluations of the patient and findings by clinical and other staff involved in the care of the patient

- Documentation of all complications, hospital-acquired infections, and unfavorable reactions to drugs and anesthesia

- Properly executed consent forms for procedures and treatments

- All practitioners' diagnostic and therapeutic orders, nursing documentation and care plans, reports of treatment, medication records, radiology, and laboratory reports, vital signs, and other information necessary to monitor the patient's condition

- Discharge summary with outcome of hospitalization, disposition of case, and provisions for follow-up care

- Final diagnosis

- Physician's attestation sheet, the accuracy of which must be attested to by the signature of a licensed attending physician, which includes the patient's age, sex, principal and other diagnoses, and principal and other procedures performed. The certification to be included on the physician's attestation sheet is to be signed and dated by a licensed attending physician and read as follows: "I certify that the narrative descriptions of the principal and secondary diagnoses and the major procedures performed are accurate and complete to the best of my knowledge."[121]

Maternity patient's medical records must also include

- Copy or abstract of the prenatal record, if existing, including a maternal history and physical examination as well as the results of maternal and fetal risk assessment and ongoing assessments of fetal growth and development and maternal health

- Results of a current physical examination

- Labor and birth information and postpartum assessment[122]

Newborn's records must be cross-referenced with the mother's and include

- Newborn physical assessment, including Apgar scores, presence or absence of three cord vessels, description of maternal-newborn interaction, ability to feed, eye prophylaxis, vital signs, and accommodation to extrauterine life

- Orders for newborn screening tests

---

121. *Id.* tit. 405 § 10.
122. *Id.* tit. 405 § 21.

- Infant footprint and mother's fingerprint or other comparable positive newborn patient identification[123]

NORTH CAROLINA

North Carolina's hospital licensing rules, North Carolina Administrative Code tit. 10, r. 3C.1404 (Feb. 1976), prescribe the minimum requirements for medical records as sufficient recorded information to justify the diagnosis, verify the treatment, and warrant the end results, including

- Identification data (name, address, age, sex, marital status)
- Date of admission
- Date of discharge
- Personal and family history
- Chief complaint
- History of present illness
- Physical examination
- Special examination, if any, such as consultations, clinical laboratory, x ray
- Provisional or admitting diagnosis
- Medical treatment
- Surgical record, including
  - Anesthesia record
  - Preoperative diagnosis
  - Operative procedure and findings
  - Postoperative diagnosis
  - Tissue diagnosis (on all specimens examined)
- Progress and nurses' notes
- Temperature chart, including pulse and respiration, medications
- Final diagnosis
- Summary and condition on discharge
- In case of death—autopsy findings, if performed

---

123. *Id.*

Nursing home records must contain

- Identification data

    - Name

    - Address

    - Age, sex, and marital status

    - Name, address, and telephone number of next of kin and/or legal guardian

- Admission data, including

    - Medical history and physical examination

    - Hospital discharge summary

    - Admission diagnosis

    - Rehabilitation potential

- Transfer form

- Diagnostic reports

- Consultation reports

- Physician's orders

- Physician's progress notes

- Medical and treatment records, which include laboratory, x-ray, dental examination, physical therapy reports, etc.

- Graphic sheet

- Medication administration sheet

- Diabetic sheets

- Patient assessment and progress notes by various disciplines

- Miscellaneous, such as consent and release forms, copy of transfer forms to the receiving institution, discharge order or release of liability for the facility if the patient or resident leaves against physician's orders

- Discharge summary, including admitting and final diagnosis and/or prognosis or cause of death[124]

Home health agency medical records must include

- Admission data

---

124. *Id.* tit. 10, r. 3H.0609 (Mar. 1983).

- Identification data (name, address, telephone number, date of birth, sex, marital status, social security number)
- Names of next of kin or legal guardian
- Names of other family members
- Source of referral
- Admission and discharge dates from hospital or other institution when applicable
- Names of physicians responsible for the patient's care
- Assessment of home environment
- Clinical data
  - Patient's diagnosis
  - Physician's plan of treatment, including drugs and treatments, diet, activity, and specific services and therapies required
  - Initial assessments by appropriate disciplines
  - Patient care plan utilizing problem identification, the establishment of goals, and proposed interventions
  - Progress notes containing a record of all services provided, directly and by contract, with entries dated and signed by the individual providing the service
  - Discharge summary, which includes an overall summary of services provided by the agency and the date and reason for discharge. When a specific service to a patient is terminated and other services continue, there must be documentation of the date and reason for terminating the specific service.[125]

Hospice medical records must include

- Identification data (name, address, telephone, date of birth, sex, marital status)
- Name of next of kin or legal guardian
- Names of other family members
- Religious preference and church affiliation and clergy if appropriate
- Diagnosis, as determined by attending physician
- Authorization from attending physician for hospice care
- Source of referral

---

125. *Id.* tit. 10, r. 3L.0605.

- Initial assessments

- Consent for care form

- Physician's orders for drugs, treatments and other special care, diet, activity, and other specific therapy services

- Care plan

- Clinical notes containing a record of all professional services provided directly or by contract, with entries signed by the individual providing the services

- Volunteer notes, as applicable, indicating type of contact, activities performed, and time spent

- Discharge summary to include services provided, or reason for discharge if services are terminated prior to the death of the patient

- Bereavement counseling notes[126]

  Cardiac rehabilitation program medical records must include

- Patient identification data

- Medical history and discharge summary

- Graded exercise data

- Record of oxygen uptake where appropriate

- Records of blood chemistry analysis lipid profile

- Informed consent to participate in the programs

- Reports of physical examinations

- Progress notes and response to the therapeutic plan

- Vocational questionnaire

- All records of each discipline's participation in the patient's therapeutic plan

- Discharge plans providing for postdischarge program continuity and follow-up as appropriate

- Miscellaneous records desirable for program continuity

NORTH DAKOTA

North Dakota's Hospital Licensing Rules, North Dakota Administrative Code § 33-07-01-16 (8) (1980), require that *hospital* medical records contain sufficient information to justify the diagnosis and warrant the treatment and end results. They must contain

---

126. *Id.* tit. 10, r. 3T.0902.

- Identification data

- Chief complaint, which must include a concise statement of the complaints that led the patient to consult the physician and the date of onset and duration of each

- Present illness

- Past history

- Family history

- Physical examination, including all positive and negative findings resulting from an inventory of systems

- Provisional diagnosis

- Clinical laboratory reports

- X-ray reports

- Consultations

- Treatment, medical and surgical, including all diagnostic treatment procedures

- Tissue reports, including a report of microscopic findings if hospital regulations require such an examination. If only gross examination is warranted, the record should contain a statement that the tissue has been received and a gross description.

- Progress notes

- Final diagnosis

- Discharge summary

- Nurses' notes

- Autopsy findings, when applicable

  Clinical records of residents of *long-term care facilities* must contain

- Identification and summary sheet or sheets, including

  - Resident's name, social security number, marital status, age, sex, home address, and religion

  - Names, addresses, and telephone numbers of referral agency, personal physician, dentist, and designated representative or other responsible person

  - Admitting diagnosis, final diagnosis, conditions on discharge, and disposition

- Initial medical evaluation, including medical history, physical examination, diagnosis, and estimation of restoration potential

- Authentication of hospital diagnosis, in the form of a hospital summary discharge sheet, a report from the physician who attended the resident in the hospital, or a transfer form used under a transfer agreement

- Physician's orders, including all medication, treatments, diet, restorative, and special medical procedures required for the safety and well-being of the resident

- Physician's progress notes describing significant changes in the resident's condition, written at the time of each visit

- Nurses' notes containing observations made by the nursing personnel

- Medication and treatment records, including all medications, treatments, and special procedures performed for the safety and well-being of the resident

- Laboratory and x-ray reports

- Consultation reports

- Dental reports

- Social service notes

- Resident care referral reports

OHIO

A "medical record" means "any document or combination of documents that pertains to a patient's medical history, diagnosis, prognosis, or medical condition and that is generated and maintained in the process of the patient's health care treatment in a hospital." A finalized medical record is one that is complete according to the hospital's bylaws.[127]

Ohio Administrative Code § 5122-14-01 (C)(29) (1991) defines medical records of psychiatric hospitals and psychiatric units as "the document which contains all significant clinical information pertaining to the patient."

Medical records of *maternity home residents* must include prenatal history, physical examination, and physician's orders and observations. The infant's record must contain history of gestation, delivery, and immediate postnatal period; physical examination; and physician's orders and observations.[128]

Current individual records of *residential care facilities* must include

---

127. Ohio Revised Code § 3701.74 (Baldwin 1991).
128. *Id.* § 3701-7-35.

- Legal status of the individual

- Records of accidents, injuries, seizures, and unusual incidents and the treatment or first aid measure administered for same

- All medical and dental examinations, and immunization records as appropriate to age

- Medication and treatment records, which must indicate the person who prescribed the medication and treatment and the person who administered the medication and treatment

- Records of absences from the residential facility for 24 hours or longer as well as notations of the time of the individual's return

- Most recent residential evaluation

- Individual plans and notations of progress

- Record of the individual's monies and negotiable items received and expended and the purpose of the expenditures

- Consents for services, treatments, or medications[129]

  Permanent records include

- Admission and referral records, including a photograph of the individual

- Medical and dental examinations, and immunization records as appropriate to age

- All medical and treatment records

- All records of the individual's monies and negotiable items received and expended and the purpose of the expenditures

- Discharge summaries prepared within seven days following the individual's discharge, including

  - Individual's progress during residence

  - New address of residence

  - Arrangements for future programming[130]

Medical records of *psychiatric hospitals and psychiatric units* must include

- Patient information to include

  - Name

---

129. *Id.* § 5123:2-3-16(B) (1991).
130. *Id.* § 5123:2-3-16(C) (1991).

- Home address

- Home telephone number

- Date of birth

- Sex

- Marital status

- Religion

- Race or ethnic origin

- Name, telephone number, and address of next of kin, significant others, or person to notify in case of emergency as identified by the patient or, as appropriate, guardian

- Education

- School or employment status

- Eligibility for third-party benefits

- Documentation of any necessary referrals to explore eligibility for income support such as social security disability insurance, supplemental security income, general relief, or food stamps

- Source of referral

- Legal status as a voluntary or involuntary patient

- Reason for admitting including presenting problem(s), precipitating factors, and initial diagnosis

- Previous hospitalizations

- Medical history

- Social history

- Reports of all patient assessments and examinations

- Individualized treatment plan, which must include plans for after-hospitalization care and services

- All medical orders

- Documentation of the patient's progress, and other significant patient events that could impact treatment

- Appropriate consents for treatment and for release of confidential information

- Discharge summary completed within 30 days after discharge, which must include

- Assessment of the patient's condition on admission

- Assessment of the patient's condition on discharge and reason for discharge

- Description of diagnostic and treatment services received by the patient, with reference to interventions identified on the treatment plan, and the patient's response

- All recommendations made to the patient

- Medications prescribed on discharge

- Initial and final diagnosis, both physical and psychiatric, according to The American Psychiatric Association's latest edition of the *Diagnostic and Statistical Manual of Mental Disorders,* which must be recorded in full without the use of either symbols or abbreviations.[131]

This regulation also requires all legal documents pertaining to civil commitment and guardianship to be included in the medical record.

Medical records of *health maintenance organizations* (HMOs) participating in Ohio's Medicaid program must include

- Patient's name, date of birth, sex, address, telephone number

- Next of kin, sponsor, or responsible party

- Medical history, including specific allergic reactions

- Dates of services

- Names and titles of providers of services

- Patient complaint/presenting problem

- Pertinent findings on examination, diagnosis

- Medications administered or prescribed

- Referrals and results of referrals

- Description of treatment(s), where applicable

- Recommendations for additional treatments or consultations

- Medical goods or supplies dispensed or prescribed

- Tests performed and results

- Documentation of emergency encounters and follow-up

- Hospitalization orders and discharge summaries

---

131. *Id.* § 5122-14-22 (E).

- Physician entries that are signed and dated

- Health education and medical social services provided[132]

Ohio law specifies almost identical requirements for HMOs in Montgomery County.[133]

Ohio requires notation in an HMO patient's medical record of relevant information related to an after-hours physician call and a notation in hospitalized patient's medical record indicating the reason, date, and duration of hospitalization, entry of pertinent reports from the hospitalization in the medical record, and entry of outcomes and discharge planning in the medical record.[134] In addition a copy of a standardized referral form must go in the medical record.

Alcoholism inpatient/emergency care resident records content must include

- Admission and summary sheet, containing

  - Client's full name

  - Home phone number

  - Social security and other insurance numbers

  - Welfare number, if applicable

  - Sex

  - Marital status

  - Age

  - Religion

  - Physician

  - Clergyman

  - Next of kin or other responsible person

  - Other pertinent data

  - Name, address, and telephone number of referring agency

  - Admitting problems and diagnosis

  - Admission and transfer information that may be pertinent

  - Discharge summary of the course of treatment followed and progress in facility

---

132. *Id.* § 5101:3-26-07 (1990).
133. *Id.* § 5101:3-36-07.
134. *Id.* § 5101:3-26-13.

- Duplicate copy of any information sent to other agencies at time of discharge or transfer

- Initial medical evaluation and assessment, including

  - Medical and drinking history

  - Physical examination

  - Diagnosis, problems, and an estimate of restoration potential

  - Results of laboratory findings showing results of evidence of freedom from communicable disease

  - Appropriate medical information and other services offered the client must be kept current.[135]

Nursing home individual medical records must contain

- Admission record, including

  - Name

  - Residence

  - Age

  - Sex

  - Race

  - Religion

  - Date of admission

  - Name and address of nearest relative or guardian

  - Admission diagnoses from referral record

  - Name of attending physician

- Referral record, including all records, reports, and orders that accompany the patient

- Nurses' notes. A note of the condition of the patient on admission and subsequent notes as indicated to describe changes in condition, unusual events, or accidents

- Medication record, including

  - Physician's order sheet on which orders are recorded and signed by the physician, including telephone orders

  - Nurse's treatment sheet on which all treatments or medications are

---

135. *Id.* § 3701-55-15.

recorded as given, showing what was done or given, the date and hour, and signed by the nurse giving the treatment or medication

- Physician's progress record. A sheet on which the physician may enter notes concerning changes in diagnosis or condition of the patient.[136]

OKLAHOMA

The Oklahoma Department of Health Regulation ch. 13 requires records of patient admission to include

- Full name of patient with age and sex, address, marital status, birth date, home phone number, date of admission, and admitting diagnosis

- Next of kin, with address, phone number, and relationship

- Date of admission, the admission and final diagnosis, and the name of physician

Medical records must contain sufficient information to justify the diagnosis and warrant the treatment and end results.
The *medical records* will contain

- Identification data

- Chief complaint

- Present illness

- Past history

- Family history

- Physical examination

- Provisional diagnosis

- Clinical laboratory reports

- Consultations

- Treatment, medical and surgical

- Tissue report

- Progress notes

- Final diagnosis

- Discharge summary

- Autopsy findings

---

136. *Id.* § 3701-17-19.

Emergency medical records will contain

- Patient identification

- Time and means of arrival

- History of disease or injury

- Physical findings

- Laboratory and x-ray reports, if any

- Diagnosis and therapeutic orders

- Record of treatment, including vital signs

- Disposition of the case

- Signature of the licensed registered professional nurse

- Signature of the physician

- Document patient leaving against medical advice

Outpatient medical records must contain information relative to the patient's history, physical examination, laboratory and other diagnostic tests, diagnosis, and treatment that is complete and sufficiently detailed to facilitate continuity of care.

OREGON

Oregon Administrative Rules list required contents of medical records for various classifications of healthcare facilities.[137] All healthcare facilities must maintain a medical record for every patient admitted for care.

Medical record (general requirements)

- Admitting identification data, including date of admission

- Chief complaint

- Pertinent family and personal history

- Medical history, physical examination report, and provisional diagnosis

- Physicians' orders such as medication, diets, treatments, records of periodic visits to patient, ongoing assessments, and any orders pertinent to the care of the patient

- Clinical laboratory reports and reports on any special examinations

---

137. Oregon Administrative Rules 333-86-055(1) to (12) (1986) (Long Term Care Facilities); *Id.* R. 333-92-095(1) & (2) (1985) (Nursing Homes for the Mentally Retarded).

- X-ray reports with identification (authentication) of the originator of the interpretation

- Authenticated reports of consultants

- Records of assessment and intervention, including graphic charts, medication records, and personal notes

- Summary, including final diagnosis

- Date of discharge and discharge note

- Autopsy report if applicable

- Such signed documents as required by law

All entries must be dated, timed, and authenticated. Entries must be verified by means of a unique identifier (i.e., signature, code, thumbprint, or voice print) that allows identification of the individual responsible for the entry. Verbal orders may be accepted by approved personnel and authenticated by the prescriber within 24 hours. A single signature or authentication does not suffice to cover the content of the entire record.

Medical records of *surgical patients* (in addition to general requirements):

- Preoperative history, physical examination, and diagnosis charted prior to operation

- Anesthesia record, including records of anesthesia, analgesia, and medications given in the course of operation, and postanesthetic condition

- A record of operation dictated immediately following surgery and including a complete description of the operation procedures and findings, postoperative diagnostic impression, and a description of the tissues and appliances, if any, removed

- Postanesthesia recovery progress notes

- Pathology report on tissues and appliances, if any, removed (except certain categories exempt from the pathology report)[138]

Obstetrical record (in addition to general requirements)

- Prenatal care record containing at least a serologic test for syphilis, Rh factor determination, and past obstetrical history and physical examination

- Labor and delivery record, including reasons for induction and operative procedures, if any

---

138. *Id.* § 333-505-050(4)(e).

- Records of anesthesia, analgesia, and medications given during the course of delivery

- Date and hour of birth

- Birth weight and length

- Period of gestation

- Sex

- Condition of infant on delivery

- Mother's name and hospital number

- Record of ophthalmic prophylaxis or refusal of same

- Physical examination at birth and at discharge

- Progress and nurses' notes

- Temperature

- Weight and feeding data

- Number, consistency, and color of stools

- Urinary output

- Condition of eyes and umbilical cord

- Condition and color of skin

- Motor behavior

- Type of identification placed on infant in delivery room

  Emergency room, outpatient, and clinic records must contain

- Patient identification

- Admitting diagnosis, chief complaint, and brief history of disease or injury

- Physical findings

- Laboratory, x-ray, and special examination reports. The original report must be authenticated and recorded in the patient's medical record.

- Diagnosis

- Record of treatment, including medications

- Disposition of case with instructions to patient

- Signature or authentication of attending physician

- A record of prehospital report form (when patient arrives by ambulance) must be attached to the emergency room record.

Long-term care facility (LTCF) records must contain

- Admitting diagnosis
- Identification data
  - Name
  - Previous address
  - Date and time of admission
  - Sex
  - Date of birth
  - Marital status
  - Religious preference
  - Social security number
  - Next of kin
  - Attending physician and dentist
- Medical history and physical examination
- Transfer information
- Clinical reports, x-ray results, laboratory tests
- Current physician's orders and progress notes
- Clinical observations
- Record of medication administration
- Record of treatments administered
- Releases, consent forms, receipts, valuables lists
- Discharge summary prepared promptly after patient discharge

Nursing homes for the mentally retarded patient records must include

- Identification data
  - Name
  - Previous address
  - Date and time of admission
  - Sex
  - Nationality
  - Date of birth

- Marital status

- Next of kin

- Date of discharge or death

- Treatment records (including all written orders of attending physician for medication and other services)

PENNSYLVANIA

An adequate medical record for a general or special hospital must contain data from all episodes of care and treatment of the patient, whether services were performed on an inpatient or an outpatient basis or in the emergency unit.[139] The contents must include sufficient information to identify the patient clearly, to justify the diagnosis and treatment, and to document the results accurately.[140]

If a member of the hospital's medical staff has performed a physical examination within 30 days prior to the patient's admission, a copy of the examination record may be used in lieu of an admission history and report of physical examination. An interval admission note, however, is required, including any additions to the history and changes in the physical findings.[141]

If the patient was admitted to another hospital within 30 days prior to his admission, the staff or attending physician must determine whether to record its own complete history and physical examination and, with the patient's written authorization, request his records from the other hospital as soon as possible.[142]

A medical record must include

- Notes by staff members and individuals who have been granted clinical privileges

- Consultation reports

- Nurses' notes and entries by specified professional personnel[143]

- Findings and results of any pathological or clinical laboratory examinations, radiology examinations, medical and surgical treatment, and other diagnostic or therapeutic procedures[144]

- Provisional diagnosis, primary and secondary final diagnoses, a clinical resume, and, where appropriate, necropsy reports[145]

---

139. 28 Pennsylvania Code § 115.31 (1989).
140. *Id.* § 115.32.
141. *Id.* § 115.32 (b).
142. *Id.* § 115.32 (c).
143. *Id.* § 115.32 (d).
144. *Id.* § 115.32 (e).
145. *Id.* § 115.32 (f).

The minimum standards of practice of the State Board of Medicine specify that physicians must maintain medical records for patients that accurately, legibly, and completely reflect the evaluation and treatment of the patient. They must contain information sufficient to clearly identify the patient; the person making the entry if the person is not the physician; the date of the entry; patient complaints and symptoms; clinical information; diagnoses, findings, and results of pathologic or clinical laboratory examination, radiology examination, medical and surgical treatment, and other diagnostic, corrective, or therapeutic procedures.

Medical records of *newborn services* of general and special hospitals must also include

- Obstetrical history of mother's previous pregnancies

- Description of complications of pregnancy or delivery

- List of complicating maternal disease

- Drugs taken by the mother during pregnancy, labor, and delivery

- Duration of ruptured membranes

- Maternal antenatal blood serology, rubella titer, blood typing, Rh factors, and, where indicated, a Coombs test for maternal antibodies

- Complete description of progress of labor including reasons for induction and operative procedures, if any, signed by the attending physician or his authorized delegate

- Anesthesia, analgesia, and medications given to mother and infant

- Condition of infant at birth, including the one- and five-minute Apgar scores or their equivalent, resuscitation, time of sustained respirations, details of physical abnormalities, pathological states observed, and treatments given before transfer to the nursery

- Any abnormalities of the placenta and cord vessels

- Date and hour of birth, birth weight and length, and period of gestation

- Written verification of eye prophylaxis

- Report of initial physical examination, including any abnormalities, signed by the attending physician or his authorized delegate

- Discharge physical examination, including head circumference and body length unless previously done; recommendations; and signature of attending physician or his delegate

- Listing of all diagnoses since birth, including discharge diagnosis

- Specific follow-up plans for care of infant

Ambulatory surgical facility medical records must include at least

- Patient identification

- Significant medical history and results of physical examination

- Preoperative diagnostic studies—entered before surgery—if performed

- Allergies or abnormal drug reactions

- Documentation of properly executed informed patient consent

- Entries related to anesthesia administration

- Findings and techniques of the operation, including a pathologist's report on tissue removed during surgery

- Notes by authorized staff members and individuals who have been granted clinical privileges, nurses' notes, and entries by other professional personnel

- Disposition, recommendations, and instructions given to the patient

- Significant medical advice given to a patient by telephone

- Discharge summary including discharge diagnosis

Long-term care facility medical records must contain

- Physicians' orders

- Observation and progress notes

- Nurses' notes

- Medical and nursing history and physical examination reports

- Identification information

- Admission data

- Documented evidence of assessment of patient's needs, establishment of an appropriate treatment plan, and plans of care and services provided

- Hospital diagnoses authentication—discharge summary, report from attending physician, or transfer form

- Diagnostic and therapeutic orders

- Reports of treatments

- Clinical findings

- Medication records

- Discharge summary including final diagnosis and prognosis or cause of death[146]

RHODE ISLAND

Rhode Island does not specifically define medical records, but does define "confidential health care information" as "all information relating to a patient's health care history, diagnosis, condition, treatment or evaluation obtained from a health care provider who has treated the patient."[147]

The Rules and Regulations for Licensing of Hospitals state that medical records must contain sufficient information to identify the patient and the problem, and to describe the treatment and document the results.[148] The content of all medical records, including inpatient, outpatient, ambulatory, and emergency, is to conform with the *Accreditation Manual for Hospitals,* Joint Commission on Accreditation of Hospitals (now Joint Commission on Accreditation of Healthcare Organizations).

SOUTH CAROLINA

Hospitals' or institutional medical facilities' medical records must contain

- Admission record, including

  - Name

  - Address, including county

  - Occupation

  - Age

  - Date of birth

  - Sex

  - Marital status

  - Religion

  - County of birth

  - Father's name

  - Mother's maiden name

  - Husband's or wife's name

  - Dates of military service

---

146. *Id.* § 211.5.
147. Rhode Island General Laws § 5-37.3-3 (1987).
148. 1990 Rhode Island Acts & Resolves R23-17-HOSP-25.6 and R23-17-HOSP-25.7.

- Health insurance number

- Provisional diagnosis

- Case number

- Days of care

- Social security number

- Name of the person providing information

- Name, address, and telephone number of person or persons to be notified in the event of emergency

- Name and address of referring physician

- Name, address, and telephone number of attending physician

- Date and hour of admission

- History and physical within 48 hours after admission

- Provisional or working diagnosis

- Preoperative diagnosis

- Medical treatment

- Complete surgical record, if any, including technique of operation and findings, statement of tissue and organs removed and postoperative diagnosis

- Report of anesthesia

- Nurses' notes

- Progress notes

- Gross and microscopic pathological findings

- Temperature chart, including pulse and respiration

- Medication administration record or similar document for recording of medications, treatments, and other pertinent data. Nurses must sign the record after each medication administered or treatment rendered.

- Final diagnosis and discharge summary

- Date and hour of discharge summary

- In case of death, cause and autopsy findings, if autopsy is performed

- Special examinations, if any, e.g., consultations, clinical laboratory, x-ray, and other examinations.[149]

---

149. South Carolina Code Regulations 61-6, § 601.5.A (1988).

Newborn records must contain

- History of hereditary conditions in mother's and/or father's family

- First day of the last menstrual period and estimated day of confinement

- Mother's blood group and Rh type—evidence of sensitization and/or immunization

- Serological test for syphilis (including dates performed)

- Number, duration, and outcome of previous pregnancies, with dates

- Maternal diseases (e.g., diabetes, hypertension, pre-eclampsia, infections)

- Drugs taken during pregnancy, labor, and delivery

- Results of measurement of fetal maturity and well-being (e.g., lung maturity and ultrasonography)

- Duration of ruptured membranes and labor, including length of second stage

- Method of delivery, including indications for operative or instrumental interference

- Complications of labor and delivery (e.g., hemorrhage or evidence of fetal distress), including a representative strip of the fetal EKG if recorded

- Description of placenta at delivery, including number of umbilical vessels

- Estimated amount and description of amniotic fluid

- Apgar scores at one and five minutes of age; description of resuscitation, if required; detailed descriptions of abnormalities and problems occurring from birth until transfer to the special nursery or the referral facility

- Test results and date specimen was collected for PKU and hypothyroid newborn screening test (except where the parents object for religious reasons. In such cases, file a copy of an executed "Statement of Religious Objection" Form.[150]

Nursing home records must include

- Identification data

  - Name

  - County

  - Occupation

  - Age

---

150. *Id.* § 601.5.B.

- Date of birth

- Sex

- Marital status

- Religion

- County of birth

- Father's name

- Mother's maiden name

- Husband's or wife's name

- Dates of military service

- Health insurance number

- Social security number

- Diagnosis

- Case number

- Dates of care

- Consent form for treatment signed by the patient or his representative

- Name and telephone number of attending physician

- Date and hour of admission

- Date and hour of discharge

- Signature of physician authorizing discharge

- Condition on discharge

- Name of the person providing information is desirable

- Name, address, and telephone number of person or persons to be notified in case of emergency

- Record of physical examination prior to admission or within 48 hours after admission, including

  - Medical history

  - Physical findings

  - Diagnosis

  - Physician's orders for medication, treatment, care and diet, which must be reviewed and reordered at least once every 30 days

- Record of all physician's visits subsequent to admission, including

- Date of visit

- Progress notes

- Orders for medications, treatment, care, and diet, which the physician must review and reorder at least once every 30 days

- Nursing record, including

  - Date, time, dosage, and method of administration of all medications and signature of nurse administering

  - Complete record of all safety precautions, including time, type, reason, and authority for applying

  - Record of all pertinent factors pertaining to the patient's condition

  - Date and time of all treatments and dressing

  - Incidents occurring while the patient is in the institution, including drug reactions and medication errors[151]

Requirements for the content of medical records of intermediate care facilities are almost identical.[152]

Health records of residents of intermediate care facilities—mental retardation providing sleeping accommodations for 15 or fewer residents must include

- Identification data, which includes name, marital status, age, sex, social security number, and home address

- Name, address, and telephone number of physician

- Name, address, and telephone number of referral source

- Name and address of next of kin or other responsible person

- Date and time of admission and discharge

- Record of the physician's or psychologist's findings and recommendation in the preadmission evaluation and in subsequent reevaluations[153]

SOUTH DAKOTA

Hospital and nursing home medical records must show the condition of the patient or resident from admission until discharge and include

- Identification data

---

151. *Id.* 61-17 § 702.
152. *Id.* 61-14 § 502.
153. *Id.* 61-13 § 504.

- Consent forms, except when unobtainable

- History of the patient or resident

- A current overall plan of care

- Report of the initial and periodic physical examinations, evaluations, and all plans of care with subsequent changes

- Diagnostic and therapeutic orders

- Progress notes from all disciplines, including practitioners, physical therapy, occupational therapy, and speech pathology

- Laboratory and radiology reports

- Descriptions of treatments, diet, and services provided and medications administered

- All indications of an illness or an injury including the date, the time, and the action taken regarding each

- Final diagnosis

- Discharge summary, including all discharge instructions for home care[154]

  Records for *supervised personal care facilities* must include

- Admission and discharge data

- Report of the physician's admission physical evaluation for resident

- Physician orders

- Medication entries

- Observations by personnel, resident's physician, or other persons authorized to care for the resident[155]

  Ambulatory surgery medical records must include

- Patient identification

- Chief complaint, pertinent medical and drug history, and preoperative physician's physical examination, including copies of any laboratory, x-ray, pathology, or anesthesia record and consultative reports

- Description of surgical procedures, treatments, medications administered, and observations of care provided, including complications

- Signature or initials of practitioner on each clinical entry

---

154. South Dakota Administrative Rules 44:04:09:05 (1991).
155. *Id.* R. 44:04:09:06.

- Signature of nursing personnel on notes or observations

- Condition of patient on discharge

- Instructions given to patient on release from facility

- Copy of transfer form if patient is transferred to another healthcare facility

- Operative and anesthesia consent forms

- Evidence that the patient is being discharged in the company of a responsible adult[156]

TENNESSEE

"Hospital records" means those medical histories, records, reports, summaries, diagnoses, prognoses, records of treatment and medication ordered and given, entries, x-rays, radiology interpretations, and other written or graphic data prepared, kept, made, or maintained in hospitals that pertain to hospital confinements or hospital services rendered to patients admitted to hospitals or receiving emergency room or outpatient care. Such records must also include reduction of the original records upon photographic film of convenient size. . . . Such records must not, however, include ordinary business records pertaining to patients' account or the administration of the institution.[157]

Rules of the Tennessee Department of Health and Environment, Board for Licensing Health Care Facilities specify that *inpatient* medical records must include

- Identification data

- Date and time of admission

- Date and time of transfer

- Date and time of discharge

- Attending and consulting physicians' names

- Written admission note within 24 hours of admissions

- Diagnostic and therapeutic orders

- Policy on informed consent developed by a medical staff and governing body and consistent with legal requirements

- Preanesthetic assessment documented by an anesthesiologist or attending physician prior to surgery. A postanesthetic assessment must document the presence or absence of anesthesia-related complications.

---

156. *Id.* R. 44:04:16:17.
157. Tennessee Code Annotated § 68-11-302 (5) (1990).

- Progress notes sufficient to denote the patient's status and the frequency and detail of changes, and the condition of the patient

- Operative description, including preoperative diagnosis, findings at the time of the procedure, postoperative diagnosis, techniques used, and the specimens removed

- Reports of all procedures along with tests performed and the results, authenticated by the appropriate personnel

- Nursing notes, including nursing observations, vital signs, and other pertinent information regarding the patient

- Discharge summary completed and authenticated to include

  - Provisional diagnosis

  - Primary and secondary final diagnoses

  - Clinical resume

  - Condition on discharge or transfer

  - Instructions to the patient

  - Necropsy results

- Final diagnosis recorded in an acceptable nomenclature and the time of discharge by the attending physician, dentist, or podiatrist[158]

  Emergency room medical records must include

- Identification data

- Information concerning the time of arrival, means, and by whom transported

- Pertinent history of the injury or illness to include chief complaint and onset of injuries or illness

- Significant physical findings

- Description of laboratory, x-ray, and EKG findings

- Treatment rendered

- Condition of the patient on discharge or transfer

- Diagnosis on discharge

- Instructions given to the patient or his family

- Control register listing chronologically the patient visits to the emergency

---

158. Tennessee Compilation Rules & Regulations tit. 1200, ch. 8-4-.03 (1990).

room. The record must contain at least the patient's name, date and time of arrival, and record number. The names of those dead on arrival must be entered in the register.

Medical records of *nursing homes* must contain

- Identification data and consent form
- Medical history of patient
- Report of physical examinations
- Diagnostic and therapeutic orders
- Progress notes
- Reports of special examinations and findings
- Nursing notes
- Medication record[159]

TEXAS

Texas Department of Health Hospital Licensing Standards simply state that medical records that must be preserved include

- Identification data
- The medical history of the patient
- Reports of relevant physical examinations
- Diagnostic and therapeutic orders
- Evidence of appropriate informed consent
- Clinical observations, including the results of therapy
- Reports of procedures, tests, and their results, including laboratory, pathology, and radiology reports
- Conclusions at termination of hospitalization or evaluation/treatment[160]

  Special care facilities' medical records must include

- Identification data, including
  - Full name
  - Sex

---

159. *Id*. tit. 1200 ch. 8-6-.07 (a).
160. Texas Department of Health, Hospital Licensing Standards ch. 1 § 22 (1991).

- Date of birth
- Usual occupation
- Social security number
- Family/friend name, address, and telephone number
- Physician names and telephone numbers, including emergency numbers

- Medical history and physical exam reports
- Any physician orders and progress notes
- Any documentation of the resident's change in health condition requiring emergency procedures and/or health services provided by facility personnel
- If appropriate, documentation of assistance with medications as stated in pharmacy services
- Other documents or reports related to the care of the resident as required by facility policy
- If appropriate, documentation of nursing services provided and nursing staff observation as required by facility policy
- A separation or discharge report completed at the time of the resident's discharge. The report must include date of departure, destination, reason for leaving, resident's health status, referral information, if any, and how to be contacted, if appropriate.

UTAH

In Utah, all medical records must contain

- Identification data
- Medical history
- Relevant physical examination
- Diagnoses including principal, provisional, final, and associate diagnoses
- Laboratory reports
- X-ray reports
- Evidence of informed consent or the reason it is unattainable
- Diagnostic and therapeutic orders by physicians and other authorized practitioners

- Medical staff orders for medications and treatments

- Anesthesia record

- Pathology report

- Clinical observations including progress notes, consultation reports, and nursing notes

- Discharge summary

- Autopsy findings

- Reports of procedures, tests, and results. If this includes reports from any facilities outside the hospital, the facilities must be identified on the report.

- Physician identification[161]

Obstetrical records must also include

- Admission history and physical examination

- Labor notes

- Obstetrical anesthesia record

- Delivery records

- Operative report, where indicated

- Discharge summary for complicated deliveries. In the case of an uncomplicated delivery, a final progress note may be substituted for the discharge summary.

- Record of administration of Rh immune globulin[162]

Newborn infant records must also include

- Copy of the maternal history from the mother's record, including

  - Relevant family history

  - Serological test for syphilis

  - Rh status

  - Analgesia

  - Anesthesia

  - Length of labor

---

161. Utah Administrative Rules 432-100-7.407 (1990).
162. *Id.* R. 432-100-7.408.

- Type of delivery

- Date and hour of birth, period of gestation, sex, reactions after birth, delivery room care, temperature, weight, time of first urination, and number, character, and consistency of stools

- PKU instruction and reports, including number of screening kit

- Record of ophthalmic prophylaxis

- If the infant is discharged to any person other than the infant's parents, then the hospital must record the name and address of such person and where the infant will be taken.[163]

Emergency room records (to be integrated into the patient's overall record or record identification system) will also contain

- Patient identification

- Time and means of arrival

- Emergency care given to patient prior to arrival

- Short history

- Physical findings

- Lab and x-ray reports, if performed

- Diagnosis

- Record of treatment

- Prognosis

- Disposition of case

- Discharge instructions

- Signature of physician rendering service

- When a patient leaves against medical advice, a statement to that effect[164]

Outpatient records must contain all information required for inpatient records, plus discharge instructions.[165]

Nursing care facility records must include

- Admission record (face sheet), including

  - Patient's name

163. *Id*. R. 432-100-7.409.
164. *Id*. R. 432-100-7.410.
165. *Id*. R. 432-100-7.411.

- Social security number

- Age at admission

- Name

- Address

- Telephone number of spouse, guardian, or person or agency responsible for the patient

- Name, address, and telephone number of attending physician

- Admission and subsequent diagnoses and any allergies

- Reports of physical examinations signed and dated by the physician

- Signed and dated physician orders for drugs, treatments, and diet

- Signed and dated nurses' notes including but not limited to

  - Records made by nurse assistants regarding the daily care of the patient

  - Informative progress notes by licensed nurses to record changes in the patient's condition. Progress notes must describe the patient's needs and response to care and treatment and must be in accord with the plan of care.

  - Documentation of administration of all PRN medications and the reason for withholding scheduled medications

  - Documentation of use of restraints in accordance with facility policy including type of restraint, reason for use, situation surrounding the application, and removal. The use of postural support must be described in the facility policy.

  - Documentation of oxygen administration

- Temperature, pulse, respirations, blood pressure, height, and weight notations, when indicated

- Laboratory reports of all tests prescribed and completed

- Reports of all x rays prescribed and completed

- Adequate records of the course of all therapeutic treatments

- Discharge summary, which contains a brief narrative of conditions and diagnoses of the patient and final disposition

- A copy of the transfer form when the patient is transferred to another healthcare facility

- Patient care plan[166]

Patient records for *mental disease facilities* must contain, in addition to the information in the records immediately above

- Identifying data that is recorded on standardized forms, including

  - Patient's name

  - Home address

  - Home telephone number

  - Date of birth

  - Sex

  - Race or ethnic origin

  - Next of kin

  - Education

  - Marital status

  - Type and place of last employment

  - Date of admission

  - Legal status, including relevant legal documents

  - Other identifying data as indicated

  - Date the information was gathered

  - Names and signatures of the staff members gathering the information

- Information for review and evaluation of treatment provided to the patient

- Documentation of patient and family involvement in the treatment program

- Prognosis

- Information on any unusual occurrences, such as treatment complications, accidents or injuries to or inflicted by the patient, procedures that place the patient at risk, absence without leave (AWOL)

- Physical and mental diagnoses using a recognized diagnostic coding system

---

166. *Id*. R. 432-150-6.106.

- Progress notes written by the physician, psychiatrist, nurse, and others significantly involved in active treatment. Progress notes should contain an ongoing assessment of the patient as well as

  - Documentation that supports implementation of the patient care plan and the patient's progress toward meeting these planned goals and objectives

  - Documentation of all treatment and services rendered to the patient

  - Chronological documentation of the patient's clinical course

  - Descriptions of changes in the patient's condition

  - Descriptions of patient response to treatment, the outcome of treatment, and the response of significant others to these changes

- Reports of laboratory, radiologic, or other diagnostic procedures, and reports of medical/surgical procedures when performed

- Correspondence and/or signed and dated notations of telephone calls concerning the patient's treatment

- A written plan for discharge including information about the following:

  - Patient preferences/choices regarding location and plans for discharge

  - Family relationships and involvement with the patient

  - Physical and psychiatric needs

  - Realistic financial needs

  - Housing needs

  - Employment needs

  - Educational/vocational needs

  - Social needs

  - Accessibility of community resources

  - Designated and documented responsibility of the patient or family for follow-up or aftercare

- Discharge summary signed by the physician and entered into the patient record within 60 calendar days from the date of discharge

- Reports of all assessments

- Consents for release of information, the actual date the information was released, and the signature of the staff member who released the information

- Pertinent prior records available from outside sources[167]

Patient records of *small healthcare facilities* must include

- Admission record (face sheet), including the patient's name; social security number; age at admission; name, address, telephone number of spouse, guardian, or person or agency responsible for the patient; name, address, and telephone number of attending physician

- Admission and subsequent diagnoses and any allergies

- Reports of physical examinations signed and dated by the physician

- Signed and dated physician orders for drugs, treatments, and diet

- Signed and dated progress notes including but not limited to

  - Records made by staff regarding the daily care of the patient

  - Informative progress notes by appropriate staff regarding changes in the patient's condition. Progress notes must describe the patient's needs and response to care and treatment and must be in accord with the plan of care.

  - Documentation of administration of all PRN medications and the reason for withholding scheduled medications

  - Documentation of use of restraints in accordance with facility policy including type of restraint, reason for use, time of application, and removal. The use of postural support must be detailed in facility policy.

  - Documentation of oxygen administration

- Temperature, pulse, respiration, blood pressure, height and weight notations, when required

- Laboratory reports of all tests prescribed and completed

- Reports of all x rays prescribed and completed

- Adequate records of the course of all therapeutic treatments

- Discharge summary, including a brief narrative of conditions and diagnoses of the patient and final disposition

- Copy of the transfer form when the patient is transferred to another healthcare facility

- Patient care plan[168]

---

167. *Id.* R. 432-151-6.100.
168. *Id.* R. 432-200-6.106.

Residential healthcare facilities—limited capacity patient records must contain

- Admission record (face sheet), including

  - Patient's name

  - Social security number

  - Age at admission

  - Name, address, telephone number of spouse, guardian, or person or agency responsible for the patient

  - Name, address, and telephone number of attending physician

- Admission diagnoses and reason for admission

- Any known allergies

- Temperature, pulse, respiration, blood pressure, height and weight notations, when required

- Physician's assessment

- If entrusted to the facility, a record of the resident's cash resources and valuables[169]

Freestanding *ambulatory surgical center* individual medical records must contain

- Admission record (face sheet), including

  - Patient's name

  - Social security number

  - Age at admission

  - Name, address, telephone number of spouse, guardian, or person or agency responsible for the patient

  - Name, address, and telephone number of attending physician

- A current physical examination and history, including allergies and abnormal drug reactions

- Informed consent signed by the patient or, if applicable, the patient's representative

- Complete findings and techniques of the operation

---

169. *Id.* R. 432-300-2.302.

- Signed and dated physician's orders for drugs and treatments

- Signed and dated nurses' notes regarding care of the patient. Nursing notes must include vital signs, medications, treatments, and other pertinent information.

- Discharge summary, which contains a brief narrative of conditions and diagnoses of the patient's final disposition, to include instructions given to the patient and/or responsible person

- Pathologist's report of human tissue removed during the surgical procedure, if any

- Reports of laboratory and x-ray procedures performed; consultations and any other preoperative diagnostic studies

- Preanesthesia evaluation[170]

Specialty hospitals—chemical dependency/substance abuse must maintain records containing

- Patient assessment, which must include a medical, psychosocial, substance abuse, and treatment history

- Individual treatment plan based on the patient assessment, including goals and methods of treatment. The plan must be reviewed and updated quarterly for outpatient care and every week for inpatient care.

- Progress notes, including description and date of service, with a summary of client programs signed by the therapist or service provider

- Discharge summary, including final evaluation of treatment and goals attained and signed by the therapist[171]

VERMONT

According to the State Hospital Licensure Regulations, Vermont Administrative Procedure Bulletin art. 2 § 3-946, a medical record must contain

- Identification data

- Complaint

- Personal and family history

- History of present illness

- Physical examination

---

170. *Id.* R. 432-500-6.103.
171. *Id.* R. 432-102-7.407. *See Id.* R. 432-550-6.104 (contents of records of birthing centers); *Id.* R. 422-600-6.104 (contents of records of abortion clinics); *Id.* R. 432-700-3.703 (contents of records of home health agencies); *Id.* R. 432-750-4 (contents of records of hospices).

- Special examinations

- Clinical laboratory reports

- X-ray and other examinations

- Provisional or working diagnosis

- Medical or surgical treatments

- Gross and microscopic pathology findings

- Progress notes

- Final diagnosis

- Condition on discharge

- Follow-up

- Autopsy findings

Residential care home licensing regulations provide that Level III (homes serving persons requiring both personal and nursing care) and Level IV (homes serving persons only needing personal care) *residential care homes* must keep the following records:

- Resident register

- Resident record, which includes

    - Resident's name

    - Emergency notification numbers

    - Name, address, and telephone number of responsible person, if any

    - Physician's name, address, and telephone number

    - Instructions in case of resident's death

    - Accident reports

    - Signed contract delineating a description of the services and charges

    - Medication documentation

- For Level III homes, the record must also contain

    - Initial assessment

    - Annual reassessment

    - Physician's admission statement and current orders

    - Staff progress notes, including changes in the resident's condition and/or illness, and action taken

- Reports of physician visits

- Signed telephone orders and treatment documentation

- Written report when a fire occurs in the home, regardless of size or damage, is to be submitted to the licensing agency and the Department of Labor and Industry within 24 hours.

- A written report of any accident or illness that involves physician follow-up, emergency room treatment, or admission to a hospital must be placed in the resident's folder and, for Level IV, a copy sent within 48 hours to the licensing agency.

- A report of any unexplained absence of a resident from a home must be reported to the police and responsible person, if any. The report must be provided to the licensing agency within 24 hours of disappearance.

- A written report of any breakdown to the home's physical plant (plumbing, heat, water supply, etc.), or supplied service, which disrupts the normal course of operation

According to the state nursing home regulations, *nursing homes* must maintain

- Resident register

- Admission and discharge records

- Record of medical history, examination, and diagnosis

- Physician's order record

- Physician's progress record

- Nursing record (including records of medication, treatment, and nurse's observation)

- Narcotic and barbiturate records

VIRGINIA

The Rules and Regulations for the Licensure of Hospitals in Virginia, Department of Health, state that the content of medical records must conform with the standards of the *Accreditation Manual for Hospitals* of the Joint Commission on Accreditation of Hospitals (now of Healthcare Organizations).[172]

The Rules and Regulations for the Licensure of Nursing Homes in Virginia provide that medical records in *nursing homes* must include

- Patient identification

---

172. Virginia Regulations Regulating Hospitals & Nursing Home Licensure & Inspection, part II § 208.5 (1982).

- Designation of physician having primary responsibility for the patient's care

- Admitting information, including recent patient history, physical examination, and diagnosis

- Physician orders, including all medications, treatments, diet, restorative, and special medical procedures required

- Physician progress notes written at the time of each visit

- Documented evidence of assessment of patient's needs, establishment of an appropriate treatment plan, and plans of care and services provided

- Nurses' notes

- Medication and treatment record, including all medications, treatments, and special procedures performed

- Pertinent copies of radiology, laboratory, and other consultation reports

- Discharge summary[173]

WASHINGTON

Washington Department of Social & Health Services Hospital Rules and Regulations, Washington Administrative Code § 248-18-440 (6) (1986), requires hospitals to include the following, when relevant, in a medical record for each inpatient or outpatient except referred outpatient diagnostic services and outpatient emergency care services:

- Admission data, including

  - Identifying and sociological data

  - Full name, address, and telephone number of the patient's next of kin or, when indicated, another person who may legally exercise control over the person of the patient

  - Date of the patient's admission

  - Name(s) of the patient's attending physician(s)

  - Admitting (provisional) diagnosis or medical problem

- Report on any medical history obtained from the patient

- Report(s) on the findings of physical examination(s) performed on the patient

---

173. *Id.* § 24.9 (1980).

- Any known allergies of the patient or known idiosyncratic reactions to a drug or other agent

- Authenticated orders for any drug or other therapy administered to a patient and for any diet served to a patient. Authenticated orders entered in the patient's record must include any standing medical orders used in the care and treatment of the patient except standing medical emergency orders.

- Authenticated orders for any restraint of the patient

- Reports on all roentgenologic examinations, clinical laboratory tests or examinations, macroscopic and microscopic examinations of tissue, and other diagnostic procedures or examinations performed upon the patient or specimens taken from the patient. Note that x-ray films, laboratory slides, tissue specimens, medical photographs, and other comparable materials obtained through procedures employed in diagnosing a patient's condition or assessing his clinical course are regarded as original clinical evidence and are not considered to be medical records.

- An entry on each administration of therapy (including drug therapy) to the patient

- Entries on nursing services to the patient. Nursing entries must include

  - Report on all significant nursing observations and assessments of the patient's condition or response to care and treatment

  - Nursing interventions

  - Other significant direct nursing care including all administration of drugs or other therapy

  - Time and reason for each notification of a physician or patient's family regarding a significant change in the patient's condition

  - Record of other significant nursing action on behalf of the patient

- An entry on any significant health education, training, or instruction related to the patient's health care that was provided to the patient or his family

- An entry on any social services provided the patient

- An entry regarding any adverse drug reaction of the patient and any other untoward incident or accident involving the patient that occurred during hospitalization or on an occasion of the patient's visit to the hospital for outpatient services

- Operative reports on all surgery

- An entry or report on each anesthetic administered

- Reports on consultations

- For any woman who gave birth in the hospital, reports regarding her labor, delivery, and postpartum period

- For any infant born in or en route to the hospital, the date and time of birth, condition at birth or upon arrival, sex and weight

- Progress notes

- In the event of an inpatient leaving without medical approval, an entry on any known events leading to the patient's decision to leave, a record of notification of the physician, and the time of departure

- Discharge data, including final diagnosis and any associated or secondary diagnoses or complications and the titles of all operations performed. For any inpatient whose hospitalization exceeded 48 hours, except a normal newborn or normal obstetrical patient, there must be a discharge summary that recapitulates significant clinical findings and events during the patient's hospitalization, describes the patient's condition upon discharge or transfer, and summarizes any recommendations and arrangements for future care.

- An entry on any transmittal of medical and related data to a healthcare facility or agency or other community resource to which the patient was referred or transferred

- In the event of the patient's death in the hospital

  - Pronouncement of death

  - Authorization for autopsy

  - Report on the autopsy findings (if performed)

  - Entry on release of the body

- Written consents, authorizations, or releases given by the patient or by a person or agency who can legally exercise control over the patient

WEST VIRGINIA

West Virginia defines hospital records as

those medical histories, records, reports, summaries, diagnoses and prognoses, records of treatment and medication ordered and given, notes, entries, X-rays, and other written or graphic data prepared, kept, made or maintained in hospitals that pertain to hospital confinements or hospital services rendered to patients admitted to hospitals or receiving emergency room or outpatient care. Such records must not, however, include ordinary business records pertaining to patients' accounts or the administration of the institution.[174]

West Virginia Regulations for Hospital Licensure specify what comprises a complete medical record:

- Patient identification

- Date

- Complaints

- History of present illness

- Personal and family history

- Physical examination

- Physician's orders including dietary orders, special examinations, and consultations

- Clinical laboratory, x-ray, and other examinations

- Provisional or working diagnosis

- Treatment and medications given

- Surgical reports including operative and anesthesia records

- Gross and microscopic pathology findings

- Progress notes

- Final diagnosis

- Condition on discharge

- Discharge summary

- Autopsy findings, if performed[175]

The same regulation provides for a short-form record for patients staying in the hospital less than 48 hours other than maternity or newborn patients. The short-form record may contain only that information necessary for proper diagnosis and treatment.[176]

WISCONSIN

Wisconsin defines "patient health care records" as "all records related to the health of a patient prepared by or under the supervision of a health care

---

174. West Virginia Code § 57-5-4a (1990).
175. West Virginia Legislature, Title 64 West Virginia Legislative Rules Department of Health: Hospital Licensure, series 12 § 10.3.1.b (1987).
176. *Id.* § 10.3.1.d.

provider except records relating to treatment of individuals for mental illness, developmental disabilities, alcoholism or drug dependence, records of chemical tests for intoxication administered or fetal monitor tracings."[177] The law requires that inpatient records include the patient's occupation and the industry in which the inpatient is employed so that if his health problems are related to his occupation, his physician can ensure that his record contains information about these occupations and any potential health hazards related to these occupations. The same must be done if the inpatient's health problems are related to his parents' occupations.[178]

Wisconsin's Health and Social Services Regulations, Wisconsin Administrative Code § HSS 124.14 (3) (Feb. 1, 1988), mandate that the medical record contain

- Accurate patient identification data

- Concise statement of complaints, including the chief complaint that led the patient to seek medical care and the date of onset and duration of each

- Health history, containing a description of present illness, past history of illness, and pertinent family and social history

- Statement about the results of the physical examination, including all positive and negative findings resulting from an inventory of systems

- Provisional diagnosis

- All diagnostic and therapeutic orders

- All clinical laboratory, x-ray reports, and other diagnostic reports

- Consultation reports containing a written opinion by the consultant that reflects, when appropriate, an actual examination of the patient and the patient's medical record

- Except in an emergency, an appropriate history and physical workup recorded in the medical record of every patient before surgery

- Operative report describing techniques and findings, written or dictated immediately following surgery and signed by the surgeon

- Tissue reports, including a report of microscopic findings if hospital regulations require that microscopic examination be done. If only macroscopic examination is warranted, a statement that the tissue has been received and a macroscopic description of the findings provided by the laboratory must be filed in the medical record.

- Physician and nonphysician notes providing a chronological picture of

---

177. Wisconsin Statutes § 146.81 (1990).
178. *Id.* § 146.815.

the patient's progress that is sufficient to delineate the course and the results of treatment

- Definitive final diagnosis expressed in the terminology of a recognized system of disease nomenclature

- Discharge summary including the final diagnosis, the reason for hospitalization, the significant findings, the procedures performed, the condition of the patient on discharge, and any specific instructions given the patient or family or both the patient and family

- Autopsy findings when an autopsy is performed

Maternal medical records must contain

- Prenatal history and findings

- Labor and delivery record, including anesthesia

- Physician's progress record

- Physician's order sheet

- Medicine and treatment sheet, including nurses' notes

- Any laboratory and x-ray reports

- Any medical consultant's notes

- Estimate of blood loss

Newborn medical records include

- Record of pertinent maternal data, type of labor and delivery, and the condition of the infant at birth

- Record of physical examinations

- Progress sheet recording medicines and treatments, weights, feedings, and temperatures

- Notes of any medical consultant

- In the case of a fetal death, the weight and length of the fetus recorded on the delivery record

Except for persons admitted to *nursing homes* for short-term care, each nursing home resident's medical record must contain

- Identification and summary sheet

- Physician's documentation

  - An admission medical evaluation by a physician or physician extender, including

- Summary of prior treatment
- Current medical findings
- Diagnoses at the time of admission to the facility
- Resident's rehabilitation potential
- Results of physical examination
- Level of care

- All physician's orders including, when applicable, orders concerning

  - Admission to the facility
  - Medications and treatments
  - Diets
  - Rehabilitative services
  - Limitations on activities
  - Restraint orders
  - Discharge or transfer

- Physician progress notes following each visit
- Annual physical examination, if required
- Alternate visit schedule and justification for such alternate visits

- Nursing service documentation

  - History and assessment of the resident's nursing needs
  - Nursing care plans
  - Nursing notes are required as follows:

    - For residents requiring skilled care, a narrative nursing note must be required as often as needed to document the resident's condition, but at least weekly.
    - For residents not requiring skilled care, a narrative nursing note must be required as often as needed to document the resident's condition, but at least every other week.

  - Documentation describing

    - The general physical and mental condition of the resident, including any unusual symptoms or actions
    - All incidents or accidents including time, place, details of incident or accident, action taken, and follow-up care

- The administration of all medications, the need for PRN medications and the resident's response, refusal to take medication, omission of medications, errors in the administration of medications, and drug reactions

- Food and fluid intake, when the monitoring of intake is necessary

- Any unusual occurrences of appetite, or refusal or reluctance to accept diets

- Summary of restorative nursing measures provided

- Summary of the use of physical and chemical restraints

- Other nonroutine nursing care given

- Condition of a resident on discharge

- Time of death, the physician called, and the person to whom the body was released

- Social service records

  - Social history of the resident

  - Notes regarding pertinent social data and action taken

- Activities records. Documentation of activities programming, a history and assessment, a summary of attendance, and quarterly progress notes

- Rehabilitative services

  - Evaluation of the rehabilitative needs of the resident

  - Progress notes detailing treatment given, evaluation, and progress

- Dietary assessment. Record of the dietary assessment

- Records of all dental services

- Records of all diagnostic tests performed during the resident's stay in the facility

- Plan of care

- Authorization or consent. A photocopy of any court order or other document authorizing another person to speak or act on behalf of the resident and any resident consent form required by law, except that if the authorization or consent form exceeds one page in length an accurate summary may be substituted in the resident record and the complete authorization or consent form must in this case be maintained under regulations requiring the facility to keep copies of court orders or other documents authorizing another to act on behalf of the resident. The summary must include

- The name and address of the guardian or other person having authority to speak or act on behalf of the resident

- The date on which the authorization or consent takes effect and the date on which it expires

- The express legal nature of the authorization or consent and any limitations on it

- Any other factors reasonably necessary to clarify the scope and extent of the authorization or consent

- Discharge or transfer information. Documents, prepared on a resident's discharge or transfer from the facility, summarizing, when appropriate

  - Current medical findings and condition

  - Final diagnoses

  - Rehabilitation potential

  - A summary of the course of treatment

  - Nursing and dietary information

  - Ambulation status

  - Administrative and social information

  - Needed continued care and instructions[179]

Records of residents of *facilities for the developmentally disabled* must contain all information relevant to admission and to the resident's care and treatment, including the following:

- Admission information. Information obtained on admission, including

  - Name, date of admission, birth date and place, citizenship status, marital status, and social security number

  - Father's name and birthplace and mother's maiden name and birthplace

  - Names and addresses of parents, legal guardian, and next of kin

  - Sex, race, height, weight, color of hair, color of eyes, identifying marks, and recent photograph

  - Reason for admission or referral

  - Type and status of admission

  - Legal competency status

---

179. *Id.* § HSS 132.45 (5) (b).

- Language spoken or understood

- Sources of support, including social security, veterans' benefits, and insurance

- Religious affiliation, if any

- Medical evaluation results, including current medical findings, a summary of prior treatment, the diagnosis at time of admission, the resident's habilitative or rehabilitative potential and level of care, and results of physical examination

- Any physician's concurrence concerning admission to the facility

- Preadmission evaluation reports. Any report or summary of an evaluation conducted by the interdisciplinary team or a team member prior to an individual's admission to the facility and reports of any other relevant medical histories or evaluations conducted prior to the individual's admission

- Authorizations or consents. A photocopy of any court order or other document authorizing another person to speak or act on behalf of the resident and any resident consent form required under this chapter, except that if the authorization or consent form exceeds one page in length an accurate summary may be substituted in the resident record and the complete authorization or consent form must in this case be maintained. The summary must include

  - Name and address of the guardian or other person having authority to speak or act on behalf of the resident

  - Date on which the authorization or consent takes effect and the date on which it expires

  - Express legal nature of the authorization or consent and any limitations on it

  - Any other factors reasonably necessary to clarify the scope and extent of the authorization or consent

- Resident care planning documentation, including

  - Comprehensive evaluation of the resident and written training and habilitation objectives

  - Annual review of the resident's program by the interdisciplinary team

  - In measurable terms, documentation by the qualified mental retardation professional of the resident's performance in relation to the objectives contained in the individual program plan

  - Professional and special programs and service plans, evaluations, and progress notes

- Direct care staff notes reflecting the projected and actual outcome of the resident's habilitation or rehabilitation program

- Medical service documentation. Documentation of medical services and treatments provided to the resident, including

  - Physician orders for

    - Medications and treatments

    - Diets

    - Special or professional services

    - Limitations on activities

  - Restraint orders

  - Discharge or transfer records

  - Physician progress notes following each physician visit

  - Report on the resident's annual physical examination

- Nursing service documentation. Documentation of nursing needs and the nursing services provided, including

  - Nursing care component of the individual program plan reviewed and revised annually

  - Nursing notes as needed to document the resident's condition

  - Other nursing documentation describing

    - General physical and mental condition of the resident, including any unusual symptoms or behavior

    - All incidents or accidents, including time, place, details of the incident or accident, action taken, and follow-up care

    - Functional training and habilitation

    - Administration of all medications, the need for as-needed administration of medications, and the effect that the medication has on the resident's condition; the resident's refusal to take medication, omission of medications, errors in the administration of medications, and drug reactions

    - Height and weight

    - Food and fluid intake, when the monitoring of intake is necessary

    - Any unusual occurrences of appetite or refusal or reluctance to accept diets

- Rehabilitative nursing measures provided

- The use of restraints

- Immunizations and other nonroutine nursing care given

- Any family visits and contacts

- Condition of a resident on discharge

- Time of death, the physician called, and the person to whom the body was released

- Social service documentation. Social service records and any notes regarding pertinent social data and action taken to meet the social service needs of residents

- Special and professional services documentation. Progress notes documenting consultations and services provided by psychologists, speech pathologists and audiologists, and occupational and physical therapists

- Dental records, as follows

  - Permanent dental record for each resident

  - Documentation of an oral examination at the time of admission or prior to admission

  - Dental summary progress reports as needed

- Nutritional assessment of the resident, the nutritional component of the resident's individual program plan, and records of diet modifications

- Discharge or transfer information. Documents prepared when a resident is discharged or transferred from the facility, including

  - Summary of habilitative, rehabilitative, medical, emotional, social, and cognitive findings and progress

  - Summary and current status report on special and professional treatment services

  - Summary of need for continued care and plans for care

  - Nursing and nutritional information

  - Administrative and social information

  - An up-to-date statement of the resident's account

  - In the case of a transfer, written documentation of the reason for transfer[180]

---

180. *Id.* § HSS 134.47 (4).

WYOMING

According to the Wyoming Public Hospital Records Management Manual, Wyoming State Archives & Historical Department, Records Disposal Manual for Wyoming County Hospitals (1987), permanent medical records include, but are not limited to

- Admission and discharge records
- Attending physician(s)
- Record of diagnosis and operations
- Operative reports
- Pathology reports
- Discharge summaries

CHAPTER 2

Who Owns
Medical Records?

Ownership Generally

What should healthcare facilities tell patients who demand their medical records, stating that the records are *theirs?* Healthcare records, in fact, do not belong to patients. However, patients may have rights with regard to these records.

Hospitals own their own records, including medical records, but some states give patients the right to review or copy their medical records. In other words, while the healthcare facility owns the record, and consequently has the right to physical possession and control, the patient has a right to the information contained therein. Many states have statutes specifying that the healthcare facility owns its medical records. Some states, such as Mississippi, add that the facility's ownership is subject to the patient's right of access to the medical information contained in the record.

Even if the state statute or an administrative regulation does not specify who owns medical records, in the absence of a statute or court decision to the contrary, a facility may safely assume that it, not the patient, owns the medical records. Similarly, physicians practicing in a private office rather than in a healthcare institution own their medical records, subject to rights of access by patients.

Because neither patients nor their authorized representatives have the right to physical possession of the records, hospitals and private physicians should not permit anyone to remove the records from their control unless a court order so requires.

When a patient changes physicians (for example, when a physician leaves practice), the previous physician should transfer the records, or copies or summaries thereof, to the current physician, although no strict legal duty to do so exists. However, hospitals that transfer patients to other facilities, or physicians who send patients to specialists, have a legal obligation to provide the receiving facilities or physicians with all medical information from the records that is necessary to treat those patients.

Federal Laws

All medical records in federal healthcare facilities belong to the United States, subject to patients' rights to access.

State Laws

ALABAMA

Rules of Alabama State Board of Health Division of Licensure and Certification provide that medical records of patients are the physical property of the hospital and control of them rests with the hospital administrator.[1]

ALASKA

Alaska Statute § 18.20.085 (1990), pertaining to hospital record retention, implies that hospitals own medical records. Other statutes indicate that patients have the right to access the information therein.

ARIZONA

Arizona Compilation Administrative Rules and Regulations § 9-10-221 (1992) stipulates that only authorized personnel have access to medical records and that written consent of the patient or legal guardian is required for release of medical record information. Arizona's retention requirements imply that records are the property of the facility with patients having reasonable access thereto.

ARKANSAS

Arkansas' rules covering medical records, Arkansas Register .0601 E, provide that medical records shall not be removed from the hospital environment except on the issuance of a subpoena, thereby strongly implying that the hospital owns its medical records. The language of these rules (that written consent of the patient or legal guardian shall be presented as authority for release) implies that the patient has a right of access to the information therein.

CALIFORNIA

In California, the facility owns the medical record, including x-ray films. However, California law considers that the facility maintains the information documented within the medical record for the benefit of the patient.[2]

---

1. Alabama Administrative Code r. 420—5-7.07(d) (1990).
2. California Code Regulations tit. 22, § 70751(b) (1991).

In addition to general acute care hospitals, Title 22 regulations specify that healthcare records are the property of the following various other types of facilities:

- Acute psychiatric hospitals[3]

- Intermediate care facilities[4]

- Primary care clinics[5]

- Psychology clinics[6]

- Chemical dependency recovery hospitals[7]

COLORADO

Colorado Revised Statutes § 18-4-412 (1990) makes it a class 5 felony for anyone, without proper authorization, to knowingly obtain a medical record or medical information with the intent to appropriate it to his own use or another's, who steals or discloses to an unauthorized person medical information or a medical record, or who, without authority, copies such. This statute implies that the record belongs to the healthcare facility, with the patient having a right to confidentiality. Similarly, *id.* § 25-1-801 requires the facility to provide copies of records in its "custody" to patients.

CONNECTICUT

The Connecticut Public Health Code does not specify who owns medical records, but its language implies that they are the property of the facility.

DELAWARE

Delaware does not specify who owns medical records, but its laws are consistent with the general view that facilities have physical custody of medical records with patients having a right of access to the information therein.

DISTRICT OF COLUMBIA

The District of Columbia does not specify who owns medical records, but nothing in its laws indicates that they are not the property of the facility.

---

3. *Id.* § 71551(b).
4. *Id.* § 73928(b).
5. *Id.* § 75055(i).
6. *Id.* § 75343(i).
7. *Id.* § 79351(b).

FLORIDA

Florida Administrative Code § 10D-28.110(10)(f)(2) (1991) provides that clinical records are the property of the facility and are maintained for the benefit of the patient, staff, and facility.

GEORGIA

Under Georgia Code § 31-33-3 (1990), records are owned by the healthcare provider, subject to access thereto by the patient.

HAWAII

Hawaii Revised Statutes § 622-51 (1990), which states that "medical records" means records of patients kept by a medical facility, and § 622-58, governing retention of medical records, imply that the facility "owns" the records with patients having a right of access to the information therein.

IDAHO

Idaho Code 39-1392d (1990)'s reference to patient access to the official hospital chart implies that medical records are the property of the hospital.

ILLINOIS

The Illinois Medical Record Association states that the medical record is the property of the hospital and is maintained for the benefit of the patient, the medical staff, and the hospital.

INDIANA

The original health record of the patient is the property of the provider and may be used by the provider without written authorization for legitimate business purposes.[8]

IOWA

The language of Iowa Administrative Code r. 441-81.9(3) (1990), that all records of nursing facilities shall be retained in the facility on change of ownership, implies that such records are the physical property of the facility as does the language of IAC 481-51.6(1) with regard to hospital medical records.

---

8. Indiana Code § 16-4-8-8 (West 1991).

KANSAS

Kansas Administrative Regulations 28-34-9a(6) (1990) provides that medical records are the property of the hospital and shall not be removed from the hospital except as authorized by the hospital or for purposes of litigation when authorized by Kansas law or court order.

KENTUCKY

The medical record is the property of the health facility[9] and may not be taken from the hospital except by court order or by physicians or dentists for consultation.

LOUISIANA

Louisiana Revised Statutes § 1299.96 (West 1990) states that medical records of a patient maintained in a healthcare provider's office are property and business records of the healthcare provider.

MAINE

Code of Maine Rules, Regulations Governing the Licensing and Functioning of General and Specialty Hospitals, ch. XII G (1972), states that medical records generally are not removed from the hospital environment except on subpoena, which certainly indicates that they are the physical property of the facility.

MARYLAND

Maryland Health-General Code Annotated § 4-301 (1990), governing disclosure of medical records, speaks of providers "having custody" of medical records.

MASSACHUSETTS

In a discussion of "records of hospitals or clinics," Massachusetts General Laws ch. 111, § 70 (1991), gives custody to the facility but provides for inspection by a patient.

MICHIGAN

Michigan Administrative Code r. 325.1028 (1987) of the Michigan Department of Public Health Rules and Minimum Standards for Hospitals requires that the hospital keep medical records, implying that they are the physical property of the facility.

---

9. 902 Kentucky Administrative Regulations 20:016(11)(c) (1991).

MINNESOTA

Minnesota Statutes § 145.32 (1992), requirements for permanent retention of portions of hospital medical records, implies that records belong to the facility. However, it also provides for patient access to such records.

MISSISSIPPI

Mississippi statutes provide that hospital records are the property of the hospital subject to reasonable access on good cause shown by the patient, his or her personal representative or heirs, attending medical personnel, and duly authorized nominees, and on payment of any reasonable charges for such access.[10]

MISSOURI

Medical records are the property of the hospital and may not be taken from the premises except by court order, subpoena, for microfilming, or for off-site storage approved by the governing body.[11]

MONTANA

Montana law does not specify who owns medical records, but Chapter 23-4 of the *Montana Health Association Consent Manual* states that the hospital has the obligation to retain possession of the record. It may, however, release x rays for not more than 30 days to doctors who require them for back-up care (*id.* ch. 23-4.1A). Nothing in the minimum standards for all healthcare facilities—medical records[12] changes the general rule giving the facility the right to physical possession of the record.

NEBRASKA

Nebraska Administrative Rules and Regulations 175-9-003.04 (1979) implies that records are the physical property of the hospital when it states that they shall be kept confidential, available only for use by authorized persons and for examination by authorized representatives of the department.

NEVADA

Nevada has no specific provisions concerning ownership, but nothing in its regulatory scheme implies that it departs from the general rule that physical possession of the record belongs to the facility, with the patient having a right of access to the information therein.

---

10. Mississippi Code Annotated § 41-9-65 (1990).
11. Missouri Code Regulations tit. 13, § 50-20.021(3)(D)6 (1990).
12. Montana Administrative Rules 16.32.308 (1984) and R. 16.32.328 (1987).

NEW HAMPSHIRE

New Hampshire Revised Statutes Annotated § 151:21 (1990), Health Facilities Licensing Law, Patients' Bill of Rights, specifies that medical information contained in the medical records at any facility licensed under Chapter 151 is the property of the patient. This language implies that the facility owns the physical record.

NEW JERSEY

New Jersey Standards for Hospital Facilities, New Jersey Administrative Code tit. 8: § 43B-7.1(c) (1984), states that medical records should not be removed from the hospital environment except on subpoena, thereby implying that they are the property of the hospital. Further, the Administrative Codes of the State Board of Medical Examiners state, in *id.* tit. 13 § 35-6.5(c) (1990), that licensees shall provide access to professional treatment records to patients or authorized representatives in certain circumstances, thereby also implying that ownership is in the facility with a right of access to the information therein held by the patient.

NEW MEXICO

The *New Mexico Hospital Association Legal Handbook,* ch. 5, ¶ B (rev. ed. 1981), states that the pieces of paper that make up hospital medical records are the property of the hospital, but that patients or third parties may have a right of access to the information in the records.

NEW YORK

New York does not specify who owns medical records, but its laws are consistent with the general rule that facilities own the records subject to a right of access to the information therein by patients.

NORTH CAROLINA

North Carolina's Administrative Code states that records of patients are the property of the hospital.[13]

NORTH DAKOTA

North Dakota Administrative Code § 33-07-01-16 (1980)'s language that medical records generally shall not be removed from the hospital environment except on subpoena implies that they are the property of the facility.

---

13. North Carolina Administrative Code tit. 10 r. 3C.1403(d) (Feb. 1976).

OHIO

Ohio Revised Code § 3701.74 (Baldwin 1991), when discussing the patient's right to examine or obtain a copy of the record, implies that hospitals own the physical record.

OKLAHOMA

Oklahoma Department of Health Regulation Chapter 13's language that only authorized personnel have access to the record, that written consent of the patient is necessary for release of medical information, and that medical records must not be removed from the hospital environment except on subpoena implies that medical records are the property of the facility, with the patient having reasonable access to the information therein.

OREGON

All medical records are the property of the healthcare facility. They may not be removed from the institution except where necessary for a judicial or administrative proceeding.[14]

Medical records are the property of the long-term care facility.[15]

PENNSYLVANIA

Medical records are the property of the hospital and may not be taken from its premises except for court purposes. Copies may be made available for authorized purposes, such as insurance claims and physician review, consistent with confidentiality requirements (28 Pennsylvania § 115.28 (1989)). *Id.* § 563.10 has similar language relating to medical records of ambulatory surgical facilities.

RHODE ISLAND

Rhode Island has no specific provisions governing ownership of medical records. Nothing in its laws would indicate that it deviates from the general rule, however, that providers own the records with patients having a right of access to the information therein.

SOUTH CAROLINA

South Carolina Code Regulations 61-16 § 601.7(A) (1990), Minimum Standards for Licensure of Hospitals and Institutional Care Facilities in South Carolina; Regulation No. 61-14 (1990), covering intermediate care facilities;

---

14. Oregon Administrative Rules 333-505-050(12) (1991).
15. *Id.* R. 333-86-055(5).

No. 61-17 (1980), governing nursing care facilities; and Regulation No. 61-13 (1980), Minimum Standards for Licensing Intermediate Care Facilities—Mental Retardation—Providing Sleeping Accommodations for 15 Residents or Less specify that the facility owns its medical records. *Id.* No. 61-16, § 601.4; *id.* No. 61-14, § 504.4; and *id.* No. 61-17, § 704.4 add that records of patients must not be taken from the hospital property except by court order. Regulation 61-13, § 502 notes that records may not be removed except by competent authorities.

SOUTH DAKOTA

Chapter 44:04:09, Medical Record Services, does not expressly state who owns medical records, but nothing indicates that South Dakota deviates from the general rule that medical records are the physical property of the facility, with the patient having a right of access to the information therein.

TENNESSEE

In Tennessee, hospital records are the hospital's property, subject, however, to court order to produce the same. The hospital also shall provide reasonable access, on good cause shown, to the patient, his personal representative or heirs, or his attending medical personnel, and on payment of any reasonable charge for such service.[16]

TEXAS

Texas does not specify who owns medical records, but nothing in its statutes or in the Hospital Licensing Standards of the Texas Department of Health indicates that any entities other than facilities own the physical records, with patients having a right of access to the information therein.

UTAH

Medical records are the property of the hospital and may not be removed from the hospital's control except by court order or subpoena.[17]

VERMONT

Vermont has no specific provisions, but nothing in its regulatory scheme would indicate a departure from the general rule that the facility owns the medical records, with patients having a right of access to the information in the records.

---

16. Tennessee Code § 68-11-304 (1990).
17. Utah Administrative Rule 432-100-7.404(D) (1990).

VIRGINIA

Virginia's Rules and Regulations for the Licensure of Hospitals in Virginia do not specifically address ownership of medical records, but nothing therein indicates that Virginia differs from the general rule that the facility owns the physical records and the patient has a right of access to the information therein.

WASHINGTON

Washington Administrative Code § 248-18-440 (1986)'s language that hospitals must establish written policies and procedures that include access to and release of data in patient's records indicates that hospitals have the physical ownership of the records with patients having a right to the information therein.

WEST VIRGINIA

West Virginia Legislature, Title 64 West Virginia Legislative Rules Department of Health: Hospital Licensure, series 12, § 10.3.1a (1987)'s language that medical records shall be retained in the hospital implies that they are the property of the facility. Similarly, West Virginia Code § 57-5-4i (1991) notes that in view of the property right of the hospital in its records, copies may be substituted in court proceedings. However, patients have the right to copy and inspect their records under *id.* § 16-29-1.

WISCONSIN

Wisconsin Administrative Code § HSS 124.14 (Feb. 1, 1988)'s language that original records may not be removed from the hospital except by authorized persons acting in accordance with a court order, a subpoena, or in accordance with contracted services implies that the records are the property of the facility. Its language further indicates that the patient has a right of access to the information therein.

WYOMING

Wyoming does not specify who owns medical records, but nothing in its laws would indicate any deviation from the general rule that the facility has the right to possess the physical record and the patient has a right of access to the information therein.

CHAPTER 3

Which Records Must You Keep and for How Long?

Why Must You Keep Records?

Healthcare providers must keep records for several reasons: because the law requires them to do so, to provide better health care, and to minimize litigation losses.

THE LAW REQUIRES YOU TO DO SO

First, all levels of government have the undoubted authority to require you to keep records. A statute, an executive order, or an agency regulation may lawfully require record keeping. The government's power to require records and reports in the area of health services is necessary to ensure the public welfare. Without records and reports, the government cannot properly fulfill this function. And if the government can require a report, the government can also inspect the report.

The government, whether acting through the courts or through an administrative agency such as a health department, also has the power to enforce sanctions for failure to maintain required records. Such sanctions may include fines, contempt citations, default judgments, and the like.

TO PROVIDE BETTER HEALTH CARE

Obviously, even if the law did not require a hospital or other healthcare facility to keep medical records, such records would still be necessary to provide proper care for patients. Cases are legion where information contained in a patient's medical record saved a patient's life. In addition, health records have important roles in research, evaluation, and education. Other records, whether administrative or financial, also are necessary to enable you to meet your goals and objectives efficiently.

TO MINIMIZE LITIGATION LOSSES

Attorneys who are involved in medical malpractice cases know that the most favorable situation for a plaintiff who is alleging medical malpractice is one in which the relevant medical records are lost, incomplete, or otherwise defective. On the other hand, good medical records that show that the plaintiff received treatment that met the standard of care are the best defense against a malpractice suit because they can demonstrate, for example, that the plaintiff's injury is nothing more than an unfortunate result of proper care. Often, malpractice attorneys will either refuse to take a case or drop one when the records fail to show malpractice. Even in the worst-case scenario, where the record shows that malpractice occurred, having a record is often still valuable. On the basis of such information, the defendant's attorney can attempt to settle the case to avoid costly litigation and the risk of an aberrant and excessive jury damage award.

Good records management must be a part of your risk management program because creating and maintaining proper records documents the health care at the time it occurs, rather than having your medical personnel rely on their imperfect memories months or years after they provided the care.

In addition, records can show that you have complied with the multitude of federal, state, and local regulatory requirements.

Which Records Do I Keep and for How Long?

Now that you're convinced that you need to keep records, you need to figure out which records and for how long. It's not hard to determine which records you need to keep. Often a federal, state, or local law or regulation will tell you which records to keep, and your experience will undoubtedly cause you to add more. However, the question of how long you must keep various records has no easy answer. The answer is easier when a law, whether a state, federal, or local statute or regulation, provides for a specific retention period. But even when a law provides for such a period, other considerations may require that you keep the record even longer. And various laws may conflict. A state regulation may, for example, provide for a longer retention period for a particular record than a federal statute does. Other laws require you to keep certain records, but contain no retention period. Sometimes you should keep records that no law or regulation mandates that you keep but other considerations do, such as sound management practices or litigation protection. Practical concerns, like the availability of resources such as space and funding, will also affect the decision of how long to retain records.

Once you determine which records to keep and for how long, establish a record retention schedule and have it approved by your lawyer and your hospital administration. Having a written retention schedule is powerful evidence that you destroyed records pursuant to your normal course of business instead of to gain an advantage in an investigation or litigation. Make certain that your schedule includes all records, even those that you want to retain permanently, and addresses retention and destruction of both original records and copies—because copies usually have the same legal significance as originals.[1] Then, make certain that you adhere to your destruction schedule and properly document the destruction of your records.[2] Of course, you should never destroy records that are involved in an investigation or in litigation, even if they are due for destruction on your retention schedule.

Statutes of Limitation

Regardless of whether a regulation specifies how long to retain a record, you must consider the effect of statutes of limitation. A statute of limitation specifies a period of time within which a plaintiff must begin a lawsuit. After the expiration of that period, the statute bars the plaintiff from bringing the suit. Statutes of limitation usually run from the date of the incident, such as the malpractice, or from the date the plaintiff learns of or reasonably should have learned of the incident, whichever is later. Thus, at a minimum, you should retain records for the period of the statute of limitations. And, because the statute may not begin to run until the prospective plaintiff learns of the causal relation between his injury and the treatment he received, you should keep the records for a longer period than the statute of limitations requires. Also, if the patient was a minor, or under some other legal disability, such as insanity, you should keep the records until the patient reaches the age of majority or becomes competent plus the period of the statute of limitations. Even if a law or regulation specifies how long you must keep a record, good risk management may dictate keeping it for the period of the statute of limitations plus an additional period to cover the situation where the statute does not begin to run until the plaintiff learns of the alleged malpractice. An attorney's help is needed to verify which statute of limitations applies and how long it runs. If the plaintiff's harm, such as an injury caused by malpractice, occurred before the effective date of the current statute of limitations, the old period of limitations may apply.

Most states have different statutes of limitations for different lawsuits (Table 3.1). A different time period may apply to suits based on contract than to a negligence action, for example. If medical malpractice does not have a separate statute of limitations, a malpractice case would be covered by the personal injury statute of limitations. Many states have different statutes of limitations when the plaintiff is a minor or otherwise incompetent. Again, because statutes of limitations are so complex, *you must consult your attorney* to make certain which statute of limitations governs your situation.

The Federal Tort Claims Act, 28 U.S.C. §§ 2671–2689 (1988), which covers medical malpractice as well as other negligent acts of federal government employees acting within the scope of their authority, has a two-year statute of limitations commencing on the date the harm happened or the plaintiff knew of or should have known of the harm. State statutes of limitation vary widely.

---

1. See Chapter 4.
2. See Chapters 13 and 14.

Table 3.1
State Statutes of Limitation

State	Contracts[3]	Wrongful Death	Medical Malpractice
Alabama	2 years § 6-5-482	2 years § 6-2-38	2 years § 6-5-482
Alaska	6 years § 09.10.050	2 years § 09.55.580	2 years § 09.10.070
Arizona	3 years § 12-543	2 years § 12-542	2 years § 12-542
Arkansas	3 years[4] § 16-56-105	3 years § 16-62-102	2 years § 16-144-203
California	2 years § 337[5]	3 years § 340(3)	3 years § 340.5
Colorado	2 years § 13-80-102	2 years § 13-80-102	2 years § 13-80-102
Connecticut	6 years § 52-576	2 years § 52-555	2 years § 52-584
Delaware	3 years Tit. 10 § 8106	2 years Tit. 18 § 6856	2 years Tit. 10 § 6856
District of Columbia	3 years § 12-301(7)	1 year § 16-2702	3 years § 12-301(8)
Florida	4 years § 95.11	2 years § 95.11	2 years § 95.11
Georgia	6 years[6] § 9-3-24	2 years § 9-3-71	2 years § 9-3-71
Hawaii	6 years § 657.1	2 years § 663-3	2 years § 657-7.3
Idaho	5 years[7] § 5-216	2 years § 5-219	2 years § 5-219

3. States may have different statutes of limitations for sales contracts and for oral as opposed to written contracts.
4. For oral contracts.
5. California Civil Procedure Code.
6. For written contracts. Oral contracts have a four-year statute of limitations.
7. Oral contracts have a four-year statute of limitations.

State Statutes of Limitation (Continued)

State	Contracts	Wrongful Death	Medical Malpractice
Illinois	10 years Ch. 110 § 13-206	2 years § 13-212	2 years § 13-212
Indiana	10 years[8] § 16-9.5-3-1	2 years § 34-1-1-2	2 years § 16-9.5-3-1
Iowa	10 years § 614.1(5)	2–6 years[9] § 1614.1(9)	2–6 years[10] § 1614.1(9)
Kansas	3 years § 60-512	2 years § 60-513(a)(5)	2 years § 60-513(a)(5)
Kentucky	15 years § 413.090	1 year § 413.180	1 year § 413.245
Louisiana	1 year Tit. 40:1299.41C	1 year Ch. 9 § 5628	1 year Ch. 9 § 5628
Maine	6 years[11] Tit. 14 § 752	3 years[12] Tit. 24 § 2902	3 years § 2902
Maryland	3 years § 5-101	3 years § 3-904	5 years[13] § 5-109
Massachusetts	3 years Ch. 260 § 4	3 years Ch. 260 § 4	3 years Ch. 260 § 4
Michigan	3 years § 600.5805(8)	3 years[14] § 600.5805(8)	2 years § 600.5805(4)

8. Oral contracts have a six-year statute of limitations. However, no claim, whether in contract or tort, may be brought against a healthcare provider based upon professional services or care rendered unless filed within two years from the date of the alleged act, omission, or neglect.
9. The action must be commenced within two years after the claimant knew, or through the exercise of reasonable diligence should have known, or received notice in writing of the existence of the injury or death for which damages are sought in the action, whichever comes first, but in no event shall any action be commenced later than six years from the date in which the action or omission occurred.
10. Same as footnote 9.
11. All civil action must be commenced within six years, ME. REV. STAT. ANN. tit. 14, § 752 (West 1990). § 751 provides for a 20-year statute of limitation on personal actions on contracts, promissory notes, and the like. ME. REV. STAT. ANN. tit. 14, § 751 (West 1990).
12. Wrongful death actions other than as a result of professional actions must be brought within 10 years. ME. REV. STAT. ANN. tit. 18A § 2.804 (West 1990).
13. After the injury or three years after discovery of the injury.
14. However, several Michigan cases hold that where medical malpractice causes the wrongful death, the statute of limitations is two years.

State Statutes of Limitation (Continued)

State	Contracts	Wrongful Death	Medical Malpractice
Minnesota	6 years § 541.05	3 years[15] § 573.02	2 years § 541.07(1)
Mississippi	3 years § 15-1-29	2 years § 15-1-36	2 years § 15-1-36
Missouri	5 years § 516.120	3 years § 537.100	2 years § 516.105
Montana	8 years § 27-2-202	3 years §§ 27-2-204 & 205	3 years § 27-2-205
Nebraska	5 years § 25-205	2 years § 30-810	2 years § 25-222
Nevada	6 years[16] § 11.190(2)	4 years[17] § 41A.097	4 years[18] § 41A.097
New Hampshire	2 years § 507-C:1	2 years[19] § 507-C:4	2 years § 507-C:4
New Jersey	6 years § 2A:14-1	2 years § 2A:31-3	2 years § 2A:14-2
New Mexico	6 years § 37-1-3	3 years §§ 41-2-1 & -2	3 years § 41-2-13
New York	6 years Civ. Prac. § 213	2 years Civ. Prac. § 208	2½ years Est. Powers & Trusts § 5-4.1
North Carolina	3 years § 1-52(1)	2 years § 153(4)	3 years § 1-15
North Dakota	6 years § 28-01-16(1)	2 years § 28-01-18(4)	2 years § 28-01-18(3)

15. However, wrongful death actions resulting from professional negligence have a two-year statute of limitations under Minn. Stat. § 541.07 (1991).
16. For written contracts. Oral contracts have a four-year statute of limitations.
17. After the date of injury or two years after the plaintiff discovers or through reasonable diligence should have discovered the injury, whichever occurs first.
18. After the date of injury or two years after the plaintiff discovers or through reasonable diligence should have discovered the injury, whichever occurs first.
19. The general wrongful death period of limitations is six years.

State Statutes of Limitation (Continued)

State	Contracts	Wrongful Death	Medical Malpractice
Ohio	15 years[20] § 2305.06	2 years § 2125.02	1 year § 2305.11
Oklahoma	5 years Tit. 12 § 95	2 years Tit. 12 § 1053	2 years Tit. 76 § 18
Oregon	6 years § 12.080	3 years § 30.020(1)	2 years § 12.110(4)
Pennsylvania	4 years Tit. 42 § 5525	2 years § 5524	2 years § 5524
Rhode Island	10 years § 9-1-13	3 years § 10-7-2	3 years § 9-1-14.1
South Carolina	3 years § 15-3-530	3 years § 15-3-530	3 years § 15-3-545(A)
South Dakota	6 years § 15-2-13	3 years § 21-5-3	2 years § 15-2-14.1
Tennessee	6 years §§ 28-3-109,	1 year 29-3-104	1 year § 29-26-116
Texas	2 years	2 years Tit. 71, art. 4590i, § 10.01	2 years
Utah	6 years § 78-12-23	2 years § 78-14-28	2 years § 78-14-4
Vermont	6 years Tit. 12 § 511	2 years Tit. 14 § 1492(a)	3 years Tit. 12 § 521
Virginia	5 years § 8.01-246	2 years § 8.01-244	2 years § 8.01-230
Washington	6 years[21] § 4.16.040	2 years § 4.16.130	3 years § 4.16.350
West Virginia	5 years § 55-2-6	2 years § 55-7-6	2 years[22] § 55-7B-4

20. For written contracts. Oral contracts have a six-year statute of limitations.
21. For written contracts. The statute of limitation for oral contracts is three years.
22. After the right to bring the action accrued if it was for personal injuries.

State Statutes of Limitation (Continued)

State	Contracts	Wrongful Death	Medical Malpractice
Wisconsin	6 years § 893.43	3 years § 893.54	3 years[23] § 893.55
Wyoming	10 years[24] § 1-3-105(a)	2 years § 1-38-102	2 years § 1-3-107

The following states commence the statute of limitations in medical malpractice cases on the date of the last treatment: Michigan, Minnesota, New York, and Virginia. The following states and territories permit the plaintiff to use the date of discovery of the malpractice to start the statute of limitations: Alabama, California, Colorado, Connecticut, Delaware, the District of Columbia, Florida, Hawaii, Idaho, Illinois, Iowa, Kansas, Kentucky, Louisiana, Maryland, Michigan,[25] Mississippi, Missouri,[26] Montana, Nebraska, Nevada, New Hampshire, New Jersey, North Carolina, North Dakota, Oklahoma, Oregon, Puerto Rico, Rhode Island, South Carolina, South Dakota, Tennessee, Utah, Vermont, Washington, West Virginia, Wisconsin, and Wyoming. Many of these states that use the time of discovery to begin the statute of limitation have an overall limit. For example, Florida law provides ". . . but in no event to exceed seven years from the date giving rise to the injury."[27]

Some states have limited the rule permitting the plaintiff to use the date of discovery to cases involving foreign objects left in the body. States and territories following the foreign body exception include Arizona, Arkansas, California, Colorado, Connecticut, Georgia, Idaho, Iowa, Maryland, Missouri, New Hampshire, New Jersey, New York, North Carolina, Ohio, South Carolina, Tennessee, Utah, Vermont, Virgin Islands, West Virginia, and Wisconsin.

Federal Retention Requirements

The federal government has many specific record-keeping requirements. However, many federal statutes and administrative regulations only imply a responsibility to keep records. Thus, if the government requires a healthcare

---

23. Wisconsin limits medical malpractice actions to three years after injury or one year after discovery.
24. Eight years for oral contracts.
25. Michigan draws a distinction between malpractice in a hospital, in which case the statute of limitations runs from the date of the injury, and other malpractice, in which the statute runs from the date of discovery.
26. In Missouri, malpractice cases are an exception to the rule that the tort claim arises at the time of injury. In malpractice cases the statute runs from the time of discovery.
27. Florida Stat. Annotated § 95.11 (West 1990).

provider to comply with a regulation, that requirement probably implies that the provider must keep a record of such compliance. If you are not certain whether you should keep such a record, check with your attorney. Some specific federal record-keeping requirements follow.

DEPARTMENT OF LABOR

Under the Federal Employees Compensation Act, hospitals and physicians that treat federal employees under the Act must maintain records of all injury cases. Such providers must give the Office of Federal Employees Compensation a history of the employee's accident, exact description of the accident; nature, location, and extent of the injury; any x-ray findings; extent of the treatment provided; and degree of impairment arising from the injury. Supplementary reports must be made at monthly intervals in cases of head or back injuries, or injuries or illnesses that require prolonged hospital care. The report must contain the examination dates, the patient's condition, physician's diagnosis, medical opinion as to the relationship between the impairment and the injury, patient's prognosis, and other findings concerning the employee.[28] This regulation does not specify a retention period.

FOOD AND DRUG ADMINISTRATION

The Food and Drug Administration imposes various record-keeping regulations on manufacturers and handlers of pharmaceuticals.[29] These records requirements pertain more to manufacturers, distributors, and wholesalers than to individual hospitals or providers.

Hospitals and other authorized dispensers of methadone must keep clinical records for three years on each patient including the dates, quantities, and batch or code mark of methadone dispensed.[30] Sponsors of methadone maintenance programs must maintain for each patient an admission evaluation and records consisting of personal and medical history, physical examinations, and other information as necessary.[31]

HEALTH CARE FINANCING ADMINISTRATION

The Health Care Financing Administration (HCFA) outlines various requirements that hospitals and other healthcare providers must meet in order to participate in Medicare.[32] These requirements apply not only to the scope of services the providers must provide but also to the recordkeeping standards they must follow.

---

28. 20 C.F.R. § 10.410 (1991).
29. 21 C.F.R. Part 211 (1991).
30. 21 C.F.R. § 291.505 (1991).
31. *Id.*
32. 42 C.F.R. Part 482 (1990).

Participating hospitals must have medical record systems. Medical records must be retained for each patient, and the hospital must have a record service that is organized and properly staffed in relation to the scope and complexity of services it offers.[33] All medical records must be kept for five years.

Additionally, HCFA requires hospitals participating in Medicare to have adequate pharmacy services to meet the needs of their patients. Pharmacy records must document the receipt and disposition of all scheduled drugs, and the pharmacy must record and report any abuses or losses of controlled substances. No retention period is specified.[34]

Medicare hospitals must also have diagnostic radiology services available that meet the needs of their patients. Radiology services must keep records of the radiologists' interpretations and data to support them for five years.[35]

If a hospital provides nuclear medicine services, the nuclear medicine service must keep signed and dated reports of nuclear medicine interpretations, consultations, and procedures for five years. The service must also keep records of the receipt and disposition of all radiopharmaceuticals, but no retention period for these records is specified.[36]

If a hospital provides surgical services, HCFA requires the surgical service to keep records containing patient histories and consent forms (except in emergency situations), a report of the surgeon's findings and techniques, and a pathology report of any tissue altered or removed.[37]

Psychiatric hospitals participating in Medicare must keep records that permit determination of the degree and intensity of the treatment provided. Medical records must stress the psychiatric components of the record, including history of and treatments provided for the patient's psychiatric condition.[38]

Home health agencies providing services under Medicare must maintain clinical records for five years after the cost report relating to the patient is submitted for reimbursement, unless state law requires a longer retention.[39]

Long-term care facilities must maintain complete and clinical records on each resident for as long as state law requires, or if there is no state law requirement, for at least five years after the resident's discharge. If the resident is a minor, the facility must keep clinical records for at least three years after the minor reaches legal age in that state.[40]

---

33. 42 C.F.R. § 482.24 (1990).
34. 42 C.F.R. § 482.25 (1990).
35. 42 C.F.R. § 482.26 (1990).
36. 42 C.F.R. § 482.53 (1990).
37. 42 C.F.R. § 482.51 (1990).
38. 42 C.F.R. § 482.61 (1990).
39. 42 C.F.R. § 484.48 (1990).
40. 42 C.F.R. § 483.75 (1990).

State Laws

ALABAMA

Under the Rules of Alabama State Board of Health Division of Licensure and Certification, the hospital administrator is responsible for the supervision, preparation, and filing of records and may delegate this responsibility to a medical records librarian or other employee.[41]

According to the Alabama rules, patients' records shall be kept current from the time of admission to the time of discharge or death and shall be stored by the hospital for a minimum of 22 years either as original records, abstracts, microfilm, or otherwise. Nurses' notes may be deleted from the permanent record.[42] The facility must properly index and file medical records for ready access.[43] Hospitals must also establish a medical records committee to be responsible for the maintenance of complete medical records,[44] and the attending physician must authenticate the records.[45]

Rules of Alabama State Board of Health Division of Licensure and Certification establish the following retention requirements: Records must be maintained of all orders, procedures, and treatments of patients. For inpatients, such records shall be made a part of the medical record. Complete reports of laboratory tests shall be kept on file with the patient's chart. Such reports must be signed or initialed by the individuals who performed the tests. The pathologist's report of any tissue examined, as required by medical staff bylaws, rules, and regulations, also must be maintained on file with the patient's chart.[46] X rays must be indexed and filed for a period of five years.[47]

Hospitals must keep records of all stock supplies of controlled narcotics, accounting for all items received and dispensed.[48]

With regard to physical medicine, the rules provide that hospitals shall maintain records of all orders, procedures, and treatment of patients. For inpatients, such records shall be made a part of the medical record.[49]

The surgical department must keep a current operating room record book listing the name of the patient, date and time of operation, operative procedures performed, name of the surgeon, name of the assistant surgeon, names of nurses assisting, type of anesthesia used, and name and title of person administering anesthesia.[50]

---

41. Alabama Administrative Code r. 420-5-7.07(a) (1990).
42. *Id.* r. 420-5-7.07(c) (1990).
43. *Id.* r. 420-5-7.07(e).
44. *Id.* r. 420-5-7.07(f).
45. *Id.* r. 420-5-7.07(f).
46. *Id.* r. 420-5-7.09.
47. *Id.* r. 420-5-7.10.
48. *Id.* r. 420-5-7.11.
49. *Id.* r. 420-5-7.14.
50. *Id.* r. 420-5-7.15.

Nursing homes are required to maintain clinical (medical) records on all patients in accordance with accepted professional standards and practices. The medical record service must have sufficient staff, facilities, and equipment to provide medical records that are completely and accurately documented, readily accessible, and systematically organized to facilitate retrieving and compiling information. The facility is responsible for developing policies and procedures governing all aspects of medical records.

The administrator may delegate overall supervisory responsibility, in writing, to a full-time employee of the facility, and the facility must employ sufficient supportive personnel competent to carry out the functions of the medical record service. If the designated record supervisor is not a registered record administrator (RRA) or an accredited record technician (ART), this person must function in consultation with a qualified person.

The medical record consultant is required to visit the facility at least quarterly, documenting the visit in a written report to the administrator, and providing and maintaining documentation of consultation and drug destruction reports. The consultant is also responsible for the training of the individual having responsibility for medical records.

The nursing home must maintain a separate, orderly file folder in the medical records of each patient. The admission record must be placed in this folder immediately on completion.

Current nurses' notes and physicians' orders must be kept at the nurses' station and be placed in the patient's file folder when completed.

Current medical records must contain at least three months of information. Documents such as histories and physicals, assessments, nursing histories, and the like will be maintained in current records at all times.

Records and reports must be originals or legible carbon copies with an original signature.

Medical records of discharged patients must be completed within 60 days. All clinical information pertaining to a patient's stay must be centralized in the patient's medical record.

Patients' medical records must be indexed according to name of patient and final diagnosis, to facilitate retrieval of statistical information for research or administrative action. The final diagnosis should be coded on the medical records (discharge summary).

Medical records must be retained for a period of not less than five years from date of discharge, or, in the case of a minor, three years after the patient becomes of age under state law.[51]

Nursing home pharmacies must maintain readily available records of receipt and disposition for all controlled drugs that provide sufficient detail to enable an accurate reconciliation.[52] The pharmacist must determine and re-

---

51. *Id.* r. 420-5-10-.16 (1988).
52. *Id.* r. 420-5-10-.10.

port, at least monthly, the status of all drug records and must report discrepancies found in the drug records to the director of nurses and to the administrator. The pharmacist is required to assist in the development and implementation of an effective control procedure.

Control records of Schedule II and III drugs must be maintained listing the following on individual patient records: name of patient; date, type, and strength of drug; dose, time administered; physician's name; signature of person administering the dose; and balance on hand.

An individual medication record may serve as a record of receipt and disposition of controlled drugs listed in Schedule IV and V, drugs not subject to frequent abuse, and noncontrolled drugs.

Destruction of controlled substances must be accomplished on the premises. Pharmacy records must include name and address of facility, date of destruction, method used in destruction, prescription number, name of drug store from which the medicine was dispensed, patient's name, name and strength of drug destroyed, amount destroyed, and reason for destruction.

A destruction form for each patient's medications requiring destruction may be completed and placed in the patient's completed medical record, or a destruction form listing all controlled substances destroyed may be completed and retained in a facility file. The original copy of the destruction record must be maintained by the facility and a copy kept by the pharmacist.

Records of destruction maintained in a patient's medical record must be retained for as long as the record is kept. If a separate file of destruction records is maintained, those records must be retained for a period of not less than two years.

ALASKA

Alaska Statutes § 18.20.085 (1990) provides that unless otherwise specified by the Department of Health and Social Services, a hospital shall retain and preserve records that relate directly to the care and treatment of a patient for a period of seven years following the discharge of the patient. However, the records of a patient less than 19 years of age shall be kept until at least two years after the patient has reached the age of 19 years or until seven years following the discharge of the patient, whichever is longer. Records consisting of x-ray film are required to be retained for five years.

The Department of Health and Social Services has defined by regulation the types of records and the information required in medical records and may specify records and information to be retained for longer periods than those set out above.

Hospitals must maintain records in a form and manner acceptable to the Department of Health and Social Services, and such reports from them must be made as requested:

- Record of admissions and discharges, including total patient days, average length of stay, and number of autopsies performed. Separate data must be maintained for adults and children (excluding newborns) and for newborn infants (excluding stillbirths).

- Register of births

- Register of deaths

- Register of operations

- Register of outpatients

- Official original records of birth, death, and stillbirth required by laws are the prime responsibility of the attending physician. The hospital is responsible for the completeness and accuracy of the data furnished from its records, and for the prompt filing of the original with the proper U.S. commissioner by the attending physician, in accordance with instructions by the Bureau of Vital Statistics, when so requested.[53]

Medical staffs are required to maintain complete records on investigational drugs, including protocol and side effects.[54]

Medical staffs are also required to adopt bylaws and rules that provide for the appointment of committees, including executive, credentials, medical records, tissue and transfusion, infection control, pharmacy and therapeutics, and utilization review committees. These committees must keep written minutes of their meetings, including committee activities, recommendations, and election of officers, with minutes and records of attendance for at least five years.[55]

Facilities providing health care to Medicaid recipients must retain all fiscal, patient care, and related records for three years following the year in which services were provided, unless the Department of Health and Social Services requests retention for a longer period.[56]

Pharmacists must maintain bound record books for the dispensing of controlled substances, containing the name and address of the purchaser, the name and quantity of the controlled substance purchased, the date of each purchase, and the name or initials of the pharmacist or pharmacy intern who dispensed the substance.

ARIZONA

Arizona statutes require hospitals to have a medical record department under the direction of a qualified person and with adequate staff and facilities to

---

53. Alaska Administrative Code tit. 7 § 12.770(h) and (f)(2) (April 1984).
54. *Id.* § 12.110(c)(5).
55. *Id.* § 12.210.
56. *Id.* § 43.005.

maintain a medical record for every person receiving treatment as an inpatient, outpatient, or on an emergency basis in any unit of a hospital. The records must be available to other units engaged in care and treatment of the patient, but only authorized personnel may have access to the records.[57]

For licensing purposes, hospital medical records must be readily retrievable for a period of not less than three years, except that Arizona law requires retention of statistics and vital records, i.e., records concerning births and deaths, for 10 years.[58] The Arizona Department of Health Services recommends that if a healthcare facility anticipates that its records might be used in a criminal case, it should retain the records for the seven-year criminal statute of limitations. The Arizona Department of Library, Archives and Public Records, however, recommends a 10-year retention period.

Arizona also requires that results of laboratory tests be reported to the physician and entered in the patient's chart.[59] The individual performing the examination must record his or her observations concurrently with the performance of each step in the examination of specimens and record the actual results of all control procedures. Records must identify the individual performing the examination. Such records, as well as duplicate copies of laboratory reports, must be retained in the laboratory area for a period of at least one year after the date the results are reported.

The portion of the regulations titled Records, Maintenance, Availability, Retention[60] states

> Records of observations, where appropriate, shall be made concurrently with the performance of each step in the examination of specimens. The actual results of all control procedures shall be recorded. Records shall be initialed or signed by the individual performing the examination. Such records as well as duplicate copies of laboratory reports shall be retained for a period of at least one year after the date the results are reported except as otherwise prescribed by law and shall be made available for inspection by representatives of the Department.

Hospitals must maintain records for each specimen examined, containing the following information:

- Laboratory number or other identification

- Name and other identification of the person from whom the specimen was taken, if available

- Name of the licensed physician or other person or laboratory who submitted the specimen

- Date the specimen was collected by the physician or other authorized person

57. Arizona Compilation Administrative Rules and Regulations § R9-10-221 (1982).
58. Id. § 36-343.
59. Id. § 9-10-222.
60. Id. § 9-14-110.

- Date the specimen was received in the laboratory

- The condition of unsatisfactory specimens and packages, when received (e.g., broken, leaked, hemolyzed, or turbid)

- Examination requested and result in units of measurement where applicable

- Normal values for the method used where requested or indicated

- Initials or signature of the individual conducting examination[61]

No clinical interpretation, diagnosis, prognosis, or suggested treatment may appear on the laboratory report form, except that a report made by a physician may include such information. When another laboratory performs the analysis, the report must include the laboratory name, laboratory address, and name of the director of the laboratory actually performing the analysis. Each laboratory must participate in a proficiency testing program provided by the American Association of Bioanalysts or the College of American Pathologists for each authorized specialty and subspecialty. Records of such testing must be kept for two years and shall be available for examination by representatives of the Department.

In 1984, the Arizona Legislature repealed a statute, Arizona Revised Statutes Annotated § 25-103.06 (1976) (repealed by 1984 Arizona Session Laws ch. 30, § 1), which had required that copies of premarital serology results be retained for five years.

Hospitals must keep records of the donor and recipient of all blood handled and report all transfusion reactions occurring in the hospital.[62]

Quality assurance regulations require hospitals to maintain a record of quality assurance activities.[63]

Hospitals must establish a discharge planning program to provide for transfer of information between the hospital and other healthcare facilities or agencies to facilitate continuity of care.[64]

Arizona appears to have no specific requirements for nursing homes.

ARKANSAS

Arkansas Hospital Medical Regulations, Arkansas Register 0601, require facilities to maintain records in either original form or microfilm for 10 years after the most recent admission. After 10 years, the facility may destroy the medical record provided it keeps the following information for 25 years:

- Basic information, including dates of admission and discharge

---

61. *Id.* § 9-14-112 (1982).
62. *Id.* § 9-10-222 G (1982).
63. *Id.* § 9-10-225.
64. *Id.* § 9-10-225 B.

- Name of physician(s)

- Record of diagnoses, operations, or both

- Operative reports

- Tissue (pathology) reports

- Discharge summaries for all admissions

Complete medical records of minors must be retained for seven years after the age of majority is attained.

Hospitals must have written policies and procedures covering all functions of the medical record department and must review and update them annually.

CALIFORNIA

California requires hospitals to keep records on all patients admitted or accepted for treatment.[65] The hospital should have a medical record service under the supervision of a registered record administrator (RRA) or accredited records technician (ART), and should maintain legible records, either as originals or accurate reproductions. These records must be readily available.

Hospitals should keep a register of operations including the following information for each surgical procedure performed:

- Name, age, sex, and hospital admitting number of the patient

- Date and time of operation and operating room number

- Preoperative and postoperative diagnosis

- Name of surgeon, assistants, anesthetists, and scrub and circulating assistants

- Surgical procedure performed and anesthetic agent used

- Complications, if any, during the operation

Each hospital must maintain reports of unusual occurrences for the preceding two years.[66]

Hospitals must maintain medical records for a minimum of seven years following patient discharge, except for minors. Records of minors must be maintained for at least one year after the minor has reached the age of 18, but in no event for less than seven years.[67] The California Hospital Association, however, recommends that medical records, including fetal heart rate moni-

---

65. California Code Regulations tit. 22 § 70751(b) (1991).
66. *Id.* § 70333(a)(8).
67. *Id.* § 70751(c).

toring, be retained for at least 10 years following discharge of the patient for adults and at least one year after a minor reaches age 18, but in no event for less than 10 years following discharge.

In addition to general acute care hospitals, regulations specify that the following various other types of facilities must retain healthcare records and exposed x rays for a minimum of seven years (except minors as detailed previously):

- Acute psychiatric hospitals[68]
- Skilled nursing facilities[69]
- Intermediate care facilities[70]
- Home health agencies[71]
- Primary care clinics[72]
- Psychology clinics[73]
- Psychiatric health facilities[74]
- Adult day health centers[75]
- Chemical dependency recovery hospitals[76]

Each California healthcare provider must keep readily retrievable records as necessary to fully disclose the type and extent of services provided to a Medi-Cal beneficiary including

- Billings
- Treatment authorization requests
- All medical records, service reports, and orders prescribing treatment plans
- Records of medications, drugs, assistive devices or appliances prescribed, ordered for, or furnished to beneficiaries
- Copies of original purchase invoices for medication, appliances, assistive devices, written requests for laboratory testing and all reports of test results, and drugs ordered for or supplied to beneficiaries

68. *Id.* § 71551(c).
69. *Id.* § 72543(a).
70. *Id.* § 73543(a).
71. *Id.* § 74731(a).
72. *Id.* § 75055(a).
73. *Id.* § 75343(a).
74. *Id.* § 77143(a).
75. *Id.* § 78435(a).
76. *Id.* § 79351(c).

- Copies of all remittance advices that accompany reimbursement to providers for services or supplies provided to beneficiaries

- Identification of the person rendering services. Records of each service rendered by nonphysician medical practitioners must include the signature of the nonphysician medical practitioner and countersignature of the supervising physician[77]

In addition, records of institutional Medi-Cal providers must include

- Records of receipts and disbursements of personal funds of beneficiaries being held in trust by the provider

- Employment records, including shifts, schedules, and payroll records of employees

- Book records of receipts and disbursements by the provider

- Individual ledger accounts reflecting credit and debit balances for each beneficiary to whom services are provided

Medi-Cal providers must document the meeting of Code I restrictions for medical supplies and drugs as follows: A practitioner who issues a prescription for a Code I supply or drug must document in the patient's chart the patient's diagnostic or clinical condition that fulfills the Code I restriction. The dispenser must maintain readily retrievable documentation of the patient's diagnostic or clinical condition that fulfills the Code I restriction. If this Code I diagnostic or clinical condition information is transmitted to the dispenser other than by personal handwritten order from the prescriber, the dispenser must document the transmittal date and the name of the prescriber, or the employee or agent who is legally authorized to transmit such information. The documentation must be personally signed by the dispenser.

In addition to the information required for every medical record,[78] every practitioner who issues prescriptions for Medi-Cal beneficiaries is required to maintain, as part of the patient's chart, records containing the following information for each prescription:

- Name of patient

- Date prescribed

- Name, strength, and quantity of item prescribed

- Directions for use

Providers of Medi-Cal psychiatric and psychological services must also include patient logs, appointment books, or similar documents showing the

---

77. *Id.* tit. 32 § 51476 (1991).
78. As described in Chapter 1.

date and time allotted for appointments with each patient or group of patients and the time actually spent with such patients. This information is in addition to the information all providers are required to keep.

Each provider of healthcare services rendered to any beneficiary must maintain records of each such service rendered, the beneficiary to whom rendered, the date, and such additional information as the department may by regulation require. Such records must be retained by the provider for three years from the date the service was rendered.[79]

California Code Regulations tit. 22, § 70753 (1991) requires hospitals to send a transfer summary with the patient on transfer to a skilled nursing facility or intermediate care facility, or to similar distinct care units within the hospital. The transfer summary must include essential information relative to the patient's diagnosis, hospital course, medications, treatments, dietary requirements, rehabilitation potential, known allergies, and treatment plan, and must be signed by the attending physician. Acute psychiatric hospitals must send the same transfer summary (*id.* tit. 22, § 71553).

Similar transfer records must also be kept by skilled nursing facilities (*id.* tit. 22, § 72519(a)). When a patient is transferred to another facility, the skilled nursing facility must enter in the patient's health record the date, time, condition of patient, and written statement of the reason for the transfer, as well as informed written or telephone acknowledgment by the patient, patient's guardian, or authorized representative, except in an emergency.

COLORADO

Colorado's regulations, 6 Colorado Code Regulations § 1011-1, ¶ 4.9 (1977), require hospitals to keep the following records:

- Daily census

- Hospital services statistics

- Admissions and discharges analysis record

- Register of all deliveries, including live births and stillbirths

- Register of all surgeries performed (entered daily)

- Diagnostic index

- Operative index

- Physician index

- Number index

- Death register

---

79. California Welfare and Institutions Code § 14124.1 (1991).

- Patient master card file

- Register of outpatient and emergency room admissions and visits

A registered record administrator or other trained medical record practitioner must be responsible for the medical record department (*id.* ¶ 4.3).

Colorado requires that hospitals preserve medical records as originals or on microfilm for not less than 10 years after the most recent patient care use, except that records of minors must be preserved for the period of minority plus 10 years (*id.* ¶ 4.2).

CONNECTICUT

Hospitals having 100 beds or more must have a medical record department with adequate space, equipment, and personnel, including at least one registered record librarian or person with equivalent training and experience. Short-term hospitals or hospices may have a person with training, expertise, and consultation from a medical record librarian in charge.[80] Hospitals must also have a medical record audit committee. The facility must keep records of attendance and minutes of all medical staff and departmental meetings.[81]

Medical records, other than nurses' notes, must be kept for a minimum of 25 years after the patient's discharge, but may be destroyed sooner if microfilmed by a Department of Health–approved process.

Homes for the aged and rest homes must maintain records on each resident, including

- Name

- Residence

- Age

- Sex

- Nearest relative

- Religion

- Other necessary information

These records must be on forms approved by the State Department of Health.[82] These facilities' records, as well as those of children's nursing homes, originals or copies, must be kept for at least 10 years following the death or discharge of the patient.[83]

Licensed maternity hospitals must keep complete records that include information as required by the State Department of Health as well as all items

---

80. Connecticut Agencies Regulations §§ 19-13-D3(d), 19-13-D4(d) (1972).
81. *Id.* § 19-13-D4(b).
82. *Id.* § 19-13-D6(e).
83. *Id.* §§ 19-13-D6(5), 19-13-D10(6).

necessary to fill out a death certificate for the mother and a birth certificate or death certificate for the baby, together with steps for handling the case.[84]

Industrial health facilities must also keep records for each individual who receives health services, containing all medical and health-related reports and letters received from laboratories, physicians, and others. An entry must be made for every visit of such persons to the facility.

Industrial health facilities must keep noncurrent medical records and medical records of former employees for at least three years.[85] Dialysis units must keep records for a minimum of five years following the discharge of a patient.[86]

Facilities must keep records, separate from the medical records, for controlled drugs, including narcotics, for three years following the transaction recorded.[87]

DELAWARE

Delaware is currently revising its healthcare retention schedules. Previously it had followed the Guidelines of the American Hospital Association and the Joint Committee on Accreditation of Healthcare Organizations and the Medicare and Medicaid requirements. For nursing homes and related institutions, the Delaware State Board of Health Nursing Home Regulations for Skilled Care § 57.810 (1986) state that for the legal protection of the institution, records should be filed for five years before being destroyed.

DISTRICT OF COLUMBIA

District of Columbia Municipal Regulations tit. 22, § 2216.3 (1986) require a medical record to be kept for not less than 10 years following the date of the patient's discharge. Any record, other than a medical record, that might be required by the District's Public Health regulations must be kept on file for not less than three years (*id.* § 2109.2). A report of a venereal disease must be kept in the reporting person's file for not less than three years (*id.* § 205.6).

FLORIDA

Florida publishes a comprehensive General Records Schedule for Hospital Records E-1, which details the retention requirements for all different types of hospital records. Schedule E-1 requires that hospitals retain inpatient medical records, emergency room records, and outpatient/clinical records for seven years after the last entry; microfilming is optional. Schedule E-1 also requires hospitals to retain x-ray film for five years; a copy of the typewritten report should be filed in the patient's medical record.

---

84. *Id.* § 19-13-D14(e).
85. *Id.* § 19-13-D44(e).
86. *Id.* § 19-13-D55(e).
87. *Id.* § 19-13-D44 (g)(5).

Florida Administrative Code Annotated r. 10D-29.118(8) (1991) requires nursing homes to retain medical records for a minimum of five years from the date of discharge, or three years after a minor resident becomes of age under state law. Resident indexes must be retained permanently.

Florida requires dentists to maintain written dental records for four years after the patient is last examined or treated (*id*. r. 21G-17.002(2)).

Physicians are required to maintain adequate written medical records (*id*. r. 21M-26.002(3)), as mandated by Florida Statutes Annotated § 458.331(1)(m) (1990), for a period of at least two years. The Florida Administrative Code Annotated r. 21M-26.002(1) (1989) recommends that physicians keep medical records as long as needed, not only to serve patients but also to protect physicians against adverse actions.

GEORGIA

Hospitals must preserve medical records as originals, microfilms, or other usable forms in such a manner that will afford a basis for complete audit of professional information until the sixth anniversary of the patient's discharge or longer. Hospitals must keep a minor's records until the patient's twenty-seventh birthday.[88]

HAWAII

In Hawaii, healthcare providers must retain medical records in the original or reproduced form for a minimum of seven years after the last data entry, except in the case of minors. The facility must keep minors' records during the period of minority plus seven years after the minor reaches the age of majority.[89] Exempted from the retention requirement are

- Public health mass screening records

- Pupils' health records and related school health room records

- Preschool screening program records

- Communicable disease reports and mass testing epidemiological projects and studies records, including consents

- Topical fluoride application consents

- Psychological test booklets

- Laboratory copies of reports

- Pharmacy copies of prescriptions

- Patient medication profiles

---

88. Georgia Compilation Rules and Regulations r. 290-5-6-.11 (1991).
89. Hawaii Revised Statutes § 622-58(a) (1990).

- Hospital nutritionists' special diet orders

- Similar records retained separately from the medical record but duplicated within them

- Social workers' case records

- Diagnostic or evaluative studies for the Department of Education or other state agencies

X-ray films, electroencephalogram tracings, and similar imaging records must be retained for at least seven years, after which they may be presented to the patient or destroyed, provided that the interpretations or separate reports of x-ray films, electroencephalogram tracings, and similar imaging records are basic information. Basic information (see above) must be retained for 25 years from the date of last entry, except for minors, whose records must be kept for the period of minority plus 25 years.[90]

IDAHO

Idaho Code § 39-1394 (1991) specifies retention periods for patient care records. Clinical laboratory test records and reports may be destroyed three years after the date of the test. X-ray films may be destroyed five years after the date of exposure or five years after the patient reaches the age of majority, whichever is later, *if* the hospital has written findings of a physician who has read such films.

Otherwise, Standard MR.4.6 of the *Manual* of the Joint Commission for the Accreditation of Healthcare Organizations states that the length of time medical records should be retained depends on the need for their use in continuing patient care and for legal, research, or educational purposes.

Skilled nursing and intermediate care facilities must keep records in a safe location protected from fire, theft, and water damage for not less than seven years. If the patient is a minor, the facility must preserve the record for not less than seven years following the patient's eighteenth birthday.[91]

Proprietary home health agencies must maintain clinical records for six years from the date of discharge or, in the case of minors, three years after the patient becomes of age.[92]

Health maintenance organizations (HMOs) must keep medical records for six years after the termination of the enrollee's contract.[93]

---

90. *Id.* § 622-58(d).
91. Licensing and Certification Section, Bureau of Welfare Medical Programs, Division of Welfare, Idaho Department of Health and Welfare, Statutes and Regulations Dealing With Medical Records Retention 3 (1989).
92. *Id.*
93. Idaho Code § 41-3909 (1991).

ILLINOIS

Illinois Administrative Code tit. 77, § 250.1510 (1985) recommends that hospitals employ a registered medical record administrator (RRA) or an accredited medical record technician (ART) as director of the medical record department, with professional consultation services available to him or her. The director must participate in educational programs relative to medical record activities, on-the-job training and orientation of other medical record personnel, and in-service medical record educational programs. A committee of the medical staff is responsible for reviewing medical records to ensure adequate documentation, completeness, promptness, and clinical pertinence.

The Illinois Hospital Association *Record Retention Guide for Illinois Hospitals* recommends retention of medical records for 10 to 22 years and notes that microfilming could take place at any time. The hospital should preserve the records or photographs of such records in accordance with hospital policy, based on American Hospital Association recommendations and legal opinion. Hospitals must submit reports containing such pertinent data as the Department of Public Health requires including birth, stillbirth, and death reports. (*id.* tit. 77, § 250.1520).

Skilled nursing facilities and intermediate care facilities must retain records in an inactive file for a minimum of five years after death or discharge of the resident (*id.* tit. 77, § 300.1820). The administrator should consult with legal counsel regarding the advisability of retaining records for a longer period and the procedures to be followed in the event the facility ceases operation. If the resident is transferred to another facility, a copy of the resident's clinical record, or an abstract thereof, must accompany the resident.

INDIANA

Indiana requires healthcare providers to maintain the original health records of a patient (or microfilms of those records) for at least seven years.[94]

Indiana State Board of Health Hospital Licensure Rules[95] require medical records to be filed in a safe and accessible manner in the hospital, and to be made available for inspection by a duly authorized representative of the Indiana Hospital Licensing Council (Council) or the Board of Health.

Hospital records must be kept on the nursing unit during the patient's hospitalization. Inactive records shall be stored in a fire-resistive structure, preferably fire-resistive cabinets or shelves, in such a way as to maintain confidentiality.

All original films or microfilms thereof must be stored in the hospital for a minimum of seven years. Microfilms may be substituted for original records at the discretion of the hospital after the original records have been on file for

---

94. Indiana Code Ann. § 16-4-8-12 (West 1991).
95. Indiana Administrative Code tit. 410, r. 15-1-9 (1988).

a period of at least three years. The Council may approve reduction of the three-year retention period on request. Microfilm records must be kept in a manner that assures their preservation and accessibility. X-ray films or minifications taken within the hospital must be retained in the same manner as other patient medical records.

A responsible employee of the hospital, preferably a registered record administrator (RRA) or a qualified accredited record technician (ART), must be in charge of medical records. If a full-time RRA or ART is not employed, a consultant RRA or ART must assist the person in charge of records. The person in charge of medical records, with assistance from appointed representatives of the organized medical staff, must

- Check records for completeness

- Maintain indices by patient, by disease, by procedure, by physician, and other as requested by the medical staff

- Provide assistance to physicians in their reviews and studies that involve medical records

- Provide assistance to physicians to effect completion of medical records as required in the medical staff rules and regulations

Healthcare providers must maintain a patient's x-ray film, or a microfilm copy, for at least five years.[96] At the time an x-ray film (other than a mammogram) is taken, the provider must follow one of two procedures. The first is to inform the patient in writing that his or her x-ray film will be kept on file by the provider for at least five years. If the patient would like a copy of the x-ray film during that period, the provider will give him or her a copy of the x-ray film at the actual cost to the provider. The alternate procedure is to post conspicuously in the x-ray examination area a sign informing patients that all x-ray films will be kept on file by the provider for five years. On request during that period, the provider will provide the patient a copy of his or her x-ray film at the actual cost to the provider.

At the time a mammogram is taken, the provider shall inform the patient in writing that

- The patient's mammogram will be kept on file by the provider for five years

- At the end of the five-year period, the patient will be given 30 days to claim and pick up the mammogram for her own use, at no charge.

- If the patient does not claim the mammogram within the 30-day period, the provider may destroy or otherwise dispose of the mammogram.

---

96. Indiana Code Ann. § 16-4-8-13 (West 1991).

- If the patient would like a copy of the mammogram before the expiration of the five-year period, the provider will provide her with a copy at the actual cost to the provider.

Emergency room register and patient records shall be maintained.[97]

Outpatient services' medical records must be maintained and should be integrated with inpatient records.[98]

Original laboratory reports, including the pathologist's findings on specimen examinations, must be placed in the patient's chart. Copies of these reports and records in the laboratory must include information on the daily accession of specimens, test methods employed, and quality control procedures to assure accuracy of laboratory analyses. These reports must be kept for two years.[99]

Records of the results of all radiological procedures must be recorded on the patient's charts, and copies kept on file in the department for two years.[100]

Every hospital must keep records of all admissions, deaths, surgeries, outpatient procedures, deliveries, births, and stillbirths. These records should include patient identification data, attending physician, results, and such pertinent data as is needed by the hospital. Computerized records that maintain confidentiality are acceptable.[101]

All providers participating in the Indiana Medicaid program shall maintain, for a period of three years from the date Medicaid services are provided, such medical or other records, or both, including x rays, as are necessary to fully disclose and document the extent of services provided to individuals receiving assistance under the provisions of the Indiana Medicaid program. Such medical or other records shall include, at the minimum, the following information and documentation:

- Identity of the individual to whom service was rendered

- Identity of the provider rendering said service

- Identity and position of provider employee rendering said service, if applicable

- Date service was rendered

- Diagnosis of medical condition of the individual to whom service was rendered (physicians and dentists only)

- Detailed statement describing services rendered

- Location at which services were rendered

---

97. Indiana Administrative Code tit. 410, r. 15-1-11 (1988).
98. *Id.* tit. 410, r. 15-1-12.
99. *Id.* tit. 410, r. 15-1-14.
100. *Id.* tit. 410, r. 15-1-15.
101. *Id.* tit. 410, r. 15-1-8.

- Amount claimed through the Indiana Medicaid program for each specific service rendered[102]

IOWA

Iowa Administrative Code r. 481-51.6(1) (1987) requires hospitals to keep admission records, death records, birth records, and narcotic records. Medical records must be filed and stored in an accessible manner in the hospital in accordance with the statute of limitations.

Hospitals must also submit the Hospital Price Information Survey to the Commissioner of Public Health annually. (*id.* r. 481-51.6(4)(135B)).

The hospital pharmacy must keep records of transactions for the control and accountability of drugs, including a system of controls and records for requisitioning and dispensing of supplies to nursing care units and to other departments or services of the hospital. It must also keep records of all medications and prescriptions dispensed (*id.* r. 481-51.25(2)(135B)).

The dietetic service must keep copies of menus as served for at least 30 days and include pertinent dietary records in the patient's transfer or discharge record (*id.* r. 481-51.19(135B)).

Nursing facilities must keep a resident's medical records for three years (*id.* r. 441-81.9(2)).

KANSAS

Each hospital is required to have a medical records service that is adequately directed, staffed, and equipped to enable the accurate processing, indexing, and filing of all medical records. The service must be under the direction of a registered record administrator (RRA) or an accredited record technician (ART) or a person who meets the educational or training requirements for such certification. If not, the hospital must employ such a qualified person as a consultant.

The medical staff must hold regular meetings for which records of attendance and minutes must be kept.[103] Also, each hospital is required to comply with vital statistics statutes and regulations regarding the completion and filing of birth, death, and fetal death certificates within a specified period.[104] The hospital must also keep records indicating the receipt, disposition, and other pertinent information concerning all blood and blood derivatives provided to patients.[105] Records must be kept of personnel radiation exposure monitoring.[106]

---

102. Id. tit. 470, r. 5-5-1.
103. Kansas Administrative Regulations 28-34-6(c) (1990).
104. *Id.* 28-34-3a(d).
105. *Id.* 28-34-11(q).
106. *Id.* 28-34-12(n).

Each medical record must be kept for 10 years after the date of last discharge of the patient or one year after the date that minor patients reach their majority, whichever is longer.[107]

Maternity centers are required to keep medical records in retrievable form for the greater of 10 years after the date of the last discharge of the patient or one year beyond the date that patients who are minors reach the age of 18.

KENTUCKY

Medical records must be maintained under the control of a medical record service with administrative responsibility for all medical records. Medical records must be kept for every patient admitted or receiving outpatient services for a minimum of five years from the date of discharge, or in the case of a minor, three years after the patient reaches the age of majority under state law, whichever is longer.[108] The medical records service must be directed by a registered record administrator (RRA) on either a full-time, part-time, or consultative basis, or by an accredited record technician (ART) on a full- or part-time basis.

LOUISIANA

Hospitals must retain hospital records in their original, microfilmed, or similarly reproduced form for a minimum of 10 years after the patient is discharged. Hospitals must retain graphic matter, images, x-ray films, and the like necessary to produce a diagnostic or therapeutic report, in their original, microfilmed, or similarly reproduced form for three years from the date the patient was discharged. However, the hospital must retain the records for a longer period when an attending or consulting physician of the patient, the patient or someone acting legally in his or her behalf, or legal counsel for a party having an interest affected by the patient's medical records so requests in writing (Louisiana Revised Statutes Annotated § 5628 (West 1990)).

Under *id.* § 40:1299.96 (West 1990), physicians must retain medical records in their original, microfilmed, or similarly reproduced form, for a minimum of six years from the date the physician last treats the patient. Graphic matter, images, x-ray films, and the like necessary to produce a diagnostic or therapeutic report must be retained, preserved, and properly stored by a physician in the original, microfilmed, or similarly reproduced form for a minimum period of three years from the date a patient is last treated by the physician and must be kept for longer periods when requested in writing by the patient.

---

107. *Id.* 28-34-9a(d)(1).
108. 902 Kentucky Administrative Regulations 20:016 § 3(11)(a) (1991).

MAINE

Code of Maine Rules, Regulations Governing the Licensing and Functioning of General and Specialty Hospitals, ch. XII C 1-2 (1972), requires hospitals to have medical record departments that maintain medical records, in accordance with accepted professional principles, for every patient admitted for care. The department should be staffed by a registered medical records librarian. If not, the hospital should use a qualified consultant or a trained part-time medical records librarian to organize the department, train the personnel, and make periodic visits to evaluate the records and the operation of the department.

Hospitals must preserve medical records, either in the original or by microfilm, for a period not less than the statute of limitations. The regulation also requires keeping of pharmacy transactions as well as the transactions of various departments such as outpatient, emergency, dentistry, and physical therapy, and the records of the activities of the utilization review committee. A revision of the regulations requires documentation of discharge planning activity *(id.* ch. XII B).

MARYLAND

Medical records must be maintained for not less than five years from the date of discharge or, in the case of a minor, three years after the patient becomes of age or five years, whichever is longer.[109] The same regulations apply to retention requirements for comprehensive care facilities and extended care facilities.

Hospital utilization agents must maintain the following records for each individual patient for whom any aspect of the utilization review procedure has been applied:

- Patient's name, hospital history number, source of payment, and other demographic information capable of being used to identify the patient

- Principal diagnosis or diagnoses, and the particular category of patient chosen for review in accordance with the hospital's utilization review plan

- Date or dates on which review activities were requested, and date or dates on which opinions were rendered

- Type of review carried out, nature of the criteria applied, and results of the review. In the case of disallowed services, the reasons for disallowance must be stated, as well as the name of the physician member of the agent's staff making the final disallowance determination.

---

109. Maryland Health-General Code Annotated § 4-305 (1990); Maryland Regulations Code tit. 10, §§ 10.07.02.20 F; 10.07.02.21 F (1991).

- In the case of objective second opinions, documentation must include name of the physician rendering the second opinion, physician's specialty, and nature of the opinion.

Each agent must maintain a listing of all reviewed cases suitable for the selection of a sample of all cases reviewed within each two-year certification period.[110]

Hospitals are required to maintain a separate credentialing file for each physician that contains documentation relating to the credentialing process.[111]

Comprehensive care facilities and extended care facilities must maintain an admission record consisting of a copy of the clinical record, identification, and summary sheet.[112]

Health maintenance organizations (HMOs) must keep an individual record for each patient, using a system for identifying and filing records that provides for a universal identifier and adequate space and equipment for filing and prompt retrieval. Retention periods must comply with state statutes.[113]

Hospices must establish and follow a policy in accordance with applicable law under which the hospice retains its patient records for a defined period of time and disposes of them thereafter.[114]

Home health agencies must maintain clinical records for at least 5 years from the date of discharge.[115]

MASSACHUSETTS

Hospitals or clinics subject to licensure by the Department of Public Health or supported in whole or in part by the Commonwealth must keep records, including the medical history and nurses' notes. Such records or parts thereof may be destroyed 30 years after the discharge or final treatment of the patient to whom they relate.[116]

Long-term care facilities must keep all clinical records of discharged patients for at least five years. Such facilities must employ a medical record librarian or must designate a trained employee to be responsible for ensuring that records are properly maintained, completed, and preserved.[117]

Hospitals or sanatoriums that treat tuberculosis are required to have medical record departments with a medical record librarian and adequate personnel to supervise and conduct the department.[118]

---

110. Maryland Regulations Code tit. 10, § 10.07.01.18 (1991).
111. *Id.* tit. 10, § 10.07.01.24 F.
112. *Id.* tit. 10, § 10.07.02.08.
113. *Id.* tit. 10, § 10.07.11.05.
114. *Id.* tit. 10, § 10.08.21.13.
115. *Id.* tit. 10, § 10.07.10.11.
116. Massachusetts General Laws ch. 111, § 70 (1991).
117. Massachusetts Regulations Code tit. 105, § 150.013 (1990).
118. *Id.* tit. 105, § 134.940.

Blood banks and transfusion services must record and retain the following information for at least five years:

- Transfusion request records

- Transfusion compatibility test results and release (issue) data

- Actual results observed with laboratory test as well as the final interpretation

- Records of recipient adverse reaction to transfusion

- Refrigeration temperature and blood inspection records

- Records of blood and components received from outside sources, including name and unit number of original collecting facility and, if present, name and unit number of the intermediate facility

- Records of the final disposition of blood and components

- Records of blood brought to operating room refrigerators and returned to the blood bank, including times and return inspection, unless the refrigerator is considered an extension of the blood bank and blood bank personnel do the transporting

- Records of therapeutic pheresis procedures[119]

In addition, blood banks only are required to retain

- Consent forms

- Donor history, examination, and reaction records

- Documentation of testing of components, reagents, equipment, and proficiency test materials including dates of performance, tests performed, observed results (all positive reactions must be graded), interpretations, identification of personnel performing the test, and any appropriate corrective action taken

Clinics are required to keep patient records for 30 years after final treatment of the patient.[120]

Hospices must maintain records for seven years after death or discharge of the patient.[121]

MICHIGAN

According to the Chief Medical Consultant of the Bureau of Health Facilities, Department of Public Health, Michigan does "not have any definitive information about Michigan policy on hospital record retention and

---

119. *Id*. tit. 105, § 135.902.
120. *Id*. tit. 105, § 140.301.
121. *Id*. tit. 105, § 141.209.

destruction. . . . [T]his is a topic under current discussion in both the regulatory and legislative arenas." Since 1990, the Health Care Information Act has been in the legislature, but no final action has been taken to date. Department of Public Health Rules, Michigan Administrative Code r. 325.1028(5) (1987), state that medical records must be preserved as original records, abstracts, microfilms, or otherwise and shall be retained in a way that affords a basis for a complete audit of professional information, but no retention period is specified.

Nursing homes, however, must maintain clinical records under the supervision of a full-time employee for a minimum of six years from the date of discharge or, in the case of a minor, three years after the individual comes of age under state law, whichever is longer (*id.* r. 325.21102 (1987)).

MINNESOTA

Minnesota Hospital Licensing and Operation Rules, Minnesota Rules 4640.1100 (1991), require hospitals to maintain the following records in a form and manner acceptable to the commissioner of health:

- Record of admissions and discharges, including total patient days, average length of stay, and number of autopsies performed. Separate data must be maintained for adults and children, excluding newborns, and newborn infants, excluding stillbirths.

- Register of births

- Register of deaths

- Register of operations

- Register of outpatients

Individual permanent medical records must be kept permanently. Other portions of the record, including any miscellaneous documents, papers, and correspondence, may be destroyed after seven years without transfer to photographic film. However, all portions of records relating to minors must be kept for seven years following the age of majority.[122]

Hospitals must maintain a record for all narcotics administered, containing the date, hour, name of patient, name of physician, kind of narcotic, and name of person by whom administered.[123]

On or before January 31 of each year, hospitals must file with the commissioner of health the annual hospital statistical report covering patient service data. On or before the tenth of each month, the hospital administrator must file with the commissioner a report of all births and deaths or stillbirths occurring in the institution during the previous month. Also, the attending

---

122. Minnesota Statutes § 145.32 (1990).
123. Minnesota Rules 4640.1200 (1991).

physician and the hospital must report by mail to the Minnesota Department of Health, Section of Maternal and Child Health, within three days after the death any death associated with pregnancy, including abortion and extra-uterine pregnancy, or the puerperium (defined as a period of three months postpartum) whether or not the abortion or extrauterine pregnancy is the actual cause of death.[124]

Every illegitimate birth must also be reported to the commissioner of human services within 24 hours after the birth.[125]

Minnesota Rules 9505.0205 (1991) requires providers receiving medical assistance payments to maintain medical, healthcare, and financial records, including appointment books and billing transmittal forms, for five years. Also, adult foster care homes must store personal records on residents for four years after discharge of the resident (*id.* r. 9555.6245).

MISSISSIPPI

All hospitals and their personnel must make and maintain accurate records.[126]

As to the retention period, hospitals must retain, preserve, and properly store records for such periods of reasonable duration as may be prescribed by the rules and regulations of the licensing authority.[127] Such rules may provide for different retention periods for the various parts of hospital records, and for different medical conditions, and may require that the hospital make an abstract of data from records. However, hospitals must retain complete records for a period of at least seven years for patients discharged at death, 10 years for adult patients of sound mind at the time of discharge, and for the period of minority or other disability, such as insanity, plus an additional seven years, but not to exceed 28 years.

If a patient dies in a hospital or within 30 days of being discharged from a hospital and if the hospital knows or has reason to know that the patient left one or more survivors under disability (such as being minors or incompetent), who are or claim to be entitled to damages for wrongful death of the patient, the hospital must maintain the patient's records for the period of the disability of the survivors plus seven years, not to exceed 28 years.

The facility may retire x-ray films four years after the date of exposure if the radiologist has made written and signed findings and those findings are kept for the same period as other hospital records. However, before the facility may retire x-ray films or graphic data, it must notify the patient or the patient's representative by certified letter. The patient or his or her representative has 60 days to request the facility to retain the material for the same retention period as hospital records. The hospital must abide by such a request.

---

124. *Id.* r. 4640.1300.
125. *Id.* r. 4640.1400, Subpart 1.
126. Mississippi Code Ann. § 41-9-63 (1990).
127. *Id.* § 41-9-69.

MISSOURI

The chief executive officer or chief operating officer of a hospital must appoint a director of medical record services who is a qualified registered record administrator (RRA), accredited record technician (ART), or who has demonstrated competence and knowledge of medical record services and who is supervised by a consultant who is an RRA or ART.[128] The hospital must also have a mechanism for the review and evaluation of medical record services on a regular basis.[129]

Hospitals must maintain medical records as required by the statute of limitations, but may preserve them longer for clinical, educational, statistical, or administrative purposes.[130] Medical malpractice cases must be brought within two years of the date of the occurrence of the act of neglect complained of with two exceptions: (1) a minor less than 10 years of age has until his or her twelfth birthday to bring action, and (2) in cases in which the negligence was permitting any foreign object to remain in a living person's body, the action must be brought within two years of either the discovery of such negligence or the date on which the patient, in the exercise of ordinary care, should have discovered such negligence, whichever occurs first. In no event must any action for damages for malpractice be commenced after 10 years from the date of the act of neglect complained of.[131]

Nursing homes must maintain records of medication destruction in the facility including

- Resident's name

- Date

- Name, strength, and quantity of the medication

- Prescription number

- Signatures of the participating parties[132]

Records of medication released to the family or resident on discharge or to the pharmacy also must be maintained in the facility and must include the same information.[133] Intermediate care and skilled nursing care facilities must also keep separate records of Schedule II medication for one year including the name of the resident and physician, the prescription number, the medication, and the signature of the person administering the drug.[134] These facilities must keep complete and accurate records of each resident in the facility,

---

128. Missouri Code Regulations tit. 13 § 50-20.021(D)(1) (1990).
129. *Id.* § 50-20.021(D)(16).
130. *Id.* § 50-20.021(D)(15).
131. Missouri Revised Statutes § 516.105 (1990).
132. Missouri Code Regulations tit. 13, § 15-14.042(66) (1991).
133. *Id.* § 15-14.042(67).
134. *Id.* § 15-14.042(68).

from admission to discharge or death, for five years after the resident leaves the facility or reaches age 21, whichever is longer.[135] When the home purges records, it must maintain a minimum of three months' documentation, as well as the most recent report of physical examination and administrative information, with access to past records readily available in the medical record department of the facility.[136]

MONTANA

The Administrative Rules of Montana require hospitals to maintain a patient's entire medical record, in either original or microfilmed form, for not less than 10 years following the date of a patient's discharge or death, or, in the case of minors, for not less than 10 years following the attainment of the age of majority or the patient's death, if earlier.[137] Diagnostic imaging film and electrodiagnostic tracings must be kept for five years; their interpretations must be kept for the same period as medical records. The rule concerning core records does not prohibit retention beyond the periods described nor does it prohibit retention of the entire record.

The healthcare facility may abridge the record following the dates established previously to form a core medical record. The facility should maintain the core medical record permanently, but must retain it for not less than 10 years beyond the periods provided. A core record must contain

- Identification data including name, maiden name if relevant, address, date of birth, sex, and, if available, social security number

- Medical history

- Physical examination report

- Consultation reports

- Report of operation

- Pathology report

- Discharge summary, except that for newborns and others for whom no discharge summary is available, the final progress note must be retained

- Autopsy findings, if relevant

   Records for each maternity patient must also include

- Prenatal record

- Labor notes

---

135. *Id.* § 15-14.042(103). See Missouri Revised Statutes § 198.052 (1990).
136. Missouri Code Regulations tit. 13, § 15-14.042(111) (1991).
137. Montana Administrative Rules 16.32.328(1) (1986).

- Obstetrical notes

- Delivery record

  Records for each newborn must also include

- Observations of newborn after birth

- Delivery room care of newborn

- Physical examinations performed on newborn

- Temperature of newborn

- Weight of newborn

- Time of newborn's first urination

- Number, character, and consistency of newborn's stool

- Type of feeding administered to newborn

- Phenylketonuria report

- Name of person to whom newborn is released

The rule concerning core records does not prohibit retention beyond the periods described or prohibit retention of the entire record.[138]

Healthcare facilities, other than hospitals, must maintain patients' or residents' health records for not less than five years following the date of their discharge or death.[139]

NEBRASKA

Hospitals must keep medical records in original, microfilm, or other approved copy for at least 10 years following discharge. In the case of minors, the hospital must keep the record until three years after the minor has reached the age of majority.[140]

Intermediate care facilities must keep resident medical records for as long as the resident remains at the facility and for at least five years thereafter, or in the case of a minor, five years after the resident comes of age.[141]

Skilled nursing facilities must maintain clinical records for each resident, although no retention period is specified.[142]

Health clinics must maintain client records for not less than five years,[143]

---

138. *Id.* R. 16.32.328.
139. *Id.* R. 16.32.308.
140. Nebraska Administrative Rules and Regulations 175-9-003.04A6 (1979).
141. *Id.* 175-8-003.04A3.
142. *Id.* 175-12-003.04.
143. *Id.* 175-7-004.04.

and drug treatment centers must maintain resident records for not less than ten years.[144]

Residential care facilities must maintain resident records for at least three years after the resident's departure.[145]

Clinical records of home health agencies must be maintained in a retrievable form for at least five years after the last discharge of the patient. For minors, the agency must keep the record for at least five years after the patient comes of age.[146]

NEVADA

Healthcare providers must retain the healthcare records of patients as part of regularly maintained records for five years after their receipt or production.[147]

All superintendents, managers, or others in charge of hospitals or other healthcare institutions to which persons resort for treatment of diseases or are committed by process of law, must make a record of all the personal and statistical particulars relative to the inmates of their institutions at the time of their admission. If the person is admitted for medical treatment of disease, the physician in charge must specify in the record the nature of the disease and where, in the doctor's opinion, the patient contracted it.[148]

Hospitals without their own long-term facilities are required to have a written transfer agreement with extended or long-term care facilities.[149] All extended care, long-term care, and psychiatric care facilities must have transfer agreements with general hospitals. The transfer agreements must be in writing and on file at each facility concerned, and must provide for transfer of patients between facilities whenever the need is medically determined, and exchange of appropriate medical and administrative information between facilities.

All facilities must obtain a patient's essential nonmedical social service information for diagnosis, observation, and treatment, and this information must become a part of the patient's written record.[150]

Nevada Revised Statutes Annotated § 453.246 (Michie 1991) requires persons registered to dispense controlled substances to keep records as required by federal and state law and state regulations. Hospitals, long-term care facilities, nursing homes, and extended care facilities must keep records of all pharmacy transactions, correlated with other applicable hospital records.[151]

---

144. *Id*. 175-6.
145. *Id*. 175-11-007.078.
146. *Id*. 174-14-006.011.
147. Nevada Revised Statutes Annotated § 629.051 (Michie 1991).
148. *Id*. § 439.230.
149. Nevada Administrative Code ch. 449 § 331(2) (1986).
150. *Id*. ch. 449 § 352(2).
151. *Id*. ch. 449 § 340(2) (1986).

Pharmacies must keep records of prescription refills on the back of the original prescription.[152]

Hospitals, long-term care facilities, nursing homes, and extended care facilities must maintain narcotic records that list the following information separately for each type and strength of narcotic:

- Prescription number

- Amount received

- Date received

- Date and time administered

- Dose

- Patient's name

- Physician's name

- Signature of person administering

- Balance remaining[153]

Hospitals, long-term care facilities, nursing homes, and extended care facilities must also maintain records of recording thermometers to verify that the performance of each autoclave is in accordance with established sterilization standards. Autoclaving results must be checked at least monthly by periodic bacteriological tests. Autoclave records must be preserved for one year.[154]

NEW HAMPSHIRE

Health facilities must keep current, written files on each resident on active file in the facility until the resident is discharged. Both hospitals and health facilities must maintain medical records for a period of seven years (from the date of the resident's discharge in the case of health facilities). Hospitals must retain children's records to the age of majority plus seven years. Each hospital must have a written policy in regard to the disposition of records.[155] X-ray film must be stored for at least seven years and then may be destroyed.[156]

Sheltered care facilities and nursing homes must retain resident records in the facility until seven years from the date of the resident's discharge.[157] Outpatient clinics must store clinical records for seven years after discharge.

---

152. Nevada Revised Statutes Ann. § 453.258 (Michie 1991).
153. Nevada Administrative Code ch. 449 § 343(8) (1986).
154. Id. ch. 449, § 325(5).
155. New Hampshire Code of Administrative Regulations [Department of Health and Human Services Regulation He-P] 802.11 and 803.06 (1986).
156. Id. 802.08(B)(5).
157. Id. 804.04(b) and 803.06.

Minors' records must be kept until one year after reaching age 18 but in no case less than seven years after discharge.[158] Residential treatment and rehabilitation facilities have the same retention period, except that minor's records must be kept no less than three years.[159] Home healthcare providers must retain records for seven years after discharge. In the case of minors, records must be kept until one year after reaching age 18, but in no case less than seven years.[160]

NEW JERSEY

New Jersey's Standards for Hospital Facilities requires hospitals to include in their bylaws requirements regarding the maintenance of complete medical records and the establishment of an acceptable format for retaining all necessary data.[161]

Hospitals must also have medical record departments under the supervision of a medical record librarian or other person qualified by education, training, and experience. Hospitals must employ such additional personnel as necessary for the efficient conduct of the department. If a professionally qualified person is not available on a full-time basis, the facility must employ a registered medical record librarian on a part-time or consultant basis. The consultant must make regular visits to evaluate maintenance of records and to advise on the operation of the service.

Facilities must preserve medical records, either in the original or by microfilm, for a period of not less than 10 years following the most recent discharge of the patient or until the discharged patient reaches the age of 23, whichever is the longer period. Hospitals must keep x-ray films for five years.[162] The Administrative Codes of the State Board of Medical Examiners of New Jersey[163] require retention of treatment records for a period of seven years from the date of the most recent entry.

Hospitals must maintain such additional records as required to fully document their operations and to provide statistical data required by the Department of Health, including

- Record of admissions and discharge

- Case and clinical reports

- Daily census

- Register of births

---

158. *Id.* 806.10(e).
159. *Id.* 807(d).
160. *Id.* 809.07.
161. New Jersey Administrative Code tit. 8, § 43B-6.2(a)9 (1984).
162. *Id.* tit. 8, § 43B-7.1(b)(3).
163. *Id.* tit. 13, § 35-6.5(b).

- Register of operative procedures

- Narcotic register

- Death records

- Autopsy records

- Consultations

- Record of emergency and clinic services

Hospitals must forward a summary report of their activities to the Department of Health within three months of the end of each calendar year.[164]

NEW MEXICO

New Mexico Statutes Annotated § 14-6-2 (Michie 1991) requires hospitals to retain all records directly relating to the care and treatment of a patient for 10 years following his or her last discharge. Laboratory test records and reports may be destroyed one year after the date of the test if a copy is placed in the patient's record; otherwise they must be retained for four years. X-ray films may be destroyed four years after exposure if the hospital record contains written findings of a radiologist who read them. A patient may recover his x rays three years after exposure.

The New Mexico Hospital Association Legal Handbook, ch. 3, ¶ 3 (rev. ed. 1991), adds that the provider should not distinguish between x rays, laboratory reports, electrocardiograms, and other records such as fetal monitor strips. Because all such records are possible legal evidence, they should be kept for a minimum of four years. The Association suggests that fetal monitor strips be kept longer than four years if the delivery had any complications that might give rise to a malpractice claim. In addition, the facility may want to provide for longer retention periods for records of treatment of pregnant women, use of investigational drugs, experimentation, artificial insemination cases involving poor results, and similar subjects.

New Mexico Statutes Annotated § 30-44-5 (Michie 1991) makes it a crime to fail to retain for five years medical and business records relating to the Medicaid reimbursement.

NEW YORK

Hospitals must have a department that has administrative responsibility for medical records and must maintain a comprehensive medical record for every patient, whether an inpatient, ambulatory patient, emergency patient, or outpatient. Medical records must be complete, legibly and accurately written, properly filed and retained, and accessible. The hospital must use a system of

---

164. *Id.* § 43B-7.3 (1984).

author identification and record maintenance that ensures the integrity of the authentication and protects the security of all record entries.[165]

The facility must retain the records in their original or legally reproduced form for a period of at least six years from the date of discharge or three years after the patient's age of majority (18 years), whichever is longer, or at least six years after death.[166]

NORTH CAROLINA

North Carolina Administrative Code tit. 10 r. 03C.1405 (Feb. 1976) requires all original medical records or photographs of such records to be preserved or retained for at least the period outlined in the North Carolina Statute of Limitations and in accordance with the hospital policy based on American Hospital Association recommendations and guidance of the hospital's legal advisers.

North Carolina's Vital Statistics Statute, North Carolina General Statute § 130A-117 (1991), however, requires all persons in charge of hospitals to maintain for not less than three years records of personal data concerning each person admitted or confined to the institution and to make these records available for inspection by the State Registrar on request. Such records must include information required for certificates of birth, death, and spontaneous fetal death.

Nursing homes must have a full-time employee designated responsible for medical record services. If that employee is not qualified by education or experience, a registered record administrator (RRA) or an accredited record technician (ART) must consult to ensure compliance with the regulations.[167] Licensed facilities' policies must ensure that either the original or a copy of each patient's or resident's medical record is retained in the facility regardless of change of ownership or administrator, in accordance with North Carolina statutes of limitations for both adults and minors.[168]

Hospices must retain medical records for not less than five years.[169]

NORTH DAKOTA

North Dakota's Hospital Licensing Rules, North Dakota Administrative Code § 33-07-01-16 (1980), require the governing board of a hospital to establish and implement procedures to ensure that the hospital has a medical record department with administrative responsibility for maintaining medical records in accordance with accepted medical record principles for every patient admitted for care in the hospital.

---

165. New York Compilation of Codes, Rules and Regulations tit. 405 § 10 (1988).
166. *Id.* § 10(a)(3).
167. North Carolina Administrative Code tit. 10 r. 3H .0606 (Mar. 1983).
168. *Id.* tit. 10 r. 03H .0607.
169. *Id.* tit. 10 r. 03T .0902.

The hospital must preserve records, either in original or any other method of preservation, for 25 years from the date of discharge, except for the records of deceased patients, which need only be retained for seven years after the date of death. Records may be retained longer if the governing body determines that they have a research, legal, or medical value.

If the department is not headed by a registered record administrator (RRA) or an accredited record technician (ART), a qualified consultant must organize the department, train the personnel, and make periodic visits to evaluate the records and the department's operation.

All clinical information pertaining to a patient's stay must be centralized in the patient's records and the original of all reports filed therein.

Long-term care facilities must retain their clinical records, either in the original or by any other method of preservation, such as microfilm, for 10 years after discharge or seven years after the death of deceased residents. Records of minors must be retained for the period of minority and 10 years after discharge. Such facilities should receive consultation at least annually from an ART or RRA, if such a qualified person is not in charge of the records.

OHIO

Every hospital must disclose to the Department of Health the following data for nongovernmental patients (i.e., those that do not have their charges paid by various government programs):

- Total number of patients discharged

- Mean, median, and range of total hospital charges

- Mean, median, and range of length of stay

- Number of admissions for the emergency room, by transfer from another hospital, and from other sources

- Number of nongovernmental patients falling within diagnosis related group numbers 468, 469, and 470, as defined in 42 C.F.R. Part 412[170]

Hospitals must make this information available for inspection and copying by the public, but under no circumstances must a hospital include the name or social security number of a patient or physician in this data.

Nursing homes must keep the following records:

- Individual medical records on each patient

- All records required by federal and state laws and regulations as to the purchase, dispensing, administering, and disposition of all narcotic and barbiturate drugs including unused portions

---

170. Ohio Revised Code § 3727.11(B) (Baldwin 1991).

- An annual report to be submitted to the Director of Health

- Records of all patients admitted to or discharged from the home including any additional information necessary to complete the annual report[171]

Rest homes must keep a record on each resident including

- Name

- Residence

- Age

- Sex

- Race

- Religion

- Nearest relative and guardian

Such homes must also keep records of medications, treatments, and unusual events or accidents involving residents and the name, address, and hours of duty of all persons who work in the home. All these records and reports must be available for inspection at all times by the director or his representative.

Maternity hospitals must keep medical records of each maternity patient and each infant for not less than two years, as well as a log of all deliveries in chronological order, including items pertinent to the delivery, patient's condition, course of labor and delivery, and disposition of newborn infant. Newborn infants with special problems must be identified in a special log as prescribed by the Director of Health.[172] Maternity hospitals are required to keep all records and reports for not less than two years.[173]

Maternity homes must keep medical records for not less than two years.[174]

Resident records of alcoholism inpatient/emergency care facilities must be kept for at least three years after discharge.[175]

All long-term care facilities participating in the Title XIX program must keep financial, statistical, and medical records for the longer of seven years or six years after the fiscal audit.[176]

Residential care facilities under the Department of Mental Retardation and Developmental Disabilities must develop a record retention schedule for all service and medical records.[177]

---

171. Ohio Administrative Code § 3701-17-19 (1989).
172. *Id.* § 3701-7-24.
173. *Id.* § 3701-7-35.
174. Ohio Revised Code § 3701-7-35 (Baldwin 1991).
175. Ohio Administrative Code § 3701-55-15 (1989).
176. *Id.* § 5101:3-3-26.
177. *Id.* § 5123:2-3-16.

OKLAHOMA

According to the Oklahoma Department of Health, healthcare facilities must retain medical records for a minimum of five years beyond the date the patient was last seen or a minimum of three years beyond the date of the patient's death.[178]

The Oklahoma Medicaid Program Integrity Act requires providers to maintain, at their principal place of Medicaid business, all required records for at least six years from the date of claimed provision of any goods or services to the Medicaid recipient and to make these records accessible to the attorney general for investigation concerning whether any person may have committed welfare fraud.[179]

Oklahoma requires hospitals in which abortions are performed and abortion hospitals to keep records of abortion patients, including

- Admission and discharge notes

- Histories

- Results of tests and examinations

- Nurses' worksheets

- Social service records

- Progress notes

- Certifications of medical necessity, nonviability, or nonavailability

- Abortion reports

- Complication reports[180]

Such records must remain in the permanent files of the hospital for not less than seven years.

OREGON

Oregon Administrative Rules 333-505-050(8) (1991) state that the following records will be maintained and kept permanently (for a period of at least 10 years from the date of last discharge, *id*. R. 333-505-050(13), except as otherwise noted) in written or computerized form:

- Patient's register, containing admission and discharges

- Patient's master index

- Register of all deliveries, including live births and stillbirths

---

178. Oklahoma Department of Health Regulation ch. 13, ¶ 13.13 A.
179. Oklahoma Statutes Annotated tit. 56, § 1004 (West 1990).
180. *Id*. tit. 63, § 1-739.

- Register of all deaths

- Register of operations

- Register of outpatients (seven years)

- Emergency room register (seven years)

To ensure the quality of record retention, Oregon also requires visits, at least annually, by a qualified medical record consultant (a registered record administrator [RRA] or an accredited record technician [ART]) unless an individual qualified as an RRA or ART is the director of the medical records department.

The attending physician is responsible for completing the medical record and must do so within four weeks of the patient's discharge (*id*. 333-505-050(9)(a)). Completion of the medical records in a long-term care facility is the responsibility of the administrator (*id*. 333-86-055(1)).

If the patient is transferred to another healthcare or long-term care facility, transfer information must accompany the patient and must include

- Facility from which transferred

- Name of physician to assume care

- Date and time of discharge

- Current medical findings, nursing assessment, history and physical, and diagnosis

- Orders from physician for immediate care of patient

- Operative report and tuberculosis test, if applicable

- Any other information germane to patient's condition (*id*. R. 333-505-050(9)(b) and R. 333-86-055(10)(d))

Medical records must be filed and fully indexed (*id*. R. 333-505-050(11)), and a master index must be kept for records of patients in long-term care facilities (*id*. R. 333-86-055(12)).

Medical records in long-term care facilities must be kept for seven years after the date of last discharge of the patient (*id*. R. 333-86-055(6) (1986)).

Original clinical records, such as x rays, electrocardiograms, electroencephalograms, and radiological isotope scans must be retained for seven years after patient's last discharge (*id*. R. 333-505-050(16)).

PENNSYLVANIA

Pennsylvania has a comprehensive regulatory scheme for medical record retention. The hospital must maintain facilities and services adequate to provide medical records that are accurately documented and readily accessible to authorized persons requiring such access and that can be readily used for retrieving and compiling information.[181] A facility's medical record service must be directed, staffed, and equipped to ensure the accurate processing, indexing, and filing of all medical records.[182]

The service must be under the direction of a certified medical record practitioner. If none is available on a full-time basis, the facility must employ a certified person on a part-time or consulting basis. At least one full-time or part-time employee must provide regular medical record service,[183] and the hospital must also have education programs and written job descriptions for such personnel.[184]

The hospital must keep medical records, whether originals, reproductions, or microfilm, for seven years following discharge of the patient. The facility must keep minors' records until their majority and then for seven years or as long as the facility keeps the records of adult patients.[185]

The hospital must have a medical record committee to periodically review such records.[186]

Hospital pharmacies must maintain a system of records and bookkeeping in accordance with the policies of the hospital in order to maintain adequate control over the requisitioning and dispensing of all drugs and pharmaceutical supplies and over patient billing for such. Records for drugs dispensed must be maintained in the pharmacy, and records of drugs administered must be maintained in the patient's medical records. Copies of records of all adverse drug reactions and drug sensitivities must be maintained in the pharmacy for two years.[187]

Ambulatory surgical facilities must have a written policy regarding the retention of records. Medical records must be kept for a minimum of seven years following discharge of a patient unless the patient is a minor, in which case the facility must keep records on file until the patient's majority and then for seven years or as long as records of adult patients are maintained.[188]

The minimum standards of practice of the State Board of Medicine specify that physicians must retain patient medical records for at least seven years from the date of the last medical service for which a medical record entry is required. Medical records of minors must be maintained until one year after the minor reaches majority, even if this means that the record is retained for more than seven years.[189]

181. 28 Pennsylvania Code § 115.1 (1989).
182. *Id.* § 115.2.
183. *Id.* § 115.3.
184. *Id.* §§ 115.5 and .6.
185. *Id.* § 115.23.
186. *Id.* § 115.34.
187. *Id.* § 113.23.
188. *Id.* § 563.6.
189. 49 Pennsylvania Code § 16.95 (1989).

Pennsylvania requires long-term care facilities to keep records for a minimum of seven years following a patient's discharge or death.[190] Home healthcare agencies must retain clinical records for seven years.[191]

Hospitals under the prospective payment system must retain complete, accurate, and auditable medical and fiscal records for medical assistance patients for four years,[192] as must private psychiatric hospitals.[193]

RHODE ISLAND

The Rules and Regulations for the Licensing of Hospitals require medical records to be under the direction of a registered medical record administrator (RRA) who is certified by the American Medical Record Association or who possesses equivalent training and experience. The director may be full- or part-time or a consultant as required by the scope of service. The hospital must staff and equip the department to facilitate the accurate processing, checking, indexing, filing, and retrieval of all medical records.[194]

The regulations also require that the facility maintain records for every person treated on an inpatient, outpatient, or emergency basis and establish written policies and procedures regarding content and completion of medical records.[195]

The retention period for medical records, in either original or accurately reproduced form, is five years following discharge of the patient, in accordance with the vital statistics provision of the General Laws of Rhode Island.[196] Facilities must maintain a minor's record for at least five years after the minor reaches the age of 18.[197]

SOUTH CAROLINA

The South Carolina Department of Health and Environmental Control's Regulations, South Carolina Code Regulations 61-16 (1982) (Minimum Standards for Licensure of Hospitals and Institutional Care Facilities in South Carolina), specify that the responsibility for supervision, filing, and indexing of medical records must be assigned to a responsible employee of the hospital who has had training in the field (*id.* § 601.2). Records must be retained for 10 years (*id.* § 601.7(A)) and may be destroyed thereafter, provided that records of minors are retained until after the expiration of the period of election following achievement of majority as prescribed by statute (one year) and that the

---

190. 28 Pennsylvania Code § 211.5 (1989).
191. *Id.* § 601.36.
192. 55 Pennsylvania Code § 1163.43 (1989).
193. *Id.* § 1151.33.
194. 1990 Rhode Island Acts and Resolves R23-17-HOSP-25.1 and .2.
195. *Id.* 25.3 and 25.4.
196. Rhode Island General Laws § 23-3-26 (1990).
197. 1990 Rhode Island Acts and Resolves R23-17-HOSP-25.9.

hospital retains an index, register, or summary cards providing certain basic information.

The South Carolina Department of Health and Environmental Control, Records Series Retention/Disposition Schedule DHEC-CHD-75(R) (1990), requires county health departments to screen records of patients who have not been treated or serviced in the preceding four years and to remove and transfer all material not needed for immediate medical or reference purposes to the State Records Center. If space is available, the records are held there for 20 years and then destroyed.

Nursing homes must store medical records in an inactive file after discharge or death of the patient and must maintain the records for 10 years after the discharge or death.

Health records of intermediate care facilities—mental retardation must be kept for five years after the resident's discharge. On discharge, the facility must complete the resident's record and file it in an inactive file.[198]

SOUTH DAKOTA

South Dakota does not specify a retention period, so a facility should keep medical records for at least the period of the statute of limitations.

The Administrative Rules of South Dakota require hospitals, supervised care facilities, and nursing homes to have a medical record department staffed with trained personnel and equipped to facilitate the accurate processing, checking, indexing, filing, and retrieval of all medical records. The individual in charge must be trained and knowledgeable in the field of medical records, and the facility must have written policies and procedures to govern the activities of the medical record department including confidentiality, safeguarding, content, continuity, completeness, and entries of medical records.[199]

TENNESSEE

Tennessee has one of the most comprehensive statutory schemes for records management.

By law, hospitals have a duty to keep "true and accurate hospital records, including records pertaining to abortions . . . complying with such methods, minimum standards, and contents thereof as may be prescribed by rules and regulations adopted by the hospital licensing board. The responsibility for supervision, filing, and indexing of medical records must be delegated to a responsible employee of the hospital."[200]

Tennessee's Department of Health and Environment, Board for Licensing Health Care Facilities, Tennessee Compilation Rules and Regulations tit. 1200,

---

198. South Carolina Code Regs. 61-13, § 503 (1980).
199. South Dakota Administrative Rules 44:04:09:02-:03 and :06 (1991).
200. Tennessee Code Annotated § 68-11-303 (1990).

ch. 8-4-.03(1)(a) (1990), adds that the supervision of medical record services must be delegated to a qualified medical record practitioner, either a registered record administrator (RRA) or an accredited record technician (ART), or other person qualified by work experience.

Hospitals are required to keep records relating to patient care for 10 years following discharge of the patient or his or her death. However, in cases involving patients under mental disability or minority, the hospital must keep records for the period of disability or minority plus one year or 10 years following the discharge of the patient, whichever is longer.[201]

The facility may retire x-ray film four years after the date of exposure, provided the written findings or interpretations of a radiologist who read the film are retained for the period required for medical records as stated in the preceding paragraph.[202]

Hospitals may retain records, either as originals or reproductions, for a longer period than the period of retention or as required by a court.[203]

The hospital may, unless otherwise required by law, court order, or applicable rules or regulations, retire any business records at such times as in its judgment may conform to sound business practices and the reasonable accommodation of other interested parties.[204]

Willful violation of these records management statutes is a misdemeanor, but no hospital or employee may be civilly liable for such a violation except for actual damages in a civil action for willful or reckless or wanton acts or omissions.[205]

Rules and regulations of the Department of Health and Environment governing nursing homes require these facilities to maintain medical records for a minimum of 10 years following the patient's discharge or death within the nursing home. For patients with mental disability or minors, the nursing home must maintain the record for the period of minority or known mental disability plus one year, or 10 years following the discharge of the patient, whichever is longer. It may retire x-ray film four years after the date of exposure, provided the written findings by a radiologist who has read and signed such reports are retained for the same period as other records, above.[206]

TEXAS

A hospital may authorize the disposal of any medical record on or after the tenth anniversary of the date on which the patient who is the subject of the record was last treated in the hospital. If the patient was less than 18 years old when last treated, the hospital may dispose of his or her records on or after

---

201. Tennessee Code Annotated § 68-11-305 (1990).
202. *Id.* § 68-11-305(b).
203. *Id.* § 68-11-307.
204. *Id.* § 68-11-309.
205. *Id.* § 68-11-311.
206. Tennessee Compilation Rules and Regulations tit. 1200, ch. 8-06-.07 (1990).

the date of his or her twentieth birthday or on or after the tenth anniversary of the date on which the patient was last treated, whichever is later.[207] These requirements apply also to private mental hospitals,[208] municipal hospitals,[209] and hospital districts.[210]

Hospitals must preserve the following information, but may do so on microfilm:

- Identification data

- Medical history of the patient

- Reports of relevant physical examinations

- Diagnostic and therapeutic orders

- Evidence of appropriate informed consent

- Clinical observations, including results of therapy

- Reports of procedures and tests and their results, including laboratory, pathology, and radiology reports

- Conclusions at termination of hospitalization or evaluation/treatment[211]

In addition, the standards require that hospital's medical staffs be responsible for keeping complete medical records.[212]

UTAH

Utah's Health Facility Licensure Rules require every health facility to have a medical record service or department, under the direction of a person whose qualifications, authority, responsibilities, and duties are defined or approved by the administrator. A registered record administrator (RRA) or an accredited record technician (ART) must be employed at least on a part-time basis. If such employment is impossible, the hospital must have an RRA or ART consultant who visits at least quarterly and provides written reports to the chief executive officer.[213]

Each record department employee must have a written job description and participate in a continuing education program.[214] The facility must have written policies approved by the medical staff and the administration that provide for

207. Texas Health and Safety Code § 241.103 (West 1991).
208. Texas Revised Civil Statutes § 5547-96A (West 1991.
209. Texas Health and Safety Code § 262.030 (West 1991).
210. *Id.* § 281.073.
211. Texas Department of Health, Hospital Licensing Standards ch.1, § 22 (1991).
212. *Id.* ch. 1, § 7.1.1.8.
213. Utah Administrative Rules 432-100-7.401.
214. *Id.* R. 432-100-7.403.

- Duties of the director and RRA or ART

- Educational requirements for medical record personnel

- Release of information including child abuse records, psychiatric records, and drug and alcohol abuse records

- Preparation of medical records

- Filing and record storage

- Transportation of medical records

- Indexing

- Coding

- Statistical reporting

- Security and confidentiality of records

- Destruction of records

- Authorization of individuals for access or nonaccess to medical records

- Retention of medical records

- Prohibition against delegation of rubber stamp usage

- Duration or revocation of consent and releases[215]

The facility must maintain a medical record on every patient admitted to the hospital or accepted for treatment. All records must be readily available to attending physicians; the hospital, its medical staff, or authorized employees; authorized representatives of the Department of Health, for determining compliance with licensure rules; and other persons authorized by consent forms.[216] The retention period for medical records is 10 years after the last date of patient care.[217]

In addition to medical records, hospitals must maintain records of admissions, discharges, number of autopsies performed, and vital statistics including registers of births, deaths, operations, and narcotics.[218] Vital statistics must be reported including birth certificates, death certificates, and fetal death certificates.[219]

Mental retardation facilities must keep client records for at least seven years after the date of last patient care, and the records of minors until the minor reaches age 18 or the age of majority but for not less than seven years.[220]

---

215. *Id.* R. 432-100-7.414.
216. *Id.* R. 432-100-7.404 A.
217. *Id.* R. 432-100-7.406 A.
218. *Id.* R. 432-100-7.412.
219. *Id.* R. 432-100-7.413.
220. *Id.* R. 432-154-4.203.

Small healthcare facilities must maintain medical records for at least seven years after the last date of patient care and records of minors until the minor reaches age 18 or the age of majority plus an additional two years. In no case may the facility maintain the record less than seven years.[221]

Residential healthcare facilities—limited capacity must maintain residents' records for at least seven years following discharge.[222]

Freestanding ambulatory surgical centers must keep records for at least seven years after the last date of patient care except for records of minors, which must be kept until the minor reaches age 18 or the age of majority plus an additional two years.[223]

Birthing centers must keep records for five years after the last date of client care. Records of minors, including records of newborn infants, must be retained for three years after the minor reaches legal age, but in no case less than five years.[224]

Abortion clinics and end-stage renal disease facilities must maintain medical records for at least seven years after the last date of patient care, and records of minors until the minor reaches age 18 or the age of majority plus an additional two years. In no case may the facility maintain the record less than seven years.[225] Home health agencies must keep records for seven years.[226]

VERMONT

According to the Vermont State Hospital Licensing Regulations, Vermont Administrative Procedures Bulletin art. 2 § 3-496, hospitals must maintain medical records for 10 years following the patient's discharge.

Hospitals must keep accounting records of all operating procedures on a monthly basis. Complete operating and financial statements must be compiled at least annually and then kept on file for 20 years.[227] The licensee must file an annual report with the State Board of Health containing

- Total number of admissions during the year

- Total number of discharges during the year

- Total number of deaths during the year

- Bed capacity

- Average length of stay

- Number of major operations

---

221. *Id*. R. 423-6.102.
222. *Id*. R. 432-300-2.302.
223. *Id*. R. 432-500-6.104.
224. *Id*. R. 432-550-6.101.
225. *Id*. R. 423-600-6.104 and R. 650-3.206.
226. *Id*. R. 432-700-3.705.
227. Vermont Administrative Procedures Bulletin art. 2 § 3-941.

- Number of minor operations

- Number of outpatient visits

- Number of autopsies

- Maternity statistics

- Any changes in structure, services, or both within the past year

- Any changes anticipated in the next year

The hospital must also provide the agency with a copy of its published annual report.[228]

Within seven days, hospitals and physicians must report all deaths of fetuses of 20 or more weeks of gestation or, if gestational age is unknown, of a weight of 400 or more grams (15 or more ounces). All therapeutic or induced abortions also must be reported to the commissioner.[229]

Level III and Level IV residential care homes must keep resident records on file for at least seven years after the date of discharge or death of the resident, whichever occurs first.[230] Such homes must also report fires to the licensing agency and the Department of Labor and Industry within 24 hours. Level IV facilities must report to the licensing agency any accidents or illness that require physician follow-up and emergency room treatment or admission to a hospital. All homes must file these reports in the resident's folder.

Homes must also report unexplained absences of residents to the police and responsible persons and follow up with a report to the licensing agency within 24 hours. Finally, these homes must report breakdowns of their physical plants that disrupt normal operations.[231]

Nursing homes must keep residents' records for at least six years following discharge or death.[232] Licensed nursing personnel must be responsible for the maintenance of medical records, and the facility must submit a semiannual statistical report to the licensing agency as of December 31 and June 30 each year, due prior to February 1 and August 1, respectively. Nursing homes must also report all fires and provide health examination certificates for all employees.[233]

VIRGINIA

Hospitals must staff and equip their medical record departments to facilitate the accurate processing, checking, indexing, filing, and retrieval of all medi-

---

228. *Id.* § 3-492.
229. Vermont Statutes Ann. tit. 18 § 5222(a)(1) (1991).
230. Vermont Agency of Human Services, Level III and IV Residential Care Home Licensing Regulations § VI-9(c) (1987).
231. *Id.* § VI-9(b)(5) and (6).
232. Vermont Department of Rehabilitation and Aging, State of Vermont Nursing Home Regulations § 3-29 (1986).
233. *Id.* § 3-28.

cal records and must establish written policies and procedures regarding content and completion of medical records.

The regulations mandate that hospitals preserve either originals or accurate reproductions for a minimum of five years following the patient's discharge, except for minor patients. Records of minors must be kept for at least five years after the patient reaches the age of 18. Birth and death information must be kept for 10 years.[234]

The same retention period applies to nursing homes.[235] Nursing homes must place overall responsibility for ensuring that medical records are maintained, completed, and preserved on a full-time employee with work experience or training that is consistent with the nature and complexity of the record system.[236]

WASHINGTON

Hospitals are required by regulation to have a well-defined medical record system and the facilities, staff, equipment, and supplies necessary for the development, maintenance, control, analysis, use, and preservation of patient care data and medical records in accordance with recognized principles of medical records management and applicable state laws and regulations. The medical record service must be directed, staffed, and equipped to ensure timely, complete, and accurate checking, processing, indexing, filing, and preservation of medical records, and the compilation, maintenance, and distribution of patient care statistics.[237] The hospital must have written policies and procedures concerning the medical record system including format, access to and release of data, retention, preservation, and destruction.

Hospitals are required to retain all medical records that relate directly to the care and treatment of a patient for not less than 10 years following the patient's most recent discharge. Hospitals must keep a minor's records not less than three years following the minor's attainment of age 18 or 10 years following discharge, whichever is longer. Reports on referred outpatient diagnostic services must be kept for at least two years; master patient index card (or equivalent) for at least the same period as the medical records to which it pertains; data in inpatient and outpatient registers for at least three years; data in emergency services registers for at least the same period as the medical record; and data in the operation register, the disease and operation indexes, the physicians' index, and annual reports on analyses of hospital services for at least three years. A hospital may elect to preserve an emer-

234. Virginia Regulations for the Regulation of Hospital and Nursing Home Licensure and Inspection, part II, § 208 (1985).
235. *Id.* § 24.5.
236. *Id.* § 24.10.
237. Washington Revised Code § 70.41.190 (1990).

gency service register for only three years after the last entry if it includes all outpatient emergency care patients in the master patient index.[238]

Hospitals must maintain current registers including inpatient registers, one or more outpatient registers, an emergency service register, and an operations register. Further, hospitals must prepare daily inpatient census reports on admissions to inpatient services, births, and discharges including deaths and transfers to another healthcare facility as well as regular monthly or more frequent reports on admissions to outpatient services and the number of emergency care patients. For patients to whom the hospital provides only referred outpatient diagnostic services, the hospital may maintain a simple record system providing for the identification, filing, and retrieval of authenticated reports on all tests or examinations provided to patients who received referred outpatient diagnostic services.[239]

WEST VIRGINIA

West Virginia Regulations for Hospital Licensure, West Virginia Legislature, Title 64 W. Va. Legislative Rules Department of Health, Hospital Licensure, series 12 § 10.3.1e (1987), state that records must be preserved in the original form or by microfilm or electronic data process without specifying a retention period, thus implying that retention must be permanent. Hospitals must maintain a medical record department under the supervision of a medical record librarian or other person qualified by training and experience (*id.* § 10.3.1).

WISCONSIN

Health and Social Services Regulations in the Wisconsin Administrative Code, Wisconsin Administrative Code § HSS 124.14 (2) (Feb. 1, 1988), require that hospitals have a medical record service with administrative responsibility for all medical records maintained by the hospital with either a registered medical record administrator (RRA) or an accredited record technician (ART) in charge. If such a person is not in charge, a consultant who is so qualified must organize the service, train the personnel, and make periodic visits to evaluate the records and operation of the service (*id.* HSS § 124.14(2)(d)2.a).

The regulations require a written policy for the preservation of medical records, either in the original or on microfilm. The hospital may determine the retention period based on historical research and legal, teaching, and patient care needs, but it must keep medical records for at least five years (*id.* § HSS 124.14(c)).

Skilled care nursing homes must designate a full-time employee as the person responsible for the medical record service (*id.* § HSS 132.45). This employee must be a graduate of a school of medical record science, accred-

---

238. Washington Administrative Code § 248-18-440 (1986).
239. *Id.* 248-18-440 (1986).

ited jointly by the Council on Medical Education of the American Medical Association and the American Medical Record Association. Alternatively, the facility may receive regular consultation from a person with such credentials. Intermediate care facilities must have an employee assigned responsibility for maintaining, completing, and preserving medical records. The facility must maintain an original medical record and legible copies of court orders or other documents authorizing another person to speak or act on behalf of the resident for at least five years following a resident's discharge or death. Facilities for the developmentally disabled must keep medical records, court orders, or other documents authorizing another to speak for the resident and resident consent documents for the same period (*id.* § HSS 134.47).

Each hospital, clinic, or other facility in which induced abortions are performed must report to the Department of Health information concerning patients.[240]

WYOMING

According to the Wyoming State Archives and Historical Department *Records Disposal Manual for Wyoming County Hospitals* (1987), patient medical records are to be maintained for 30 years, then destroyed. However, administrative and discharge records, diagnoses of operations, operative reports, pathology reports, and discharge summaries are to be kept permanently. Nursing histories and care plans are to be kept for three years. Nuclear medicine records and blood bank laboratory reports must be kept for five years. Facilities must keep emergency care records, donor records, and outpatient records for 10 years. Incident reports have an eight-year retention schedule.

The Records Management Archives, Records Management, and Micrographics Service of Wyoming notes the following recent changes for publicly funded hospitals:

- Patient registration forms, duplicates—destroy at discretion

- Patient continuing care records—retain 5 years, then destroy if no litigation is pending

- X-ray index file cards—retain 5 years, then destroy

Abortions must be reported without disclosing the identity of the patient. The physician must send such reports to the administrator of the division of health and medical services within 20 days after performing the abortion.[241]

---

240. Wisconsin Statutes § 69.186 (1990).
241. Wyoming Statutes § 35-6-107 (1991).

PART II

How Do You Keep Your Medical Records?

Now that we know what medical records you must keep and for how long, you must make sure that you use the right media and store the records properly. You must also be careful that you don't harm their effectiveness by making improper corrections. Chapters 4, 5, and 6 will discuss these issues.

CHAPTER 4

Which Media Can You Use to Maintain Medical Records?

Media Generally

Some states, by statute or by administrative regulation, specify which media are permissible for medical records. Others do not. Regardless of whether your state specifically authorizes the use of particular media, you must carefully consider whether a particular medium is permissible and whether it is admissible in evidence. Records that are not admissible in evidence do not help you very much. If an inadmissible record shows that one of your staff physicians provided proper care to a patient who is suing for malpractice, the record won't help you avoid liability.

The dynamic nature of today's information technology provides both an opportunity and a challenge with regard to healthcare record retention. New diagnostic equipment, new information storage equipment, and the need for better documentation of patient care to avoid malpractice losses together have revolutionized medical and other healthcare record retention. How do we retain this critical information, considering the possibility of litigation that might require us to produce the record as well as the practical and financial aspects of maintaining the records?

In most states, when you record information, such as patient examination data, on a computer or other electronic device, its output, such as a hardcopy printout, becomes the original physical record of that examination and thereby becomes a part of the patient's medical records, subject to the same retention requirements.

If the output, such as the printout, is visually intelligible, you may retain it in that form in the regular course of your business. The situation is more complicated when the output is not visually intelligible, such as a magnetic tape. In such cases, any future use of the data, as in a court case, would require turning the data into a written or visually understandable form. Should you retain the unintelligible "original" or reproduce the output in an intelligible form and store it? The answer depends, in part, on your state law. Under federal and many state laws, you can reproduce data from an unintelligible form and use it as evidence. The law calls such evidence "duplicate originals."[1]

---

1. Federal Rules of Evidence 1001(4).

Again, you must create and store the data in conformance with your established procedures in the normal course of your business. Your personnel must, of course, properly operate the recording devices for such information to be admissible in court.

Microfilming is permissible in almost all states and with the U.S. government.[2] You must, however, be certain that your staff conducts microfilming during the regular course of business and "in good faith," that is, not only of records that are involved in an investigation or litigation. You should also be certain that you can produce a readable copy of the microfilmed records. Microfilm is most appropriate for bulky records of uniform size that do not require frequent access.

Computer-stored data is likewise generally admissible into evidence if the record was made at or within a reasonable period of time after the event or transaction it memorialized and in the regular course of business and if the procedure, including the printout, was reliable. Optical storage media have aspects of both microfilm and computer stored data. Optically stored data is hard to alter, as is microfilm; but, like magnetic computer data, optically stored data cannot be read without being translated into visually readable form. Consequently, the evidentiary advantage microfilm has over computer generated-data, its unalterability, should result in unalterable optical storage data's admissibility. State statutes or evidence codes that refer to "any other information storage device" or similar language should encompass optical storage systems. Federal Rules of Evidence Rule 1001(4)'s definition of "duplicate" includes "other equivalent techniques which accurately reproduces the original." Federal Rules of Evidence Rule 1001(4) would seem to authorize the use of optical storage systems. Check with your attorney before adopting a new record storage medium.

Federal Laws

28 U.S.C. § 1732 (1988) governs business and public records. The statute provides that if any business, institution, member of a profession or calling, or any department or agency of government in the regular course of business keeps any memorandum, writing, entry, print, or representation of any act, transaction, occurrence, or event, and in the regular course of business records, copies, or reproduces the original by any photographic, photostatic, microfilm, microcard, miniature photographic, or other process that accurately reproduces the original, the entity may destroy the original unless its preservation is required by law (*id.*). Such reproduction is admissible in evidence to the same extent as the original was.[3]

42 U.S.C. § 2112(a) (1988) provides that when a statute requires indefinite

---

2. 28 U.S.C. § 1732 (1988).
3. Federal Rules of Evidence 1001(5).

retention of a record, the retention of a photographic, microphotographic, or other reproduction suffices.

44 U.S.C. § 3312 (1988) provides that photographs or microphotographs made in compliance with federal regulations have the same effect as the originals and are originals for the purposes of admissibility in evidence.

The Public Health Service permits microfilming or other adequate copies of records required of grantees.[4] The Internal Revenue Service also permits the use of microfilm.[5]

The Food and Drug Administration,[6] the Occupational Safety and Health Administration,[7] and the Veterans Administration[8] also permit microfilming of records.

State Laws

ALABAMA

Alabama's rules of the State Board of Health Division of Licensure and Certification permit patients' records to be stored either as original records, abstracts, microfilm, or otherwise.[9]

ALASKA

The medical record retention requirements of the Alaska Administrative Code speak of "originals or accurate reproductions of the originals of records, including x-rays, must be retained in a form which is legible and readily available. . . ."[10]

ARIZONA

Arizona permits microfilming of records that may be used in court regardless of whether the hard copy is extant.[11]

ARKANSAS

Hospital records must be retained in either original form or microfilm. Required indexes may be kept on punch cards or print-out sheets kept in books in hospitals using automatic data processing. Rule 1003 of the Arkansas Rules of Evidence states that a copy is admissible to the same extent as an original

---

4. *See* 45 C.F.R. § 74.20 (1990).
5. Revenue Procedure 81-46; Revenue Ruling 75-265, 1967-1 CB 576.
6. 21 C.F.R. § 58.195(g) (1991).
7. 29 C.F.R. § 1910.20(2) (1991) (except x rays, which must be kept in their original form).
8. 38 C.F.R. § 17 (1991).
9. Alabama Administrative Code r. 420-5.7.07(c) (1990).
10. Alaska Administrative Code tit. 7 §§ 12.425 and 12.530 (1984).
11. *See* Arizona Revised Statutes Annotated § 12-2262 (1991).

unless a genuine question exists as to the authenticity of the original. Rule 1001 (4) defines "duplicates" as counterparts of the original made by photography, including enlargements or miniatures, or by other equivalent techniques that accurately reproduce the original.

CALIFORNIA

California law permits the use of microfilm.[12] In addition, California's administrative code, which requires hospitals to keep medical records either as originals "or [as] accurate reproductions," would seem to authorize any medium that reproduces records accurately and legibly.[13]

In addition to general acute care hospitals, California's administrative code specifies that the following other types of facilities are to keep records either as originals or accurate reproductions that are maintained in a legible and readily retrievable form:

- Acute psychiatric hospitals[14]

- Skilled nursing facilities[15]

- Intermediate care facilities[16]

- Home health agencies[17]

- Primary care clinics[18]

- Psychology clinics[19]

- Psychiatric health facilities[20]

- Chemical dependency recovery hospitals[21]

COLORADO

Hospitals may preserve records either as originals or on microfilm.[22]

CONNECTICUT

Connecticut permits microfilming of medical records.[23]

---

12. California Evidence Code § 1550 (West 1991).
13. California Code Regulations tit. 22, § 70751(a) (1988).
14. *Id.* § 71551(a).
15. *Id.* § 72543(a).
16. *Id.* § 73543(a).
17. *Id.* § 74731(b).
18. *Id.* § 75055(a).
19. *Id.* § 75343(a).
20. *Id.* § 77143(a).
21. *Id.* § 79351(a).
22. 6 Colorado Code Regs. § 1011, ¶ 4.2 (1977).
23. Connecticut Agencies Regulations § 19-13-D4b (6) (1972).

DELAWARE

Delaware does not provide any specific rules for permissible media for medical records. (*See* Chapter 17 for media for general business records, which should cover medical records as well.)

DISTRICT OF COLUMBIA

The District of Columbia's regulations provides that medical records can be kept in the form of the original record or in the form of a microfilm or photostatic copy.[24]

FLORIDA

Florida permits microfilming of records, provided that records are microfilmed in accordance with Florida's Administrative Code.[25]

GEORGIA

Georgia permits medical records to be preserved as originals, microfilms, or other usable forms.[26]

HAWAII

Hawaii's evidence code permits medical records to be computerized or minified by the use of microfilm or other similar photographic process, provided that the method used creates an unalterable record.[27]

IDAHO

Hospitals may preserve records relating to the care and treatment of a patient in microfilm or other photographically reproduced form.[28] The statute considers such copies as originals for evidentiary purposes.[29]

ILLINOIS

Illinois does not specify authorized media for medical records, but copies made under the business records statutes, including microfilm, should be permissible (*see* Chapter 17).

---

24. District of Columbia Municipal Regulations tit. 22, § 2216.3 (1986).
25. Florida Administrative Code Annotated r. 1B-26.0021 (1986); General Records Schedule E-1 (1988).
26. Georgia Compilation Rules and Regulations r. 290-5-6-.11(h) (1991).
27. Hawaii Revised Statutes § 622-58(a) (1990).
28. Idaho Code § 39-1394(a) (1991).
29. *Id.*

INDIANA

Indiana's Hospital Licensure Rules permit the use of microfilm or computerized records that maintain confidentiality.[30]

IOWA

Iowa Code does not specify any authorized media for medical records, but its business records laws would seem to permit microfilm and similar media (*see* Chapter 17).

KANSAS

Medical records may be microfilmed after completion.[31]

KENTUCKY

Medical records may be microfilmed or otherwise photographically reproduced in Kentucky.[32]

LOUISIANA

Hospitals may, in their discretion, microfilm, or similarly reproduce any hospital record or part thereof in order to efficiently store and preserve it.[33]

MAINE

Records may be preserved either in the original or by microfilm.[34] Maine Revised Statutes Annotated tit. 16, § 456 (West 1989) authorizes hospitals to make photographic or microphotographic copies.

MARYLAND

Maryland does not specify any different requirements for acceptable media for medical records than for business records (*see* Chapter 17).

MASSACHUSETTS

Massachusetts provides for photographic or microphotographic copies of medical records.[35]

---

30. Indiana Administrative Code tit. 410, r. 15-1-8(2) (1986), r. 15-1-9(1) (1988), and r. 15-1-9(2)(b)(1) (1988).
31. Kansas Administrative Regulations 28-34-9a(d)(5) (1990).
32. Kentucky Revised Statutes Annotated § 422.105 (1990).
33. Louisiana Revised Statutes Annotated § 2144 (1990).
34. Code of Maine Rules, Regulations Governing the Licensure of General and Specialty Hospitals in the State of Maine, ch. XII B (1972).
35. 111 Massachusetts General Laws ch. 233, § 70 (1991).

MICHIGAN

Hospitals may preserve medical records as originals, abstracts, microfilms, or otherwise.[36]

MINNESOTA

Minnesota Statute 145.30 (1990) permits the transfer and recording of any or all of the original files and records of the hospital dealing with the case history, physical examination, and daily hospital records of individual patients, including any miscellaneous documents, on photographic film of convenient size.

MISSISSIPPI

Mississippi Code Annotated § 41-9-77 (1990) permits reproduction of any hospital record or part thereof on film or other material by microfilming, photographing, photostating, or other appropriate process. Such are deemed originals for all purposes, including admission into evidence. A facsimile, exemplification, or copy of such reproduction or copy shall be deemed to be a transcript, exemplification, or copy of the original hospital record or part thereof.

MISSOURI

Missouri Code Regulations tit. 19, § 30-20.021(3)(D)15 (1990) permits hospitals to maintain medical records in the original or on microfilm. *Id.* tit. 13 § 14-15 does not specify media for long-term care facilities, but microfilm would appear to be permissible.

MONTANA

Montana Administrative Rules 16.32.308(3) (1990) permits microfilming if the healthcare facility has the equipment to reproduce records on the premises.

NEBRASKA

Nebraska law provides that provider may preserve medical records in original, microfilm, or other approved copy.[37]

NEVADA

Nevada healthcare providers may retain healthcare records on microfilm or any other recognized form of size reduction that does not adversely affect their use for inspections by the patients or the State Board of Medical Examiners.[38]

---

36. Department of Public Health Rule, Michigan Administrative Code r. 325.1028(5) (1987).
37. Nebraska Revised Statutes § 27-1003 (1989).
38. Nevada Revised Statutes § 629.051 (Michie 1991).

Nevada Administrative Code ch. 449, § 379(2) (1986) requires records to be permanent, that is, printed, typewritten, or legibly written. Medical histories may be microfilmed after three years if stored on rolls. Emergency room and outpatient records may be microfilmed after one year. If unitized jackets or cards are used, microfilming may be done at time of discharge.

NEW HAMPSHIRE

New Hampshire Code of Administrative Regulations [Department of Health and Human Services Regulation He-P] 802.11(b) (1986) requires storage of all original hospital records or "photographs" of such records, presumably authorizing microfilm or other similar means of reproduction.

NEW JERSEY

Medical records shall be preserved, either in the original or by microfilm.[39]

NEW MEXICO

Medical records may be microfilmed or otherwise photographically reproduced under New Mexico Statutes Annotated § 14-6-2.A (Michie 1991). Such reproductions are deemed originals for evidentiary purposes under the New Mexico rules of evidence.

NEW YORK

Medical records are to be maintained in their original or "legally reproduced form."[40]

NORTH CAROLINA

Medical records or "photographs" of such records shall be preserved.[41] For nursing homes, the regulations speak in terms of originals or "copies."[42]

NORTH DAKOTA

North Dakota specifies that hospital records may be preserved either in original or any other method of preservation such as microfilm.[43]

OHIO

Ohio does not specify any particular media for medical records. (*See* Chapter 17 on business record media in Ohio.)

---

39. New Jersey Administrative Code tit. 8, § 43B-7.1(b)3 (1985).
40. New York Compilation of Codes, Rules and Regulations tit. 405, § 10(3) (1988).
41. North Carolina Administrative Code tit. 10, r. 03C.1405 (Feb. 1976).
42. *Id*. tit. 10, r. 03H.0607.
43. North Dakota Administrative Code § 33-07-01-16.3 (1980).

OKLAHOMA

According to the Oklahoma Department of Health, healthcare facilities generating medical records may microfilm the medical records and destroy the original record in order to conserve space. The Department notes that federal and Oklahoma laws specify that records reconstituted from microfilm are to be considered the same as the original and that retention of the microfilmed record constitutes compliance with preservation laws. The minimum contents of a medical record to be microfilmed will be

- Identification data (name, address, age, sex, marital status)
- Date of admission
- Date of discharge
- Personal and family history
- Chief complaint
- History of present illness
- Physical examination
- Special examination, if any, such as consultation, clinical laboratory, or x ray
- Provisional or admitting diagnosis
- Medical treatment (signed or initialed by person giving the medication or treatment)
- Progress and nurses' notes
- Temperature chart, including pulse and respiration, medications
- Final diagnosis
- Summary and condition on discharge
- In case of death, autopsy findings, if performed[44]

OREGON

Oregon permits photographic, microphotographic, or photographic reproduction of records. Oregon Revised Statutes § 40.560 (1989), Oregon Rule of Evidence 1003, provides that a duplicate is admissible in evidence to the same extent as an original unless a genuine question is raised as to the authenticity of the original or, in the circumstances, it would be unfair to admit the original. *Id.* § 41.930 adds that copies of hospital records are admissible to the same extent as the original would be.

---

44. Oklahoma Department of Health Regulation ch. 13, ¶ 13.13B.

The medical record shall be legible and reproducible.[45] Records required to be kept permanently may be in written or computerized form.[46] Original medical records may be retained on paper, microfilm, or electronic or other media.[47]

Medical records for long-term care facilities shall be typewritten or written legibly in ink, and may be stored in original or microfilm.[48]

PENNSYLVANIA

Hospitals may store medical records as originals, as reproductions, or as microfilm (28 Pennsylvania Code § 115.23 (1989)). *Id.* § 115.24 states that medical records may be microfilmed immediately after completion. If done off the premises, the hospital shall take precautions to ensure the confidentiality and safekeeping of the records. The original of microfilmed medical records shall not be destroyed until the medical record department has had an opportunity to review the processed film for content. Further, *id.* § 115.26 authorizes the use of automation in the medical record service, provided that all statutory requirements are met and the information is readily available for use in patient care. This regulation expressly encourages innovations in medical record formats, compilation, and data retrieval. *Id.* § 563.7 contains similar language permitting ambulatory surgical centers to microfilm medical records, and *id.* § 563.8 also encourages automation of medical records.

RHODE ISLAND

This state permits preservation of medical records either as originals or "accurate reproductions."[49]

SOUTH CAROLINA

South Carolina Code Regulations 61-16, § 601.7 (1982), covering minimum standards for hospitals and institutional general infirmaries, states that facilities that microfilm before 10 years have expired must film the entire record.

SOUTH DAKOTA

South Dakota has no specific requirements for medical record media. (*See* the business records media requirements in Chapter 17, which would seem to authorize microfilming or similarly preserving medical records.)

---

45. Oregon Administrative Rules 333-505-050(3) (1991).
46. *Id.* 333-505-050(8).
47. *Id.* 333-505-050(13).
48. *Id.* §§ 333-86-055(5) and 333-86-055(10).
49. 1990 Rhode Island Acts and Resolves R23-17-HOSP-25.9.

TENNESSEE

Tennessee permits transfer upon photographic film of convenient size, such as microfilm, photograph, or photostat, for the purposes of medical research and professional education, or administrative convenience, of any or all original files and records of any such hospital including case history, physical examination, and daily hospital records of the individual patients thereof, including any miscellaneous documents, papers, and correspondence.[50]

Tennessee Compilation Rules and Regulations tit. 1200, ch. 8-6-.07(9) (1990) permits storage of records either as originals or on microfilm.

TEXAS

All medical records, and any other records considered by the hospital as necessary to preserve, may be microfilmed for retention.[51]

UTAH

Utah's Health Facility Licensure Rules contain no specific requirements for media for medical records, except in Utah Administrative Rule 432-550-7.100, which specifies that birthing centers may replace original medical records with microfilmed copies. However, the general business records statutes (*see* Chapter 17) would appear to authorize reproduction of medical records.

VERMONT

Vermont does not specify media for medical records, but its business records statutes (*see* Chapter 17) would appear to permit reproduction of medical records.

VIRGINIA

Virginia permits records to be preserved as either originals or accurate reproductions, presumably allowing any medium that results in an accurate copy.[52] Virginia Code Annotated § 8.01-391(C) (Michie 1991) makes microphotographic copies of hospital records admissible in evidence.

WASHINGTON

Originals or "durable, legible, direct copies" of originals of reports may be filed in patients' individual medical records.[53] Computer entries may be stored on magnetic tapes, disks, or other devices suited to the storage of data.

---

50. Tennessee Code Annotated § 53-1324 (1976).
51. Texas Department of Health and Hospital Licensing Standards tit. 1, § 22.1.4 (1991).
52. Virginia Regulations Regulating Hospital and Nursing Home Licensure and Inspection, part II, § 208.7 (1982).
53. Washington Administrative Code § 248-18-440 (1986).

WEST VIRGINIA

West Virginia's healthcare regulations provide for preservation in the original form or by microfilm or electronic data process.[54] Hospitals using automatic data processing may keep indexes on punch cards or reproduced on sheets bound in books.[55]

WISCONSIN

Medical records may be retained either as originals or in the form of microfiche.[56] In its rule interpretations for that rule, the Department of Health and Social Services, Division of Health, opined that the term "legally reproduced copy" means a duplicate copy of the original document and includes photocopies and FAX reproductions.[57]

WYOMING

Wyoming has no specific requirements for medical record media. (*See* Chapter 17 for business record media, which should apply to healthcare records as well.)

---

54. State Department of Health, Creation & Contents: West Virginia Regulations and Law for Licensing Hospitals, part IV, § 603.1(e) (1969).
55. West Virginia Legislature, tit. 64, West Virginia Legislative Rules Department of Health: Hospital Licensure, series 12, § 10.3.1.n (1987).
56. Wisconsin Administrative Code § HSS 124.14(2)(e)(1), 124.14(2)(e)(3) (Feb. 1, 1988).
57. *Id.* § HSS 124.14(2)(c) (Feb. 1, 1988).

CHAPTER 5

How to Store Medical Records

Storage Generally

Two major concerns should determine how you store your records: utility and security.

Storing records in such a manner that no one can use them is not very efficient. Many state laws and regulations provide, for example, that healthcare facilities must maintain their medical records in a manner providing easy retrievability. (*See* Connecticut's State Department of Health Regulation, Connecticut Agencies Regulations § 19-13-D3(d)(1) (1987).) Similarly, Maryland Regulations Code tit. 10, § 10.07.02.20G (1991) states that hospitals shall maintain adequate space and equipment, conveniently located, to provide for efficient processing of medical records (reviewing, indexing, filing, and prompt retrieval). Also, *see* Appendix A for Health Care Financing Administration guidelines.

You must also consider the security of your medical records. Obviously, the loss of information contained in vital medical records could have catastrophic consequences. You must protect against loss, damage, destruction, or unauthorized access or release. To do this effectively, you must consider personnel security, physical security, and system security. California and Colorado have very detailed storage specifications that you may want to examine to help you plan for security of your records.

PERSONNEL SECURITY

Probably the most effective way to ensure the security of your records is to make certain the people who work with your records safeguard them. First, a careful screening of employees who have access to critical or confidential records is a must. Once you are certain that you have responsible employees handling your records, you should promote security consciousness on the part of your staff by orienting new employees and refreshing old ones about the principles of record security and confidentiality. You should stress their responsibility for records in their possession and their duty not to disclose confidential information (*see* Part IV). Your staff should sign an agreement verifying that they understand your policies and procedures concerning records retention, security, and disclosure; that they will adhere to your policies and procedures; and that they understand that they face disciplinary action if they fail to. A sample "Medical Records Oath of Confidentiality" used in California is provided in Figure 5.1. You should provide for periodic refreshers in record security to emphasize staff accountability for information security.

You should also require your staff to have to show identification, preferably photo identification badges, to gain access to your records. Computer security, with appropriate access and passwords, is also crucial. Of course, you must have a system to recover keys and badges and delete computer access codes when your personnel no longer work for you. Your staff is more likely to remember the rules on access to and disclosure of records if you clearly mark records with warnings about any special requirements.

PHYSICAL SECURITY

Physical security is probably easier to accomplish than personnel security is. Obviously, you will need to store your medical records in fireproof or fire-resistant storage facilities with a sprinkler system. In fact, many state regulations require that you store medical records in fireproof or fire-resistant facilities.

Figure 5.1
Medical Records Oath of Confidentiality

I, _____ do hereby swear and affirm that I will not discuss, reveal, copy or in any manner disclose the contents of the medical record of any patient who has received or is receiving health care services from _____ _____ unless an appropriate and properly executed "Authorization for Release of Medical Information" form is received and it is determined that the records are to be released to a person with a legitimate interest.

I understand that medical records are confidential; that the information in a medical record is protected by both Federal and California state laws and regulations and that reading, discussing or otherwise utilizing the information within the record for other than legitimate health care purposes is grounds for immediate dismissal and possible legal action.

Sworn before me this _____ day of _____ 19___ at _____, California.

_____
Signature of Employee

_____
Signature of Administrator of Oath

You should also consider whether you need to maintain a certain temperature and humidity to prevent the records from deteriorating. Generally, a temperature of about 70 degrees and humidity between 50 and 60 percent will be safe for most records. Finally, you need to consider how to limit access. Confidential and critical records should be stored in a secure area that is kept locked unless a records custodian is actually present. California has very specific requirements for off-site storage, discussed below, that you may wish to review to help you consider how to keep your records secure.

SYSTEM SECURITY

System security is related to both personnel and physical security. Having a security-conscious staff and good physical security will not prevent loss, damage, destruction, or unauthorized disclosure of records if you do not have a good system to control access to and disclosure of your records. You need to implement a requisition and charge-out system for critical records, especially medical records. Users should requisition records. Requisitions help record custodians ensure that the requester is authorized access to the record and that the request is a proper one. Your requisition procedure should require countersignatures by supervisors of individuals such as student nurses, who would not normally have access.

Once record custodians have proper requisitions, they should require requesters to sign out the records, either on the requisition documents or on separate forms. Custodians must maintain the sign-out forms, which should contain the name of the requester, an identification of the record, the date, and the location of the file. Your policy should require requesters who have signed out records to notify their custodians of any changes in the records' location, as by use of a records transfer form.

You should also consider the security aspects of transferring records and reproducing them. Loose reproduction procedures, for example, may lead to unauthorized disclosure of confidential information.

Your procedures should also cover how your staff ensures that the release of records to other parties, such as patients, is proper. Comparing signatures on patient requests with the signature on admission documents, for example, ensures that the patients themselves are making the request, not someone else. Your staff must check the credentials or authorization of others who request records or information and specify any restrictions, such as nondisclosure to any other party, on the use of the record. You can require a third party who receives a record to sign a nondisclosure agreement.

Finally, proper destruction of records (*see* Chapter 13) is the final step in ensuring confidentiality.

Federal Laws

There are no specific federal requirements.

State Laws

ALABAMA

Alabama's hospital regulations require you to make provision for the safe storage of records. "This shall mean that records are handled in such manner as to assure safety from water or fire damage and are safeguarded from unauthorized use" (Alabama Administrative Code r. 420-5-7.07(b) (1990)).

For nursing homes, *id.* r. 420-5-10-.16 requires the facility to maintain adequate facilities and equipment, conveniently located, to provide efficient processing of medical records (reviewing, indexing, filing, and prompt retrieval), and to provide for safe storage, ensure safety from water or fire damage, and safeguard from unauthorized use.

ALASKA

Alaska Health and Social Services Regulations provide that a facility must maintain procedures to protect the information in medical records from loss, defacement, tampering, or access by unauthorized persons.[1]

ARIZONA

Arizona regulations note that a hospital may store records it does not currently need in a responsible warehouse in which the confidentiality and safety of the records are protected.[2]

ARKANSAS

According to Arkansas' rules governing medical records, Arkansas Register 0601 T, all patients' records shall be kept in two-hour fire rated enclosures and protected against undue damage from dust, vermin, water, and similar destructive agents. The facility should install a smoke detector in areas where records are filed or permanently stored. 0601 W adds that all medical records shall be secured at all times. If authorized personnel are not present, the department shall be locked.

CALIFORNIA

California requires hospitals to store records in an easily accessible manner in the hospital or an approved medical record storage facility off the hospital premises.[3] The hospital must safeguard records against loss, defacement, tampering, or use by unauthorized persons.[4]

---

1. Alaska Administrative Code tit. 7, §§ 12.425(c), 12.770(d) (1984).
2. Arizona Compilation Administrative Rules and Regulations § 9-10-221 (1982).
3. California Code Regulations tit. § 70751(f) (1988).
4. *Id.* § 70751(b).

California has guidelines for off-site storage of medical records:

- Physical plant

  - Concrete block structure with loading dock and adequate parking for vehicle maneuvering

  - The record storage center should be the sole occupant

  - Open-faced shelving with vertically adjusted shelves is recommended. Maximum height—147 inches with seismic bracing to meet uniform building codes. Bracing should be adequate to meet a static load of 3,325 pounds and to withstand an impact load of 40 pounds from a height of 18 inches.

- Protection from fire, flood, or intrusion:

  - Sprinkler system with at least 18 inches between the sprinkler head and the top of the files

  - Fire/smoke alarm systems

  - Four-hour fire walls with all openings protected by Class "A" fire doors

  - Disaster plan for flood or water damage from sprinklered rooms

  - Protection from material carried in overhead pipes

- Ambient environment

  - Temperature maintained between 65 and 75 degrees Fahrenheit

  - Relative humidity between 50 and 55%

  - Ventilation system of fresh forced air

- Fluorescent lights should be filtered to remove ultraviolet radiation. Protect records against exposure to direct sunlight.

- Minimum standards for illumination are three feet above the storage area, at least 25 footcandles of illumination. For office space, at least 50 footcandles

- Policies and procedures

  - Retrieval

    - Records are accessible 24 hours a day, seven days a week

    - Turnaround time for stat patient use: 0–1 year—20 minutes; 1–5 years—40 minutes; 5–7 years—60 minutes; 7 plus years—2 hours

    - Turnaround time for administrative/subpoena use: 0–7 years—24 hours; 7 plus years—3 days

- Confidentiality
  - In-service training of personnel
  - Document individual employee orientation to facility policies and procedures
- Retention
  - Describe the age of files in storage
  - Identify destruction dates
  - Identify records destroyed to include name of patient, date of last treatment, date of birth, date of destruction
  - Destroy by shredding, burning, or in a commercial landfill. If personnel other than facility employees with training in confidentiality destroy the records, have a supervisor with such training observe. Obtain a certificate of destruction from a commercial firm.
- Access and transport
  - Specify in policy the functional titles of persons authorized to request records
  - Specify in policy the functional titles of persons authorized access to the storage facility
  - Describe procedures for retrieval and transport, such as in sealed envelopes that are hand delivered to authorized users.
- Inventory control and indexing
  - Policies describe use of a master patient index.
  - File organization specified
  - Method to audit records in storage to determine current location and user with procedures to locate misfiles
- Physical environment
  - Service aisle must allow for passage of loading carts or vehicles. Files must terminate at least 18 inches from a wall, with no dead-end isles.
  - Adequate work space for employees in the storage area

In addition to general acute care hospitals, Title 22 regulations specify that the following various other types of facilities must store records in an easily accessible manner in the facility or in off-site health record storage, and protect the records against loss, defacement, tampering, or use by unauthorized persons. In most cases, the facility must obtain prior health department approval to store health records off-site.

- Acute psychiatric hospitals[5]

- Skilled nursing facilities[6]

- Intermediate care facilities[7]

- Home health agencies[8]

- Primary care clinics[9]

- Psychology clinics[10]

- Psychiatric health facilities[11]

- Adult day health facilities[12]

- Chemical dependency recovery hospitals[13]

COLORADO

Colorado has one of the more detailed requirements for medical record rooms. Generally, each hospital shall have an adequate medical record room or other suitable facility with adequate supplies and equipment and should store records to provide protection from loss, damage, and unauthorized use (6 Colorado Code Regulations § 1011-1 ¶ 4.1 (1977)).

Under *id.* § 4.1.1, new hospitals, or those modifying an existing hospital facility, shall have a medical record department and other medical record facilities with supplies and equipment for medical record functions and services including

- Active record storage area

- Record review and dictating room for physicians

- Work area for sorting, recording, typing, filing, and other assigned medical record functions shall be separate from the record review and dictating room. Consideration should be given to isolation of noisy equipment. Accommodations should be provided for conducting medical record business with hospital paramedical personnel or public individuals for legitimate access to medical records.

- Medical record storage area within the department

5. *Id.* § 71551(f).
6. *Id.* §§ 72543(h), (i).
7. *Id.* § 73543(g).
8. *Id.* § 74731(h).
9. *Id.* §§ 75055(g), (h).
10. *Id.* §§ 75343(g), (h).
11. *Id.* § 77143(f).
12. *Id.* § 78435(c).
13. *Id.* §§ 79351(b), (f).

- Inactive medical record storage area (may be omitted if microfilming is used).

The medical record department shall be located in an area of the hospital that is convenient to most of the professional staff (*id.*). Security measures shall be maintained by mechanical means in the absence of medical record supervision, to preserve confidentiality and to provide protection from loss, damage, and unauthorized use of the medical records (*id.* § 4.1.2).

Note that Colorado Revised Statute § 18-4-412 (1990) makes anyone who, without proper authorization, obtains, steals or discloses, or copies a medical record guilty of a felony.

CONNECTICUT

The State Department of Health Regulations merely say to store medical records in a manner providing easy retrievability. Medical record departments must have adequate space and equipment.[14]

Nursing homes must keep all parts of the patient medical record pertinent to the daily care and treatment of the patient on the nursing unit in which the patient is located. The record must be safeguarded against loss, destruction or unauthorized use.[15]

DELAWARE

No specific storage requirements.

DISTRICT OF COLUMBIA

District of Columbia Municipal Regulations tit. 22, § 2216.3 (1986) requires that medical records "be filed in a safe place."

FLORIDA

Florida Administrative Code § 10D-28.081(24) (1986) requires hospitals to provide rooms, areas, and offices for the medical records administrator for sorting, recording, microfilming, and storing records.

Id. § 10D-28.110(10)(f)(3) provides that the facility is responsible for safeguarding the information in clinical records against loss, defacement, tampering, or use by unauthorized persons. Records may be removed from the facility's jurisdiction and safekeeping only according to the facility policy or as required by law.

---

14. Connecticut Agencies Regulations §§ 19-13-D3(d)(1) and (6) (1987).
15. *Id.* §§ 19-13-D8t(o)(1) and (4).

GEORGIA

Georgia Compilation Rules and Regulations r. 290-5-6-.11 (1991) provides that patient statistics and hospital operational records shall be kept current and in such a way as to yield required information easily. *Id.* r. 290-5-6-.12 requires hospitals to provide administrative space and facilities for medical records among other services.

HAWAII

Hawaii Revised Statutes § 622-58 (1990) pertaining to retention of medical records does not specify how the facility should store the records other than authorized media.

IDAHO

Skilled nursing and intermediate care facilities shall preserve records in a safe location protected from fire, theft, and water damage.[16]

ILLINOIS

Hospitals shall maintain suitable record facilities with adequate supplies and equipment and provide for safe storage of medical records. Safe storage means to ensure safety from water seepage or fire damage and to safeguard the records from unauthorized use.[17]

INDIANA

In Indiana, medical records shall be filed in a safe and accessible manner in the hospital, and they shall be made available for inspection by a duly authorized representative of the Indiana Health Licensing Council or the Board of Health.[18] Hospital records shall be kept on the nursing unit during the patient's hospitalization.[19]

Inactive records shall be stored in a fire-resistive structure, preferably fire-resistive cabinets or shelves, in such a way as to maintain confidentiality.[20]

IOWA

Iowa Administrative Code r. 481-51.7(26) (1990) requires the following rooms or spaces for the medical records unit: medical record librarian's office or space, review and dictating room(s) or spaces, a work area for sorting, recording, or microfilming records, and a storage area for records.

---

16. *Skilled Nursing and Intermediate Care Facilities* 02.2203,04.b (1989).
17. Illinois Administrative Code § 250.1510(a) (1988).
18. Indiana Administrative Code tit. 410, r. 15-1-9 (1988).
19. *Id.* r. 15-1-9(2)(a) and (c).
20. *Id.* r. 15-1-9.

KANSAS

The medical record department shall be properly equipped to enable its personnel to function in an effective manner and to maintain medical records in such a manner that the records are readily accessible and secure from unauthorized use (Kansas Administrative Regulations § 28-34-9a(c)).

Id. § 28-34-57 requires ambulatory surgical centers to provide adequate space, facilities, and equipment for completion and storage of medical records, as does *id.* § 28-34-83 for hospital recuperation centers.

Id. § 30-22-33 requires community mental health centers to keep clinical records in locked cabinets or other secured locations.

KENTUCKY

The hospital is responsible to safeguard the record and its information against loss, defacement, and tampering. Particular attention is to be given to protection from damage by fire or water.[21]

LOUISIANA

40 Louisiana Revised Statutes Annotated § 2144 (1990), governing media, specifies that a hospital may microfilm or similarly reproduce any hospital record to accomplish efficient storage and preservation.

MAINE

Maine has no specific storage requirements.

MARYLAND

Maryland Regulations Code tit. 10, § 07.02.20G (1991) states that hospitals shall maintain adequate space and equipment, conveniently located, to provide for efficient processing of medical records (reviewing, indexing, filing, and prompt retrieval). *Id.* § 07.02.20H states that closed or inactive records shall be filed in a safe place (free from fire hazards) that provides for confidentiality and, when necessary, retrieval.

Under *id.* § 10.07.11.05E and F, health maintenance organizations (HMOs) shall maintain a system that provides for adequate space and equipment for filing and prompt retrieval of medical records and have established policies assuring that medical records are retained in safekeeping according to acceptable professional practices and state statutes.

Home health agencies shall properly safeguard clinical record information against loss, destruction, or illegal or unauthorized use.

---

21. 902 Kentucky Administrative Regulations 20:016 § 3(11)(a)3 (1991).

MASSACHUSETTS

Hospitals must have a medical record department that keeps records inviolate and preserved permanently with a system of identification and filing to ensure the rapid location of a patient's record (Massachusetts Regulations Code tit. 10, § 134.490 (1990)). Under *id.* § 150.013, all long-term care facilities shall provide conveniently located and suitably equipped areas for the recording and storage of records.

MICHIGAN

Michigan's rules only provide that hospitals may preserve medical records as originals, abstracts, microfilms, or otherwise so as to afford a basis for a complete audit of professional information without specifying the means of storing them.[22]

MINNESOTA

Minnesota's Hospital Licensing and Operation regulations, Minnesota Rules 4640.1000(2) (1991), require hospitals to provide space and equipment for the recording and completion of the record by the physician as well as for the indexing, filing, and safe storage of medical records.

Id. R. 4605.7707, pertaining to venereal disease control, requires locked files for medical records.

Nursing and boarding homes shall have a central control point for the storage of records and medications. The records are to be filed at the nurses' or attendants' station (*id.* R. 4655.3500).

MISSISSIPPI

Mississippi Code Annotated § 41-9-63 (1990) simply states that all hospitals must prepare and maintain hospital records in accordance with the minimum standards adopted by the licensing agency. *Id.* § 41-9-69 adds that hospitals will properly store their records.

MISSOURI

Hospitals must store records in such a manner as to safeguard them from loss, defacement, and tampering, and to prevent damage from fire and water. Medical records must be kept in the permanent file in the original or on microfilm[23] and maintained so as to facilitate rapid retrieval and utilization by authorized personnel.[24] Intermediate care and skilled nursing facilities shall keep medical and nursing records for current residents in each nursing unit.[25]

---

22. Michigan Administrative Code r. 325.1028 (1987).
23. Missouri Code Regulations tit. 13, § 50-20(3)(D)16 (1982).
24. *Id.* § 50-20(3)(D) 5.
25. *Id.* 15-14.042.

MONTANA

Montana Administrative Rules 16.32.308(1) (1990) requires healthcare facilities to maintain medical records by storing them in a safe manner and in a safe location. Chapter 23-4.1B of the *Montana Hospital Association Manual* amplifies this guidance by suggesting that storage be in a responsible warehouse that protects the security and safety of the records.

NEBRASKA

Home health agencies must keep records secured in locked storage.[26]
 Records of health clinic patients must be kept in locked files.[27]

NEVADA

Nevada Administrative Code ch. 449, § 403(3) (1986) requires extended care facilities and nursing homes to provide suitable storage space for safe, confidential retention of records. The facility must also provide a system of identification and filing for rapid location of records, with a designated employee responsible for maintaining completed records (*id.*).

NEW HAMPSHIRE

As to hospitals, this state only specifies that "provision shall be made for storage of all records required by these regulations" (New Hampshire Code of Administrative Regulations [Department of Health and Human Services Regulation He-P] 802.11(b) (1986)). Its rules for other facilities are a little more specific. Sheltered care facilities must store resident records in a fire-proof cabinet (*id.* 804.04(b)). In addition to the fire-proof cabinet, *id.* 805.05 requires sheltered care facilities with nursing units to protect records against loss, destruction, or unauthorized use, as does *id.* 806.10 for outpatient clinics and *id.* 803.06 for nursing homes. *Id.* 807.07(c) requires residential treatment and rehabilitation facilities to have written policies and procedures to safeguard clinical records against loss or unauthorized use. Finally, *id.* 809.07 requires home healthcare providers to safeguard records against loss or unauthorized use.

NEW JERSEY

Hospitals' medical record departments must be conveniently located and adequate in size and equipment to enable physicians to properly complete medical records. The filing equipment and storage space must be adequate to accommodate all records and to facilitate retrieval. The facility shall keep

---

26. Nebraska Administrative Rules and Regulations 175-14-006.01H (1988).
27. *Id.* 175-7-004.04.

records confidential and inaccessible to unauthorized persons.[28] Cardiac diagnostic or surgical medical records shall be safeguarded against loss, destruction, or unauthorized use.[29]

NEW MEXICO

New Mexico has no specific requirements for medical record storage.

NEW YORK

The New York Department of Health only requires, in New York Compilation Rules and Regulations tit. 405 § 10(a)(1) (1988), that records be properly filed and retained, and accessible and ensure the confidentiality of medical records.

NORTH CAROLINA

North Carolina Administrative Code tit. 10, r. 03C.1403(e) (Feb. 1976) places the responsibility on the hospital to safeguard the information in medical records against loss, tampering, or use by an unauthorized person. The medical record department shall be conveniently located, adequate in size and equipment, and the hospital must provide for safe storage of all medical records. If records are stored in a separate building, it shall be of fire-resistive construction (*id.* r. 03C.1401).

For nursing homes, *id.* tit. 10, 03H.0606 requires locating medical record work space to ensure that records are protected from unauthorized disclosure. The facility must store records in a protected or supervised environment.

NORTH DAKOTA

North Dakota does not specify any particular storage requirements.

OHIO

Ohio Administrative Code § 5123:2-3-16 (1991) specifies that residential care facilities shall maintain records in such a manner as to ensure their confidentiality and protect them from unauthorized disclosure.

Health maintenance organizations (HMOs) must have a medical records system that

- Assigns a unique identifier to each medical record

- Identifies the location of every medical record

- Places medical records in a given order and location

---

28. New Jersey Administrative Code tit. 8 § 43B-7.1 (1985).
29. *Id.* tit. 8, § 43B-17.10(c).

- Produces a specific medical record on demand
- Maintains the confidentiality of medical record information, and releases such information only in accordance with established policy
- Maintains inactive medical records in a specific place
- Permits effective professional review and medical audit processes
- Facilitates an adequate system for follow-up treatment including monitoring and follow-up of off-site referrals and inpatient stays
- Meets state and federal reporting requirements applicable to HMOs (*id.* § 5101:3-26-07)

Resident records of alcoholism inpatient/emergency care facilities shall store resident records of discharged patients in a safe place (*id.* § 3701-55-15).

OKLAHOMA

The only language pertaining to storage of medical records is the language in the Department of Health requirements that health facilities generating medical records may microfilm them and destroy the originals to conserve space.

OREGON

Oregon Administrative Rules 333-70-055(11) (1991) states that medical records shall be protected against unauthorized access, fire, water, and theft.

Nursing homes for the mentally retarded must make provisions for safe storage of all originals or photographic copies of records (*id.* R. 333-92-095(4)).

PENNSYLVANIA

General and special hospitals and ambulatory surgical centers must store medical records in such a manner as to provide protection from loss, damage, and unauthorized access.[30] Long-term care facilities must provide a locked space for medical records.[31]

RHODE ISLAND

Rhode Island's Rules and Regulations for the Licensing of Hospitals, 1990 Rhode Island Acts and Resolves R23-17-HOSP-25.8, require hospitals to make provisions for the safe storage of medical records in accordance with the standards in "Protection of Records" of the National Fire Protection Association.

---

30. 28 Pennsylvania Code §§ 115.22 and 563.5 (1989).
31. *Id.* § 205.29.

SOUTH CAROLINA

South Carolina Code Regulations 61-16, § 601.7(a) (1982), governing hospitals and institutional general infirmaries, requires that the institution make provision for storing medical records in an environment that will prevent unauthorized access and deterioration. Intermediate care facilities must keep records in a safe storage area (*id.* Regulations 61-14, § 504.1 (1980)), as must nursing care facilities, (*id.* Regulations 61-17, § 704.1 (1982)).

SOUTH DAKOTA

The medical record units of hospitals and nursing homes must include an active record storage area; record review and dictating area; work area for sorting, recording, or microfilming; and an inactive record storage area, which may be omitted if microfilming is used.[32] Supervised personal care facilities must have written policies to safeguard the residents' records against destruction, loss, and unauthorized use.

TENNESSEE

Tennessee has no specific requirements for medical record storage.

TEXAS

Texas Department of Health and Hospital Licensing Standards ch. 7, § 21 (1991) states that the medical record unit shall have: medical record administrator/technician officer or space; review and dictating room(s) or spaces; work area for sorting, recording, or microfilming records; and a storage area for records. Its standard for special care facilities requires that such facilities store records in a lockable area during nonuse and after the resident's discharge (*id.* § 22.1.4).

UTAH

Utah requires that facilities have sufficient space and equipment to enable medical record personnel to function effectively and make provision for the filing, safe storage, and easy accessibility of medical records. The records and their contents must be safeguarded against loss, defacement, tampering, fires, and floods as well as against access by unauthorized individuals.[33] Similar requirements exist for mental retardation facilities,[34] small healthcare facilities,[35] freestanding ambulatory surgical centers,[36] abortion clinics,[37] and end-stage

---

32. South Dakota Administrative Rules 44:04:14:14 (1991).
33. Health Facility Licensure Rules, Utah Administrative Rules 432-100-7.402.
34. *Id.* R. 432-152-4.203.
35. *Id.* R. 432-200-6.102.
36. *Id.* R. 432-500-6.104.
37. *Id.* R. 432-600-6.104.

renal disease centers,[38] Home health agencies[39] must develop and implement record-keeping procedures that address storage and maintain an identification system to facilitate locating records.

VERMONT

The only reference to record storage standards for Vermont hospitals requires that storage facilities for x-ray films shall be in accordance with the requirements of the National Board of Fire Underwriters and the state fire marshal.[40]

Vermont's Residential Care Home Licensing Regulations for Level III and Level IV Facilities require such facilities to store records in an orderly manner so that they are readily available for reference.[41] The regulations for nursing homes have a similar provision, adding that separate file folders shall be provided for each resident, employee, and administrative report.[42]

VIRGINIA

Hospitals shall provide for safe storage of medical records or accurate and legible reproductions in accordance with "Protection of Records" of the National Fire Protection Association.[43]

WASHINGTON

Hospitals must store medical records and other personal and medical data on patients so they are not accessible to unauthorized persons, are protected from undue deterioration or destruction, and are easily retrievable.[44]

WEST VIRGINIA

The only language regarding storage of medical records is that all medical records of services to outpatients and patients treated in the emergency room shall be maintained in the files of the medical record department.[45]

---

38. *Id.* R. 432-650-3.206.
39. *Id.* R. 432-700-3.
40. Vermont Administrative Procedure Bulletin art. 2, § 3-964(c)(6).
41. Vermont Agency of Human Services, Levels III and IV Residential Care Home Licensing Regulations § VI-9(c) (1987).
42. Vermont Department of Rehabilitation and Aging, State of Vermont Nursing Home Regulations § 3-29 (1986).
43. Virginia Regulations for the Regulation of Hospital and Nursing Home Licensure and Inspection, part II, § 208.7 (1982).
44. Washington Administrative Code § 248-18-440 (1986).
45. West Virginia Legislature, tit. 64 West Virginia Legislative Rules Department of Health: Hospital Licensure, series 12, § 10.3.1.0 (1987).

WISCONSIN

Wisconsin's rules only specify that filing equipment and space must be adequate to maintain the records and facilitate retrieval. If records are taken from the hospital, as under subpoena, measures must be taken to protect the records from loss, defacement, tampering, and unauthorized access.[46] The system for identifying and filing shall permit prompt location of each patient's medical records and filing equipment and space shall be adequate to maintain the records and facilitate retrieval.[47]

WYOMING

Wyoming has no specific requirements for storage of medical records.

---

46. Wisconsin Administrative Code § HSS 124.14(2)(b)2 (Feb. 1, 1988).
47. *Id.* § HSS 124.14(2)(e)1 and 3.

CHAPTER 6

Correcting Medical Records

What Do You Do if a Medical Record Is Inaccurate?

What do you do if you find out that a medical record is inaccurate? Certainly you can and should correct an inaccurate record. But you must be careful to make the change properly—by noting the change in the record in the proper chronological order and by noting that it is an addition or a correction.

You should not alter the original record in any way, such as by trying to erase, remove, or change the information contained therein. You must leave the original record in its original condition. Why? If it appears that you have tampered with a record, such as a medical record, the tampering can result in losing a malpractice case, even when the medical care was proper, because of the loss of credibility inherent in such an improper alteration. Modern technology can easily detect tampering. Further, if a judge or jury believes that the defendant tried to tamper with the evidence, they may increase the damages in addition to imposing other penalties such as an indictment for forgery or obstruction of justice.

Altering a medical record to avoid liability for malpractice is especially foolhardy because not all errors in treatment amount to the negligence that results in malpractice liability. And your malpractice liability insurance may be voided if you alter any pertinent records.

What you should do, if you find it necessary to correct a record, is to leave the original record intact. Draw a line through the incorrect matter, being careful to ensure that it is still legible. Make a notation in the margin indicating that the entry was erroneous and enter the correction in the record in the proper order at the time noted.

Only a few states have specific statutory or regulatory rules concerning altering medical records. Some laws, such as Florida's, make it a crime to alter, deface, or falsify a medical record; some, such as New Mexico, specify how to correct an erroneous record; and some, like Maryland, specify procedures for patients who want their records corrected.

Federal Laws

The Privacy Act, 5 U.S.C. § 552 (1992), gives an individual access to records the federal government maintains on him or her and to any pertinent information maintained in the system, and individuals may request that the government amend the records to correct any errors. The statute also provides a procedure, including a possible lawsuit, to contest a government agency's refusal to amend records. Different agencies follow different regulations under the act to allow people to obtain and correct their records. For example, the Social Security Administration requires that a request for a medical record name a representative who will review the record. Failure to name a representative may result in denial of a request for a record.[1] The Health and Human Services requirements for access to records under both the Freedom of Information and the Privacy Acts may be found at 45 C.F.R. Part 5.1 (1991).

State Laws

ALABAMA

Alabama has no specific requirements for correcting medical records.

ALASKA

7 Alaska Administrative Code tit. 7, § 12.770(d) (April 1984) specifies that facilities must maintain procedures to protect the information in medical records from loss, defacement, tampering, or access by unauthorized persons.

ARIZONA

Arizona has no specific requirements for correcting medical records.

ARKANSAS

According to Arkansas' rules governing medical records, Arkansas Register 0601 G, errors in medical records shall be corrected by drawing a single line through the incorrect data, labeling it as "error," initialing, and dating the entry.

CALIFORNIA

California has no specific procedures for correcting medical records. (*See* Chapter 5 for requirements to guard records against defacement or tampering.)

COLORADO

Colorado has no specific requirements for correcting medical records.

---

1. 20 C.F.R. § 401.410 (1991).

CONNECTICUT

Connecticut has no specific requirements for correcting medical records.

DELAWARE

Delaware has no specific requirements for correcting medical records.

DISTRICT OF COLUMBIA

The District has no specific requirements for correcting medical records.

FLORIDA

Florida Statutes tit. 395 § 0165 (1990) provides that any person who fraudulently alters, defaces, or falsifies a medical record or causes or procures these offenses is guilty of a second-degree misdemeanor.

GEORGIA

In Georgia, any person who, with intent to conceal any material fact relating to a potential claim or cause of action, knowingly and willfully destroys, alters, or falsifies any record shall be guilty of a misdemeanor.[2]

HAWAII

Hawaii has no specific requirements for correcting medical records.

IDAHO

Idaho has no specific requirements for correcting medical records.

ILLINOIS

Illinois has no specific requirements for provider correction of medical records but does give any person entitled to access to the record the right to submit a written statement to correct inaccurate information or to add new information. If the record custodian discloses the disputed information, he or she must also disclose the person's statement contesting the disputed information. The person may also seek a court order if the facility does not modify the information on request.[3]

---

2. Georgia Code Annotated § 16-10-94.1(b) (Michie 1991).
3. Illinois Revised Statute, ch. 91½, ¶ 804(c)–(d) (1991).

INDIANA

A person who intentionally destroys or falsifies records of health facilities is guilty of a class D felony.[4]

IOWA

Iowa has no specific requirements for correcting medical records.

KANSAS

According to Kansas Administrative Regulations 28-39-91 (1990), skilled nursing and intermediate care facilities shall not use erasures or white-outs, but rather shall line errors through and add the word "error." The person making the correction will sign and date the error.

KENTUCKY

902 Kentucky Administrative Regulations 20:016, § 3(11)3 (1991), requires hospitals to safeguard records and their contents from tampering.

LOUISIANA

Louisiana has no specific requirements for correcting medical records.

MAINE

Maine has no specific requirements for correcting medical records.

MARYLAND

Maryland Health-General Code Annotated § 4-401 (1991) makes it a misdemeanor for a healthcare provider to knowingly or willfully destroy, damage, alter, obliterate, or otherwise obscure a medical record, hospital report, x-ray report, or other information about a patient in an effort to conceal the information from use as evidence.

Id. § 4-302(c) establishes a procedure by which a person in interest may request an addition to or other correction of a medical record. If the facility does not make the requested change, it must give the person in interest written notice of the refusal and the reason as well as the procedure for review of the refusal. It must then permit him or her to insert a statement of disagreement in the record. The facility must provide a notice of a change or the statement of disagreement to every person to whom they previously disclosed inaccurate, incomplete, or disputed information and whom the person designates to receive such notice.

---

4. Indiana Code § 16-10-4-23 (1991).

MASSACHUSETTS

Massachusetts Regulations Code tit. 105, § 150.013(B) (1990), notes that no erasures or ink eradicator shall be used or pages removed.

MICHIGAN

Michigan Compiled Laws § 750.492a (1991) makes it a felony for a healthcare provider to intentionally or willfully place misleading or inaccurate information in medical records or intentionally or willfully alter or destroy a patient's records for the purpose of concealing responsibility for the patient's injury, sickness, or death. A reckless placing of misleading or inaccurate information is a misdemeanor. However, the supplementation of information or correction of an error in the patient's medical record or chart in a manner that reasonably discloses that the supplementation or correction was performed and that does not conceal or alter prior entries does not violate the statute.

MINNESOTA

Minnesota has no specific requirements for correction of medical records.

MISSISSIPPI

Mississippi has no specific requirements for correcting medical records.

MISSOURI

Missouri has no specific requirements for correcting medical records.

MONTANA

Montana has no specific requirements for correcting medical records.

NEBRASKA

Nebraska has no specific requirements for correcting medical records.

NEVADA

Nevada has no specific provisions concerning correcting medical records.

NEW HAMPSHIRE

New Hampshire has no specific requirements for correcting medical records.

NEW JERSEY

New Jersey has no specific requirements concerning correcting medical records.

NEW MEXICO

Chapter 3, ¶ b (rev. ed. 1991) of the *New Mexico Hospital Association Legal Handbook,* suggests you make corrections carefully and notes that physicians, administrative supervisors, or nursing supervisors should correct significant errors, such as those involving medication orders or test data. Errors should not be obliterated, erased, or destroyed so as to destroy the initial entry. Instead, draw a line through a mistake and make a correction clearly. After a claim has been made or a lawsuit filed, do not make any changes in the complainant's medical record without first consulting defense counsel.

NEW YORK

New York Compilation of Codes, Rules and Regulations tit. 405, § 18 (1988), provides that a qualified person may challenge the accuracy of information maintained in patient records and may require that the provider insert a brief written statement concerning the challenged information in the record. The statement becomes a permanent part of the record, and the provider shall release the statement whenever it releases the information.

Id. § 405.10(a)(6) notes that hospitals shall allow patients and other qualified persons to obtain access to their medical records and to add brief written statements that challenge the accuracy of the medical record documentation and become a permanent part of the record.

NORTH CAROLINA

North Carolina does not have any specific requirements for correcting medical records.

NORTH DAKOTA

North Dakota does not have any specific requirements for correcting medical records.

OHIO

Ohio Administrative Code § 5101:3-3-125 (1991), covering the resident review process, specifies that entries in medical and nursing information undergoing review are corrected by crossing through or circling the entry, writing the word "error" or "mistaken entry," and dating and signing the corrections. In situations where there is not sufficient room for the correction to be made and the correct information to be recorded on the record, e.g., medication and treatment records, a long-term care facility may develop a policy to reflect where the correction and the correct information shall be documented. Otherwise, the form may have a legend that reflects where the correction and the correct information can be found. If this requirement is not met, the entry will not be considered for review. Erasures, obliterations, the use of correcting fluid, or superimpositions used to alter medical or nursing information reviewed will invalidate the information that has been altered.

Ohio Revised Code Annotated § 2913.40 (Baldwin 1991), governing Medicaid fraud, makes it criminal to knowingly alter, falsify, destroy, conceal, or remove any records necessary to fully disclose the nature of all goods or services for which the claim was submitted or for which reimbursement was received by the person, or to do the same with regards to records that are necessary to disclose fully all income and expenditures on which rates of reimbursements were based.

OKLAHOMA

Oklahoma Statutes Annotated tit. 17, § 16 (1992), makes destroying, concealing, mutilating, or attempting to do so, the records, books, or files of any corporation doing business in Oklahoma in order to defeat, hinder, or delay an investigation, prosecution, or lawsuit a felony.

OREGON

Oregon has no specific requirements for correcting medical records.

PENNSYLVANIA

Pennsylvania has no specific requirements for correcting medical records.

RHODE ISLAND

Rhode Island has no specific requirements for correcting medical records.

SOUTH CAROLINA

South Carolina has no specific requirements for correcting medical records.

SOUTH DAKOTA

South Dakota Codified Laws Annotated § 36-4-30 (1991) makes it unprofessional conduct for physicians or surgeons to falsify the medical records of a patient or any official record regarding possession and dispensing of narcotics, barbiturates, and habit-forming drugs or regarding any phase of medical treatment of a patient.

TENNESSEE

Tennessee has no specific requirements for correcting medical records.

TEXAS

Texas has no specific requirements for correcting medical records.

UTAH

Utah has no specific requirements for correcting medical records.

VERMONT

Vermont has no specific requirements for correcting medical records.

VIRGINIA

Virginia has no specific requirements for correcting medical records.

WASHINGTON

Washington has no specific requirements for correcting medical records.

WEST VIRGINIA

West Virginia has no specific requirements for correcting medical records.

WISCONSIN

Wisconsin Statutes § 51.30 (1989-90) provides rules for modifying treatment records of patients who have been treated for mental illness, developmental disabilities, or alcoholism or drug abuse other than by private practitioners. The patient, or the parent, guardian, or person in place of a parent of a minor, or the guardian of an incompetent may challenge the accuracy, completeness, timeliness, or relevance of factual information in his or her records and may request in writing that the facility maintaining the record correct it. The facility must act on such requests within 30 days and provide reasons for denial of the request along with how to file a grievance or seek judicial review. If the request is denied, the denial will include notice to the patient that he or she has a right to insert a statement in the record challenging the accuracy or completeness of the challenged information in the record.

WYOMING

Wyoming has no specific requirements for correcting medical records.

PART III

When Should You Refuse to Release Records and When Is Disclosure Permitted?

The Fifth Amendment privilege against compulsory self-incrimination does not protect records that the government requires a healthcare provider to keep. Official records are the property of the government and, consequently, healthcare providers have to produce them on demand. Similarly, private records that the government requires healthcare providers to keep are not within the scope of the Fifth Amendment privilege, so healthcare providers must produce them on demand. Thus, if a law or regulation requires a healthcare provider to keep a record, it becomes a "public" record and the healthcare provider may not rely on the privilege against self-incrimination to keep from disclosing it.

Thus, while maintaining the confidentiality of healthcare records, state and federal law may require healthcare providers to disclose medical information on the patient's request. Similarly, the law may require healthcare providers to disclose information concerning a patient's alcohol and drug abuse or a patient's communicable diseases. A healthcare provider may also be required to disclose information for research purposes or pursuant to a court order.

Deciding whether to release records first requires the provider to determine whether the records are confidential and then whether the law permits disclosure of such confidential information. Consequently, this part of the book will review the patient's right to privacy and the laws permitting diclosure. Chapter 7 discusses patients' rights to privacy. Chapter 8 discusses disclosure of records on request of a patient, governmental agency, or others. Chapters 9 and 10, respectively, discuss disclosure of records dealing specifically with alcohol and drug abuse and records concerning communicable diseases. Chapter 11 discusses disclosure of healthcare records pursuant to a court order, and Chapter 12 discusses disclosure of healthcare records for research purposes. One should note that while many states permit disclosure of confidential information, most states require the provider to maintain confidentiality when making the disclosure.

PART

What Should You Refuse to Release/Record and When Is Disclosure Permitted?

CHAPTER 7

Patients' Rights to Privacy

Definition of the Right to Privacy

The traditional legal definition of privacy is "the right to be left alone." Modern privacy laws have expanded this definition to include an individual's right to control personal information. The United States Supreme Court has recognized a constitutional right to privacy. In addition, many statutes, such as the federal Privacy Act of 1974, have expanded individuals' right to privacy. The right to privacy is not an absolute right, however. In some situations, the public's or the government's need to know may outweigh an individual's privacy rights. Please see the American Medical Association's Confidentiality Statement in Appendix C.

Federal Laws

The Privacy Act allows patients access to their medical records and the information contained therein, but it does not apply to private hospitals and other private healthcare facilities.[1]

The Comprehensive Alcohol Abuse and Alcoholism Prevention, Treatment, and Rehabilitation Act of 1970, 42 U.S.C. § 242(a) (1988) and 21 U.S.C. § 872(e) (1988)(as amended), prohibits discrimination in the admission of alcohol abusers to any hospital or outpatient facility that receives federal funding. A similar provision of the Drug Office Abuse and Treatment Act of 1972, 42 U.S.C. § 290ee (1988) (formerly 21 U.S.C. § 1175(b)(2)(c) (1972)), prohibits discrimination in the admission of drug abusers to hospitals that receive federal funding. Both statutes establish standards for disclosure of medical records of drug abusers. Violating patients' confidentiality may result in a criminal penalty.

42 C.F.R. Part 2 (1991) requires public, nonprofit, and for-profit private entities conducting, regulating, or assisting alcohol or drug abuse programs to maintain records showing patient consent to disclosure from confidential alcohol and drug abuse patient records and documenting such disclosure to medical personnel in a medical emergency.

---

1. 5 U.S.C. §§ 552(a)(1) and 552(e) (1992).

The provisions concerning confidentiality of drug and alcohol abuse patients are applicable to Peer Review Organizations (*id.* § 476.109).

Utilization review (UR) plans must provide that identities of individual recipients in all UR records and reports are kept confidential (*id.* §§ 456.113, 456.213, and 456.313).

Section 417.115 outlines confidentiality requirements affecting federally qualified health maintenance organizations (HMOs). Each recipient of federal financial assistance must hold confidential all information obtained by its personnel about the participants in the project. The facility must not disclose information unless disclosure is authorized by the patient, necessary to treat the individual, required by law, or needed under compelling circumstances to protect the health or safety of an individual. However, information may be disclosed in summary, statistical, or other forms that do not identify particular individuals.

State Laws

ALABAMA

Alabama Administrative Code r. 420-5-7.07(h) (1990) dealing with the licensure and certification of healthcare providers states that records and information regarding patients are confidential. Access to these records shall be determined by the hospital governing board. Inspectors for licensure or surveyors for membership in professional organizations shall be permitted to review medical records as necessary for compliance.

Similarly, Rule 420-5-10-.16 makes records and information regarding patients of nursing homes confidential, limiting access to designated staff members, physicians, and others having professional responsibility and to members of the state board of health.

Code of Alabama § 22-11A-14 (1991) provides that reports of sexually transmitted disease will be confidential and makes unauthorized release a misdemeanor.

Section 22-6-9 provides for confidentiality of Medicaid recipients.

Section 22-5A-6 provides for the right to privacy of long-term residential healthcare patients' complaints to the ombudsmen.

ALASKA

Alaska's Constitution sets forth a right to privacy. In Gunnerud v. State, 611 P.2d 69 (Alaska 1980), the court held that it would be an unwarranted infringement of a witness's privacy to grant access to his or her private medical records unless the material was relevant.

Alaska Administrative Code tit. 7, § 12.890(a)(7) (Jan. 1984) states that patients have the right to confidentiality of their medical records and treatments. Both Alaska's statutory law and administrative code specify that information regarding a patient may be released without consent only to

- A person authorized by court order

- Healthcare providers if a medical emergency arises

- Research projects authorized by the governing board, if provision is made to preserve anonymity in the reported results

- Other persons to whom disclosure is required by law (*id.* § 13.130. Alaska Statute §§ 47.17.010-47.17.070 (1991))

A facility may release records and information regarding a patient to the patient or to an individual for whom the patient, or legally designated representative of the patient, has given written consent to disclosure. The consent must include the

- Patient's name

- First and last dates of service authorization

- Information to be released

- Recipient of the information

- Signature of the patient or the legally designated representative of the patient[2]

Alaska Administrative code tit. 7, §§ 36.010-36.020 (April 1985) applies to the use or disclosure of information concerning applicants and recipients of services from the division of family and youth services and requires safeguarding of information about such clients, including medical examinations.

ARIZONA

Arizona Health Care Institutions Licensure Regulation, Arizona Compilation Rules and Regulations 9-10-221 (1982), provides that medical record information shall be released only with the written consent of the patient, the legal guardian, or in accordance with law. Hospitals that have designated psychiatric or substance abuse units shall maintain confidentiality of medical records as required by Arizona Revised Statutes Annotated § 36-509 (1991) and applicable regulations.

Similarly, Arizona Compilation Rules and Regulations 9-10-221(E), concerning medical record services, provides that confidentiality of medical records shall be maintained as required by Arizona Revised Statutes Annotated § 36-509 and applicable regulations for hospitals that have designated psychiatric or substance abuse units.

---

2. Alaska Statute § 18.23.065 (1991).

Id. § 36-509(A), concerning confidential records, states

- All information and records obtained in the course of evaluation, examination, or treatment shall be kept confidential and not as public records, except as the requirements of a hearing pursuant to this chapter may necessitate a different procedure. Pursuant to rules established by the department, information and records may only be disclosed to

  - Physicians and providers of health, mental health, or social and welfare services involved in caring for, treating, or rehabilitating the patient

  - Individuals to whom the patient has given consent to have information disclosed

  - Persons legally representing the patient. In such case, the department's rules shall not delay complete disclosure.

  - Persons authorized by a court order

  - Persons doing research or maintaining health statistics, provided that the department establishes such rules for the conduct of research as will ensure the anonymity of the patient

  - The state department of corrections in cases where prisoners confined to the state prison are patients in the state hospital on authorized transfer either by voluntary admission or by order of the court

  - Governmental or law enforcement agencies when necessary to secure the return of a patient who is on unauthorized absence from any agency where the patient was undergoing evaluation and treatment

  - Family members actively participating in the patient's care, treatment, or supervision. An agency or treating professional may only release information relating to the person's diagnosis, prognosis, need for hospitalization, anticipated length of stay, discharge plan, medication, medication side effects, and short-term and long-term treatment goals (*id.* § 36-509(A)(1)-(8)).

- An agency shall release information pursuant to the paragraph immediately above only after the treating professional or his designee interviews the person undergoing treatment or evaluation to determine whether release is in that person's best interests. A decision to release or withhold information is subject to review pursuant to § 36-517.01 (*id.* § 36-509(B)). The treating agency shall record the name of any person to whom information is given.

Several other Arizona statutes provide for confidentiality. For example, § 32-1451.01 provides that patient records and the like kept by the board of medical examiners are confidential and not to be released to the public. Nursing care institution requirements for service delivery specify that each patient shall be assured confidential handling of personal and medical records (*id.* § 36-447.17). The release of such records shall be by written consent of the patient or responsible party, except as otherwise required or permitted by law. Similarly, § 36-448.08 gives residents of adult care homes the right to have medical and financial records kept in confidence.

ARKANSAS

Medical records are confidential. Only personnel authorized by the administrator shall have access to the records. Written consent of the patient is necessary to authorize release of medical records.[3] Medical records cannot be removed from the hospital except on issuance of a subpoena by a court with authority to issue such an order.[4]

All laboratory notifications of communicable diseases are confidential and shall not be open to inspection by anyone except public health personnel.[5] Similarly, any reports, information, or records of a physician misconduct proceeding before the Arkansas State Medical Board are strictly confidential,[6] as are those of peer review boards.[7]

In addition, the identity of persons voluntarily participating in the Department of Health acquired immune deficiency syndrome (AIDS) testing program must be kept secret.[8]

CALIFORNIA

California's Confidentiality of Medical Information Act, California Civil Code § 56.10 (Deering 1992), confirms patients' rights to privacy in their medical records by governing the release of patient-identifiable information by healthcare providers. The Health and Safety Code § 1795.12 (Deering 1992) provides for patient or patient representative access on request and payment of reasonable clerical costs. Violation of this section may result in disciplinary action by the licensing authority. The California Civil Code § 56.10(c) also provides for permissive access by healthcare providers; insurers to the extent necessary to obtain payment; credentialing committees; licensing or accrediting bodies (however, in such cases, the facility may not permit identifiable patient information to be removed unless expressly permitted or required by

---

3. Arkansas Register 0601 U (Medical Records).
4. *Id.* 0601(V) and 0601(W).
5. Arkansas Code Annotated § 20-16-504 (Michie 1992).
6. *Id.* § 17-93-104.
7. *Id.* § 20-9-503.
8. *Id.* § 20-15-901.

law); the county coroner; researchers; and employers, if the medical treatment was at the prior request and payment of the employer (*id.* § 56.10(a)). The code also provides for mandatory disclosure to authorized representatives of patients when the patient has executed a valid release. Violations of this statute constitute a misdemeanor if the patient is harmed by the unauthorized release (*id.* § 1798.57). In addition, the patient may recover actual damages, punitive damages not to exceed $3,000, and attorney's fees not to exceed $1,000 (*id.* § 56.35).

Recipients of medical information under California Civil Code § 56.10 may not further disclose it without a new authorization (*id.* § 56.13). But unless a patient specifically requests in writing to the contrary, a provider may release at its discretion any of the following information, upon an inquiry concerning a specific patient:

- Patient's name, address, age, and sex

- General description of the reason for treatment (whether an injury, a burn, poisoning, or some unrelated condition)

- General nature of the injury, burn, poisoning, or other condition

- General condition of the patient

- Any information that is not medical information (*id.* § 56.05(c))

Similarly, the Welfare and Institutions Code § 5328 (Deering 1992) covers psychiatric records. In such cases, patient authorization requires the approval of a physician, psychologist, or social worker. Mandatory disclosure is required

- Between qualified professionals when providing services, in referrals, and in conservatorship hearings

- To the extent necessary to make an insurance claim

- To persons designated by the conservator

- For research

- To courts and law enforcement agencies as needed to protect public officials

- To the patient's attorney

- To probation officers

- To county patients' rights advocates with patient authorization

- To law enforcement officials if the patient is a victim or has committed a crime in the facility

Whenever a facility discloses such information, the facility shall promptly cause to be entered into the patient's medical record the date and circumstances under which such disclosure was made; the names and relationships to the patient, if any, of persons or agencies to whom such disclosure was made; and the specific information disclosed (*id.* § 5328.06).

Permissive disclosure of information, not access to the records, is allowed to the family or persons designated by the patient or without designation if the patient is unable to give consent.

Section 4514 has similar provisions for records of the developmentally disabled. Facilities must record the circumstances of the disclosure in the patient's record (*id.* § 4516).

California Unemployment Insurance Code § 2714 (Deering 1992) specifies that all medical records obtained by the department shall be confidential and shall not be published or be open to public inspection in any manner revealing the identity of the claimant or the nature or cause of his or her disability. Such records are not admissible in evidence in any action or special proceeding other than one directly connected with and limited to the administration of public social services. The department may reveal its records to the Director of Social Services or his or her representatives, and may reveal the identity only of the claimant to the Department of Rehabilitation, but the information shall remain confidential and shall not be disclosed.

California Code of Regulations tit. 22, § 70707(b)(8) (1992) provides that anyone not directly connected with a patient's care must obtain written permission of the patient before any medical records are made available.

In addition to general acute care hospitals, regulations specify that the following other types of facilities must maintain confidentiality of patient records:

- Acute psychiatric hospitals (*id.* § 71551(a))

- Skilled nursing facilities (*id.* § 72543(b))

- Intermediate care facilities (*id.* § 73543(b))

- Home health agencies (*id.* § 74731(c))

- Primary care clinics (*id.* § 75055(b))

- Psychology clinics (*id.* § 75343(b))

- Psychiatric health facilities (*id.* § 77143(a))

- Adult day health facilities (*id.* § 78433)

- Chemical dependency recovery hospitals (*id.* § 79347(b))

COLORADO

Colorado does not permit a person responsible for the diagnosis or treatment of venereal diseases or addiction to or use of drugs, in the case of minors, to release records of such diagnosis or treatment to a parent, guardian, or other person other than the minor or his designated representative (Colorado Revised Statutes § 25-1-801(d) (1991)). Similarly, records relating to illegitimate children may not be disclosed except as required by a court or by the department or local board of health (*id.* § 25-3-204). Section 25-1-120 specifies that among the rights of patients of nursing and intermediate care facilities is the right to privacy in treatment, including confidentiality in the treatment of personal and medical records. Section 27-10-120 provides that records pertaining to the care and treatment of the mentally ill are also confidential. Finally, § 18-4-412 makes it a felony to knowingly obtain, steal, disclose to an unauthorized person, or copy a medical record or medical information without proper authorization. The statute defines "proper authorization" as

> a written authorization signed by the patient or his duly designated representative or an appropriate order of court or authorized possession pursuant to law or regulation for claims processing, possession for medical audit or quality assurance purposes, possession by a consulting physician to the patient, or possession by hospital personnel for record-keeping and billing purposes.

CONNECTICUT

Patients' rights to confidentiality generally are provided for in Connecticut General Statute 19a-550, titled, "Patient's Bill of Rights." Section 19a-550 provides that any patient of a nursing home or chronic disease hospital is assured confidential treatment of his personal and medical records and may approve or refuse their release to any individual outside the facility, except in case of his transfer to another healthcare institution or as required by law or third-party payment contract.

A number of other Connecticut statutes provide for confidentiality of healthcare information. For example, § 19a-25 makes records procured by the Department of Health Services (or by staff committees of facilities accredited by that department in connection with studies of morbidity and mortality) confidential, and restricts their use to medical or scientific research.

Sections 19a-853 and 19a-585, discussed in Chapter 10, provide for confidentiality of human immunodeficiency virus (HIV)–related information. Similarly, section 17a-630 provides for confidentiality of alcohol and drug abuse patients.

Information showing that a doctor consulted with, examined, or treated a minor for venereal disease is confidential (*id.* § 19a-216). In addition, records of applicants for enrollment and enrolled patients in community drug abuse treatment programs are confidential (*id.* § 17a-630(b)–(c)), as are records showing that a minor requested or received treatment and rehabilitation for drug dependence (*id.* § 17a-630(d)).

State Department of Health Regulations, Connecticut Agencies Regulations § 19-13-D44 (1990) makes industrial health facilities' records confidential, except for cases involving claims under the Workman's Compensation Act, as authorized by law, to responsible individuals when such disclosure is in the employee's best interest or when authorized by the employee.

DELAWARE

Delaware Code Annotated tit. 16, § 1121(6) (1991), governing the rights of patients in sanatoria, rest homes, nursing homes, boarding homes, and related institutions, specifies that such facilities shall treat personal and medical records confidentially and not make them public without the consent of the patient or resident.

Information and records held by the Division of Public Health relating to known or suspected sexually transmitted diseases, including human immunodeficiency virus (HIV) infection, are confidential, as are reports of venereal disease cases (*id.* § 702), and may only be released in limited circumstances (*id.* tit. 16, §§ 711 and 712).

Clinical records of mental health patients, *id.* tit. 16, § 5161, and health information obtained by health maintenance organizations (HMOs) (*id.* tit. 16, § 9113), are confidential.

DISTRICT OF COLUMBIA

Any publication by any medical utilization review committee, peer review committee, medical staff committee, or tissue review committee shall keep confidential the identity of any patient whose condition, care, or treatment was a part thereof (District of Columbia (D.C.) Code Annotated § 32-504 (1991)).

Section 32-255(a) governs the confidentiality of medical records and information at D.C. General Hospital. It provides that medical records and other information, or materials, or both pertaining to any patient shall not be disclosed for any reason other than the medical care of the patient without the informed written consent of the patient or his or her legally authorized representative. Each request must be specific; blanket consent may not be secured.

Section 6-2002 prohibits disclosure of mental health information by any mental health professional or facility to any person, including an employer.

FLORIDA

Florida Statutes ch. 110.123(9) (1991) ensures the confidentiality of patient medical records and medical claim records of state employees, former employees, and eligible dependents in the custody or control of the state group insurance program.

Chapter 119.07 provides extensive rights, restrictions, and exceptions to the availability of public records for inspection by any person desiring them.

Chapter 119.07(3) exempts all records that are confidential as provided by law, including certain patient records obtained by the Department of Health and Rehabilitative Services pursuant to other statutes.

Chapters 110.123(3), 110.1091, and 112.0455 provide that patient medical records and medical claim records of state employees, former employees, and eligible dependents in the custody or control of the state group insurance program are confidential and exempt from the provisions of Chapter 119.07(1). Such records shall not be furnished to any person other than the employee or his or her legal representative, except upon written authorization of the employee (*id.* ch. 110.123(9)), but may be furnished in any civil or criminal action, unless otherwise prohibited by law, on the issuance of a subpoena from a court of competent jurisdiction and proper notice to the employee or his or her legal representative by the party seeking such records (*id.*). Nursing home patient records are similarly confidential and exempt from public disclosure (*id.* ch. 400.321(1)).

Florida Administrative Code Annotated r. 10D-28.110(10)(f)(5) (1990) provides that hospitals may not release clinical record information without the written consent of the patient, family, or other legally responsible party. Rule 10D-28.110(10)(f)(4) directs hospitals to protect the confidentiality of clinical information and communication between staff and patients.

Rule 10D-28.158(3) provides that hospital patient records shall have a privileged and confidential status and shall not be disclosed without the consent of the person to whom they pertain, but appropriate disclosure may be made without such consent to

- Hospital personnel for use in connection with the treatment of the patient

- Hospital personnel only for internal hospital administrative purposes associated with the treatment

- The Hospital Cost Containment Board

Rule 10D-29.082(2) provides that nursing home clinical records are confidential and may not be released without written permission of the patient or guardian, except to persons or agencies with a legitimate professional need or regulatory authority. Similarly, § 21G-17.001(1) provides that dental records are confidential and may not be released unless authorized by the patient in writing.

GEORGIA

No physician, hospital, or healthcare facility shall be required to release any medical information concerning a patient except to the Department of Human Resources and its subelements, unless the patient, his or her parents, or guardian authorizes such release in writing; the patient waives any privilege; a law, statute, or regulation requires release; a court orders release; or the records are subpoenaed (Georgia Code Annotated § 24-9-40 (Michie 1991)). This section does not apply to psychiatrists or to hospitals in which the patient is or has been treated solely for mental illness.

Section 24-9-47 makes acquired immune deficiency syndrome (AIDS) information confidential and specifies the limited circumstances under which such information may be disclosed.

As discussed in Chapter 10, records of medical review committees are confidential (*id.* § 31-7-143).

Data concerning the diagnosis, treatment, or health of anyone enrolled in a health maintenance organization (HMO) is confidential and may not be disclosed except upon consent of the enrollee or pursuant to statute or court order or in the event of a claim or litigation between the enrollee and the HMO (*id.* § 33-21-23).

Section 26-5-17 provides for confidentiality of records, names, and communications of drug dependent persons who seek or obtain treatment, therapeutic advice, or counsel from any licensed program. Further, any communication such person has with an authorized employee or license holder is confidential.

HAWAII

Hawaii's retention of medical records statute requires medical records to be retained "in a manner that will preserve the confidentiality of the information in the record."[9]

IDAHO

Idaho Code § 54-1814 (1991) lists failure to safeguard the confidentiality of medical records or other medical information pertaining to identifiable patients as a ground for medical discipline.

Section 39-308 makes records of treatment facilities for alcoholism confidential and privileged to the patient.

Similarly, all reports of reportable diseases made to the Department of Health and Welfare are confidential (*id.* § 39-606, effective July 1, 1993).

Section 39-1310, also effective July 1, 1993, makes confidential all information received by the licensing agency that would identify individual residents or patients.

All written records of interviews; all reports, statements, minutes, memoranda, charts, and the contents thereof; and all physical materials relating to research, discipline, or medical study of any in-hospital medical staff committees or medical society are confidential, with some exceptions (*id.* § 39-1392b). Records of in-hospital medical staff committees and recognized medical societies for the purpose of reducing morbidity and mortality and enforcing

---

9. Hawaii Revised Statutes § 622-58 (1991).

and improving the standards of medical practice are confidential (*id.* § 39-1392). Section 39-1393, effective July 1, 1993, provides for limited confidentiality of information used for disciplinary actions by the medical staff of licensed acute care hospitals. Section 39-1394(d) requires that the method used to destroy the record be in keeping with its confidential nature.

Finally, § 6-1008 provides for confidentiality in the proceedings of medical malpractice panels.

ILLINOIS

Every patient has the right to confidentiality in healthcare information under Illinois Revised Statutes, ch. 111 ½, ¶ 5403(c) (1988). Healthcare providers may not disclose the nature or details of services provided to patients without written consent from the patient or the patient's guardian. Under ¶ 5404, no provider may require a patient to waive his privacy rights as a condition of receiving care. And, where two or more patient confidentiality statutes conflict, the more stringent applies (*id.* ch. 110, ¶ 8-2002). Thus, the more stringent rules of ch. 111 ½, ¶ 6358-2, providing for keeping drug and alcohol abuse patient records strictly confidential (ch. 111 ½, ¶ 693.30(c)), requiring strict confidentiality for reporting of sexually transmissible diseases, including acquired immune deficiency syndrome (AIDS) (ch. 91 ½, ¶ 802(1)), the Mental Health and Developmental Disabilities Confidentiality Act, which prohibits disclosure that a named person is a recipient of mental health care, would apply over the general confidentiality provision of ch. 111 ½, ¶ 5403 (c).

Illinois Administrative Code tit. 77, § 250.1510(b)(5) (1991), recommends that hospitals issue definite policies and procedures pertaining to the use of medical records and the release of medical record information and that they safeguard records from unauthorized use (*id.* § 250.1510).

INDIANA

Indiana Code § 16-4-8-8 (Supp. 1991) provides that the original health record of the patient is the property of the provider and thus may be used by the provider without specific written authorization for legitimate business purposes. However, the provider shall at all times protect the confidentiality of the record and may only disclose the identity of the patient when it is essential to the provider's business use, to quality assurance, or to peer review.

Inactive records shall be stored in such a way as to maintain confidentiality.[10]

IOWA

Iowa provides for confidentiality of medical records in several places. Iowa Code § 22.7 (1991) makes certain public records confidential, including hospital records, medical records, and professional counselor records of the

---

10. Indiana Administrative Code tit. 410, r. 15-1-9(2)(b) (1988).

condition, diagnosis, care, or treatment of a patient or former patient or a counselee or former counselee, including outpatients.

Section 229.25 requires hospitals or other facilities treating mentally ill persons to keep records relating to the examination, custody, care, and treatment of any person in that hospital or facility confidential, with three exceptions:

- When the information is requested by a licensed physician, attorney, or advocate who provides the facility's chief medical officer with a written waiver signed by the patient

- When the information is sought by a court order

- When the person who is hospitalized or the patient's guardian, if the person is a minor or is not legally competent, signs an informed consent release specifying the person or agency to whom the facility is to send the information

The chief medical officer may release such records for research purposes so long as he or she does not disclose patients' names or identities. He may also release appropriate information to the spouse of a patient if he deems it to be in the best interests of the patient and the spouse.

Section 125.93 makes substance abusers' involuntary commitment or treatment records confidential, consistent with the federal confidentiality laws.

Under §§ 135.40–135.41, certain records of in-hospital committees and medical societies are confidential. Records of acquired immune deficiency syndrome (AIDS) testing (*id.* §§ 141.10 and 141.23) and communicable disease reports are also confidential (*id.* § 139.2).

Section 514B.30 prohibits officers, directors, trustees, partners, and employees of health maintenance organizations (HMOs) from testifying to or making public disclosure of privileged communications and may not release the names of its membership list of enrollees.

Iowa Administrative Code r. 441-81.13(5) (1990) specifies that residents of nursing facilities have the right to personal privacy and confidentiality of personal and clinical records.

Rule 481-63.38(135C) guarantees residents of residential care facilities for the mentally handicapped confidential treatment of all information contained in their medical, personal, and financial records. Rule 481-57.40(135C) has identical provisions governing records of residential care facilities, as does Rule 481-59.49(135C) for skilled nursing facilities and Rule 481-58.44(135C) for intermediate care facilities.

The interpretive guidelines to the regulations governing confidentiality of mentally retarded patient records (*id.* § 483.410(c)(1)) define "keep confidential" as safeguarding the content of information (including video-, audio-, and computer-stored information) from unauthorized disclosure without the specific informed consent of the individual, parent of a minor child, or legal guardian, and consistent with the advocate's right of access, as required in the Developmental Disabilities Act. If the facility maintains information that is too confidential to place in the record used by all staff, it may retain the information in a secure place and make a notation in the main record of the location of the confidential record.

KANSAS

Kansas Administrative Regulations § 28-34-9a(d)(5) (1991) specifies that records shall be confidential. Only persons authorized by the hospital governing body, including individuals designated by the licensing agency to verify compliance with statutes or regulations and for disease control investigations, shall have access to the records.

KENTUCKY

902 Kentucky Administrative Regulation 20:016 § 3(11)(c) (1990) states that only authorized personnel shall be permitted access to patient records. Patient information shall be released only on authorization of the patient, the patient's guardian, or the executor of his or her estate.

All records in the possession of local health departments or the Cabinet for Human Resources that concern persons infected with sexually transmitted diseases are confidential and may only be released to the physician retained by the patient; for statistical purposes as long as no individual can be identified; with consent, if necessary to enforce the rules of the Cabinet for Human Resources relating to the control and treatment of such diseases; and to the extent necessary to protect the life or health of the named party.[11]

Section 211.463(c) provides that a private agent charged with utilization review (UR) may not disclose or publish individual medical records or any other confidential medical information in the performance of UR activities except that private review agents may, if otherwise permitted by law, provide patient information to a third party on whose behalf the private review agent is performing UR. Section 211.464(b) requires that private review agents charged with UR include in their applications a UR that includes the policies and procedures that will ensure that all applicable state and federal laws to protect the confidentiality of individual medical records are followed.

LOUISIANA

Under Louisiana Revised Statutes § 28:171 (West 1991), mental patients have a right to privacy:

> No patient in a treatment facility pursuant to this Chapter shall be deprived of any rights, benefits, or privileges guaranteed by law, the Constitution of the state of Louisiana, or the Constitution of the United States solely because of his status as a

---

11. Kentucky Revised Statutes Annotated § 214.420(2) (Baldwin 1991).

patient in a treatment facility. These rights, benefits, and privileges include, but are not limited to, civil service status; the right to vote; the right to privacy; rights relating to the granting, renewal, forfeiture, or denial of a license or permit for which the patient is otherwise eligible; and the right to enter contractual relationships and to manage property (*id.* § 28:171(A)).

The Nursing Home Residents' Bill of Rights, Louisiana Statutes § 2010.8, provides that all residents have the right to have confidentiality in the treatment of personal and medical records (*id.* § 40:2010.8(A)(8)).

Patients of professional corporations have a right to confidentiality (Louisiana Statutes §§ 12:905 and 12:906). Shareholders of such corporations shall not have access to any records or communications pertaining to medical services rendered by, or any other affairs of, the corporation, except as provided by § 12:913B.

Professional veterinary medicine corporations (*id.* §§ 12:1155 and 12:1156), professional psychology corporations (§§ 12:1134 and 12:1135), professional dental corporations (§§ 12:985 and 12:986), and professional optometry corporations (§§ 12:1115 and 12:1116 (1990)) have similar requirements.

Worker's compensation employee records are confidential (*id.* § 23:1293 (1990)).

MAINE

The Regulations for the Licensure of General and Specialty Hospitals published by the State of Maine, ch. XII, § A (1972), state that the licensing standard is that only authorized personnel have access to the record, that written consent of the patient must be presented as authority for the release of medical information, and that medical records are generally not removed from the hospital except on subpoena.

Maine has a comprehensive statute covering acquired immune deficiency syndrome (AIDS) testing,[12] which provides that no person, on penalty of termination of employment or civil liability including damages and a fine of up to $1,000 for a negligent violation and $5,000 for an intentional violation, may disclose the results of a human immunodeficiency virus (HIV) test, except as follows:

- To the subject of the test

- To his designated healthcare provider, who may only further disclose the information to other healthcare providers providing direct patient care to the subject

- To others that the subject has designated in writing

- To healthcare providers who process donated human body parts to assure medical acceptability of the gift

---

12. Maine Revised Statutes Annotated tit. 5, §§ 19201-19208 (1991).

- To certain research facilities when the test is performed in a manner by which they do not reveal the subject's identity

- To an anonymous testing site

- To other agencies responsible for the treatment or care of the subject, including the Department of Corrections, the Department of Human Services, and the Department of Mental Health and Mental Retardation

- To the Bureau of Health

- As part of the medical record when disclosure has been authorized by the subject

- Pursuant to court-ordered disclosure.

No medical record containing test results may be disclosed in any proceeding without the patient's consent except

- In proceedings under the communicable disease laws

- In proceedings under the Adult Protective Services Act

- In proceedings under child protection laws

- In proceedings under mental health laws

- Pursuant to a court order on a showing of good cause

- In utilization reviews

Healthcare providers with patient records containing HIV infection status must have a written policy providing for confidentiality that requires, at a minimum, termination of employment for any employee who violates the confidentiality policy.

MARYLAND

Maryland Health-General Code Annotated § 4-302 (1991) provides for confidentiality of medical records. Healthcare providers shall keep the medical record confidential and disclose it only as provided by law. However, this statute does not apply to information

- Not kept in the medical record of a patient or recipient that is related to the administration of the facility, including

  - Risk management

  - Quality assurance

  - Any activities of medical or dental review committees that are confidential

- Governed by the federal confidentiality of alcohol and drug abuse patient regulations

- Governed by the developmental disability confidentiality provisions

Section 8-601 provides for alcohol and drug abuse information confidentiality and specifies that the federal regulations govern disclosure and use of such records.

Maryland Code § 18-206 makes infectious or contagious disease reports (*id.* § 18-201), cancer reports (*id.* § 18-203), laboratory examination reports (*id.* § 18-205), and sentinel birth defects reports (*id.* § 18-206) confidential. Section 18-207(d) makes required monthly reports of directors of medical laboratories concerning the identity of anyone tested for human immunodeficiency virus (HIV) confidential.

Similarly, §§ 7-610 through 7-612 make developmental disability information confidential.

Code of Maryland Regulations tit. 10, § 07.10.12 (1989) requires home health agencies to have proper safeguards for clinical record information against illegal or unauthorized use. Regulations for health maintenance organizations (HMOs) have more detailed requirements, which state that all information contained in the medical records and information received from physicians, surgeons, or hospitals incidental to the doctor-patient or hospital-patient relationship shall be kept confidential and may not be disclosed without the consent of the patient, except for research or education or the Department of Health and Mental Hygiene's review (*id.* tit. 10, § 07.11.05(B)).

MASSACHUSETTS

Massachusetts General Laws ch. 214, § 1B (1992), gives a person a right against unreasonable, substantial or serious interference with his or her privacy; the person may sue for a violation thereof. In Tower v. Hirschhorn,[13] the court found that a physician's disclosure of confidential medical information to two people without the patient's consent was sufficient to find an invasion of privacy under this law.

Every patient or resident of a hospital, institution for the care of unwed mothers, clinic, infirmary, convalescent or nursing home, or home for the aged has the right to confidentiality of all records and communications.[14] This section does not prevent any third-party reimburser from inspecting and copying, in the ordinary course of determining eligibility for or entitlement to benefits, records relating to diagnosis, treatment, or other services provided to any person for which coverage, benefit, or reimbursement is claimed so long as the policy provides for such access or in connection with any peer or

---

13. 397 Mass. 581, 492 N.E. 2d 728 (1986).
14. Massachusetts General Laws ch. 111, § 70E.

utilization review. Confidential information in medical records may only be provided on written authority of the patient or the executor of his estate.[15]

Chapter 111, section 119 makes records pertaining to venereal diseases confidential, as are records of human immunodeficiency virus (HIV) tests.[16] Chapter 112, § 12G prevents physicians, healthcare facilities, nursing homes, and any other medical provider from disclosing information concerning the diagnosis, treatment, or condition of a patient in connection with the establishment of eligibility for certain medical benefits.

MICHIGAN

Under Michigan Compiled Laws § 333.6111 (1991), records of the identity, diagnosis, prognosis, and treatment of an individual maintained in connection with the performance of a licensed substance abuse treatment and rehabilitation service, a licensed prevention service, an approved service program, or an emergency medical service are confidential.[17]

Section 333.5114a, governing human immunodeficiency virus (HIV) testing, provides that such information is exempt from disclosure under the Freedom of Information Act.

Section 333.2367 requires the Department of Public Health to establish procedures to protect the confidentiality of data and records. Section 333.5111(2) requires the Department to promulgate rules to provide for the confidentiality of reports, records, and data pertaining to the testing, care, treatment, reporting, and research associated with communicable diseases and serious communicable diseases and infections. Reports of birth defects are likewise confidential (*id.* § 333.5721). Further, reports of critical health problems are available only to persons who demonstrate a need for the report or other data that is essential to health-related research (*id.* § 325.75). Further, under § 15.243, public bodies may exempt from disclosure as public records any information subject to the physician-patient or psychologist-patient privilege or medical, counseling, or psychological facts or evaluations concerning an individual if the individual's identity would be revealed by a disclosure.

Data concerning medical research projects are inadmissible in evidence and may not be disclosed except as is necessary for furthering the research (*id.* § 333.2632).

A person who permits or encourages the unauthorized dissemination of information contained in the child abuse or neglect registry is guilty of a misdemeanor and is civilly liable for the damages proximately caused by the dissemination (*id.* § 722.633).

---

15. *Id.*
16. *Id.* ch. 111, § 70F.
17. For disclosure, see chapters 8 and 9.

MINNESOTA

Minnesota Statutes § 144.651(16) (1991) assures patients and residents of healthcare facilities confidential treatment of their personal and medical records and may approve or refuse release of these records to any individual outside the facility. The facility shall notify residents when any individual outside the facility requests personal records and may select someone to accompany them when the records or information are the subject of a personal interview.

Records of treatment for alcohol and drug abuse are confidential (*id.* § 254A.09), as are records concerning drug and alcohol testing of employees (*id.* § 181.954).

Minnesota statutes make revealing a privileged communication, except as required or permitted by law, a ground for disciplinary action (e.g., *id.* §§ 147.091(1)(m) [physicians, surgeons, osteopaths] and 148.261(13) [registered and licensed practical nurses]).

Information concerning illegitimate births is confidential and may not be released except to representatives of the commissioner of health or the commissioner of human services (Minnesota Administrative Rules § 4640.1400(2) (1991)).

MISSISSIPPI

According to Mississippi Code § 41-9-67 (1991), hospital records are not public records and patients have a privilege of confidence in them.

Under § 41-83-17, private review agents may not disclose or publish individual medical records or other confidential medical information obtained in the performance of utilization review activities without the patient's authorization or a court order.

Section 41-21-97 provides for confidentiality of records of civilly committed patients.

Records of disciplinary proceedings against physicians and all patients' charts, records, emergency room records, or any other document copied in connection therewith are confidential (*id.* § 73-25-28).

Under the Mississippi Vulnerable Adults Acts, reports of abuse, neglect, or exploitation are confidential (*id.* § 43-47-7), as are domestic abuse reports (*id.* § 93-21-25).

MISSOURI

Missouri Revised Statutes § 198.032 (1990) provides for confidentiality of reports of complaints and records, including medical, social, personal, or financial records, of residents of convalescent, nursing, and boarding homes held by the Missouri Department of Social Services. Rights of residents of such facilities include the right to be ensured confidential treatment of all information contained in their records, including information contained in an automatic data bank (*id.* § 198.088(1)(6)(n)). Section 192.067 requires the

Department of Health to maintain the confidentiality of medical record information abstracted by or reported to the Department of Health.

Acquired immune deficiency syndrome (AIDS) information and records held by any person, agency, department, or political subdivision of the state are strictly confidential and shall not be disclosed, except as discussed in Chapter 10. The Department of Mental Health shall not report to the Department of Health the identity of any individual for whom human immunodeficiency virus (HIV) testing confirms HIV infection if such reporting is prohibited by federal confidentiality laws or regulations (*id.* § 191.662).

Section 191.317 provides for confidentiality of all test results and personal information obtained from any individual tested under genetics and metabolic disease programs.

Section 208.217 permits the Missouri Department of Social Services to obtain medical insurance information from health maintenance organizations (HMOs) and others. A request for data must include sufficient information to identify each person named in the request in a form compatible with the record-keeping methods of the entity. Failure to provide the requested information within 60 days subjects the entity to civil penalties. However, the Department of Social Services must establish guidelines to ensure that medical insurance information does not violate confidentiality laws (*id.*). Section 198.032 prohibits the Department of Social Services from publicly disclosing confidential medical, social, personal, or financial records of any convalescent, nursing, or boarding home resident, except in a manner that does not identify any resident or pursuant to court order. Similarly, child or nursing home resident abuse records are also confidential (*id.* § 198.032).

Records and information concerning applicants and recipients of medical assistance are confidential, and any disclosure shall be restricted to purposes directly connected with the administration of the medical assistance program (*id.* § 208.155).

Missouri Code Regulations tit. 13, 50-20.021(d)(7) (1992), notes that hospitals cannot release medical records or information without the written consent of the patient or his or her legal representative.

MONTANA

A number of Montana laws provide for confidentiality of medical records and information. Montana's constitution delineates a right to privacy.[18] Montana Code Annotated § 53-20-161 (1992) provides for confidentiality of records concerning developmentally disabled persons, as does § 53-21-166 for records concerning mental illness. Section 50-16-204 requires confidentiality of material used by peer committees, requiring such committees to protect the identity of any patient whose condition or treatment has been studied and not reveal his or her name. Section 50-19-108 makes unauthorized disclosure of

---

18. Montana Constitution article II, § 10 (1992).

information concerning serological tests for women seeking prenatal care a misdemeanor.

Reports of abortion (*id.* § 50-20-110); information on infant morbidity and mortality, specifically the identity of persons whose condition or treatment was studied (*id.* § 50-16-102); and child abuse records (*id.* § 41-3-205) are confidential. Of course, the doctor-patient privilege (*id.* § 26-1-805) protects the patient's confidentiality. Further, § 50-16-529, which specifies conditions under which patients' healthcare information may be disclosed without their authorization based on need to know, contains provisions requiring the recipient to treat the information as confidential.

Montana puts teeth into confidentiality requirements by making it a crime to willfully misrepresent one's identity or purpose (false pretenses) or to use bribery or theft to examine healthcare information (*id.* § 50-16-551).

The *Montana Hospital Association Manual,* chapters 23 and 24, speaks of maintaining records to protect their secrecy.

NEBRASKA

Revised Statutes of Nebraska §§ 44-32,171 and 44-4725 (1990) notes that data or information pertaining to the diagnosis, treatment, or health of any enrollee or applicant of a health maintenance organization (HMO) is confidential.

Section 68-1025 makes information regarding applicants for or recipients of medical assistance confidential.

Section 71-511 makes information concerning any patient or test results involving communicable diseases confidential. Similarly, laboratory notifications involving contagious diseases (*id.* § 71-502.04) and data of the cancer registry (*id.* § 81-647; Nebraska Administrative Rules and Regulations 174-5-008 (1987)) are confidential.

Nebraska Administrative Rules and Regulations 175-9-003.04A6 (1979), concerning the Nebraska Department of Health, states that medical records are confidential, privileged, and subject to inspection by authorized persons.

NEVADA

Nevada Revised Statutes § 449.720 (1991) specifies that all patients of medical facilities have the right to retain their privacy concerning their programs of medical care, including confidentiality of all communications and records concerning them.

Persons applying for or receiving treatment for alcohol or drug abuse have a right to confidentiality concerning any information relating thereto (*id.* § 458.055).

The health division may not disclose the identity of any patient, physician, or hospital involved in a required cancer report unless the party gives prior written consent (*id.* § 457.270).

Records made available under § 629.061 may not be used at a public hearing unless the patient named in the records has consented in writing, or appropriate procedures are used to protect the identity of the patient from public disclosure.

Section 108.640 allows any party legally liable or named in a claim for compensation or damages for injuries to a person the right to examine and make copies of all hospital records related to hospitalization of such injured person.

NEW HAMPSHIRE

A number of New Hampshire administrative regulations and statutes protect patients' rights to privacy. The general confidentiality statute is New Hampshire Revised Statutes Annotated § 151:13 (1991), which provides that information other than reports relating to vital statistics received by the Department of Health and Human Services, Division of Public Health Services, through inspection or otherwise, is confidential and shall not be disclosed publicly except in a proceeding involving the question of licensure or revocation of license. Hospital and Sanitaria Patients' Bill of Rights specifies that the patient shall be ensured confidential treatment of all information contained in his or her personal and clinical record, including that stored in an automatic data bank, and his or her written consent shall be required for the release of information to anyone not otherwise authorized by law to receive it (*id.* § 151:21).

Records of residents of sheltered care facilities are also confidential.[19] Clinical records of outpatient clinics, residential treatment and rehabilitation facilities, and home healthcare providers shall be safeguarded against unauthorized use.[20] Clinical laboratories must keep records and reports of tests confidential.[21]

New Hampshire Revised Statutes Annotated § 318-B:12 makes healthcare practitioners responsible for keeping separate records of receipt and disposition of controlled drugs, "so as not to breach the confidentiality of patient records."

Section 151:13 makes information other than reports relating to vital statistics received by the Department of Health and Welfare confidential and not subject to disclosure except in licensing or revocation of license proceedings.

Neither can the identity of a person tested for the human immunodeficiency virus (HIV) be disclosed (*id.* § 141-F:8. *See also* Chapters 9 and 10).

Under § 21-M:8-c, physicians and hospitals may not send the bill for the medical examination of a sexual assault victim to the victim or family of the victim and must maintain the privacy of the victim to the extent possible

---

19. New Hampshire Code Administrative Rules Hospital Department of Health and Human Services Regulations (General Hospitals) He-P 804.04(c).
20. *Id.* He-P 806.10, 807.07, and 809.07.
21. *Id.* He-P 808.12(e).

during third-party billings. Billing forms in such cases are subject to the same principles of confidentiality as other medical records.

NEW JERSEY

Both New Jersey Statutes and Administrative Regulations provide for patients' rights to confidentiality. For example, New Jersey Revised Statutes § 26:5C-5 (1991) provides for confidentiality of acquired immune deficiency syndrome (AIDS) and human immunodeficiency virus (HIV) infection information. Section 17:48D-21 provides for confidentiality of diagnostic or treatment information of enrollees in dental plans. Research data provided to the State Department of Health is confidential (*id.* § 26:1A-37.2). Reports of suspected elder abuse and all matters with respect to any complaints or investigations involving the ombudsman for the institutionalized elderly are confidential (*id.* § 52:27G-13).

Facilities must develop procedures to protect medical records from unauthorized use.[22]

The Department of Health may not disclose information it acquires during inspections in such a way as to indicate the names of the specific patients or hospital employees to whom the information pertains.[23]

NEW MEXICO

New Mexico Statutes Annotated § 26-2-12 (1992) prohibits disclosure of the record of a resident of the state who voluntarily undergoes treatment for alcoholism except on court order. Similarly, § 26-2-14 makes records on drug abuse treatment confidential.

Section 14-6-1 states that all health information that identifies specific individuals as patients is strictly confidential and is not a matter of public record or accessible to the public even though it is in the custody of a governmental agent or a licensed health facility. The custodian of such information may furnish it on request "to a governmental agency or its agent, a state educational institution, a duly organized state or county association of licensed physicians or dentists, a licensed health facility or staff committees of such facilities." Statistical studies and research reports may be published if they do not identify individual patients or otherwise violate the physician-patient privilege.

Similarly, New Mexico requires authorization by the patient for release of any information relating to a mental disorder or developmental disability from which a person well acquainted with the patient might recognize the patient, unless

---

22. New Jersey Administrative Code tit. 8, § 8:43B-7.4 (Supp. 1989). Standards for Hospital Facilities.
23. *Id.* § 43B-1.10.

- The recipient of the information is a mental health or developmental disabilities professional working with the patient when access to such information is required for the treatment.

- Disclosure is necessary to protect against a clear and substantial risk of death or serious injury.

- In the case of a minor, the disclosure to a parent or guardian is essential for the minor's treatment.

- The disclosure is to an insurer who is contractually obligated to pay expenses for the patient's treatment (*id.* § 43-1-19).

All records and files of the Health and Environment Department giving identifying information about individuals who have received or are receiving treatment, diagnostic services, or preventive care for diseases, disabilities, or physical injuries are confidential (*id.* § 24-1-20), as is all information voluntarily provided to the director or his or her agent in connection with studies designated by him or her as medical research.

According to the *New Mexico Hospital Association Legal Handbook,* ch. 5B (rev. 1981), all hospitals should treat all patient information as confidential and should not divulge it to anyone other than the patient's physician without the patient's written consent. The hospital should notify the patient of any subpoena it receives concerning his records in any case in which the patient is not a party and should not release the records unless the patient consents or the facility receives a court order. The *Handbook* notes that unauthorized release of information from the patient's medical record may give rise to civil liability.

NEW YORK

New York Public Health Law § 2803-c (McKinney 1992), Rights of Patients in Certain Medical Facilities, provides that every patient shall have the right to confidentiality in the treatment of personal and medical records. New York Social Services Law § 461-d (McKinney 1992) has a similar requirement with regard to residents in adult care facilities.

New York Compilation of Codes, Rules and Regulations tit. 10, § 405.10(a)(5) of the Department of Health, Health Facilities Series H-40 (1989), notes that hospitals shall ensure the confidentiality of patient records. Section 405.7, titled "Patients' Rights," specifies that one right is to confidentiality of all information and records pertaining to medical treatment, except as otherwise provided by law.

New York Mental Hygiene Law § 23.05 (McKinney 1992) provides for confidentiality as to all records of identity, diagnosis, prognosis, or treatment in connection with a person's receipt of substance abuse services. Similarly, § 33.13 provides for confidentiality of clinical records of clients or patients of facilities licensed or operated by the Office of Mental Health or the Office of

Mental Retardation and Developmental Disabilities and contains detailed guidance on disclosure.

New York Public Health Law § 2782 provides for confidentiality of human immunodeficiency virus (HIV)–related information and § 2306 makes information concerning sexually transmissible diseases confidential.

Reports of abuse of persons receiving care or services in residential healthcare facilities are also confidential (*id.* § 2803-d).

NORTH CAROLINA

North Carolina's physician-patient communications privilege statute states that confidential information in medical records shall be furnished only on the authorization of the patient or, if deceased, his or her executor, administrator, or next of kin or if ordered by a judge (North Carolina General Statute § 8-53 (1991)). Other provisions prohibit disclosure of specific medical information, such as records of cancer patients (*id.* § 130A-212), drug abuse patients, nursing home patients (*id.* § 131E-117), domiciliary home residents (*id.* § 131D-21), and persons identified as having the acquired immune deficiency syndrome (AIDS) virus or other communicable or reportable diseases (*id.* § 130A-143). In addition, § 131E-124 provides for confidentiality of all nursing home patients who register complaints with the department and all medical records it inspects. Any long-term care ombudsman who discloses any information obtained from a patient's medical or personal financial records without a court order or authorization in writing from the resident or legal representative is guilty of a misdemeanor (*id.* § 143-B-181.20).

The Mental Health, Developmental Disabilities, and Substance Abuse Act (*id.* § 122C-55), specifies confidentiality requirements for mental health, developmental disabilities, and substance abuse patients and limits disclosure to those situations detailed in Chapter 12.

Medical information concerning enrollees or applicants in health maintenance organizations (HMOs) is confidential (*id.* § 58-67-180).

Section 130A-12 makes all privileged patient records in the possession of the Department of Human Resources or local health departments confidential. Such records are not public records. Under § 103A-374, the State Center for Health Statistics shall take appropriate measures to protect the security of health data it collects. Medical records of individual patients are confidential and not public records open to inspection. The Center may only disclose records of individual patients that identify the individual if he or she authorized the disclosure or it is for bona fide research purposes.

North Carolina statutes also govern confidentiality of medical information in the insurance context. Section 58-2-105 makes such records in the possession of the Department of Insurance confidential, and § 58-39-45 limits access to recorded personal information to those situations detailed in the statute.[24]

---

24. *See* Chapter 13.

NORTH DAKOTA

North Dakota's Administrative Code § 33-07-01-16(a)–(c) (1990), Hospital Licensing Rules, requires that hospitals keep medical records confidential. Only authorized persons shall have access to the record, and the written consent of the patient must be presented as authority for the release of medical information. Medical records generally shall not be removed from the hospital environment except on subpoena. Section 33-07-03-13-4 specifies that all information contained in clinical records of long-term care facilities shall be treated as confidential and may be disclosed only to authorized persons.

OHIO

A number of Ohio statutes and administrative regulations provide for confidentiality. Ohio Revised Code § 3793.12 (Baldwin 1992) makes communications by a person seeking aid in good faith for alcoholism or drug dependence confidential, and § 3793.13 provides for confidentiality of records of drug abuse treatment programs.[25] Ohio Administrative Code 3701-55-15(c) (1989) amplifies this guidance by noting that all information contained in records of alcohol inpatient/emergency care patient records is confidential and the provider shall only disclose it to authorized persons.

Ohio Revised Code § 3701.241 requires the health director to develop and administer a program for confidential and anonymous acquired immune deficiency syndrome (AIDS) testing and a confidential partner notification system. Under Ohio Administrative Code 3701-3-08, communicable disease information is confidential.

All records of the Department of Mental Retardation and Developmental Disabilities, other than court journal entries or court docket entries that directly or indirectly identify a resident or former resident of an institution for the mentally retarded or person whose institutionalization has been sought, are confidential and shall not be disclosed with limited exceptions.[26] Reports of abuse of mentally retarded adults are not public records.[27] Records of those hospitalized for medical illness are confidential and may only be disclosed as specified therein.[28]

Similarly, medical records of persons covered by health maintenance organizations (HMOs) are confidential and shall not be released without the written consent of the covered person or a responsible party.[29]

Section 2305.251 of the Ohio Code provides for confidentiality of information of utilization review committees.

---

25. *See also* Chapter 8.
26. Ohio Revised Code § 5123.89.
27. *Id.* § 5123.61(j).
28. *Id.* § 5122.31.
29. *Id.*

Section 3701.041 provides for confidentiality of records of the employee assistance program (paid by warrant of the auditor of state), which refers state employees who are in need of medical, social, or other services to providers of those services.

Section 3727.14 prohibits disclosing the name or social security number of a patient or physician in data, except that § 3727.11 requires hospitals to furnish such numbers to the Department of Health.[30]

Abortion reports are confidential and shall not contain the name of the woman.[31]

OKLAHOMA

Oklahoma Statutes tit. 43A, § 1-109 (1991) makes medical records both confidential and privileged. Such information is available only to persons or agencies actively engaged in patient treatment or related administrative work. No such information shall be released to anyone not involved in treatment without a written release by the patient or, if the patient is a minor or if a guardian has been appointed, the guardian of the patient or a court order. (*id.* tit. 43A, § 1-109(A)(l)).

Similarly, birth defect information (id. tit. 63, § 1-550.2) and tumor registry information (*id.* tit. 63, § 1-551.1) are confidential and may only be divulged under limited circumstances. Child abuse reporting information is also confidential (*id.* tit. 21, § 846).

Under the Oklahoma Alcohol and Drug Abuse Services Act, all medical records and communications between doctor and patient are privileged and confidential and will not be released to anyone not involved in the treatment programs without a written release from the patient or a court order. Such information must be kept in folders clearly marked "Confidential" (*id.* tit. 43A, § 3-422.)

Nursing homes, rest homes, specialized homes, and group homes for the developmentally disabled or physically handicapped must ensure that every resident receives respect and privacy in his or her medical care program. Case discussion, consultation, examination, and treatment shall remain confidential, and personal and medical records shall be confidential (*id.* tit. 63, § 1-1918 and § 1-818.20).

Under title 63, § 2602, information about minor patients receiving services under the Health Services for Minors Act, which provides for situations in which minors may consent to health services, is not to be disseminated to any health professional, school, law enforcement agency, or official employer, without consent of the minor, except through specific legal requirements, or if the provision of information is necessary to the health of the

---

30. *See* Chapter 3.
31. Ohio Administrative Code 3701-47-03(c) (1989).

minor and the public. Statistical reporting may be done when the minor's identity is kept confidential.

Finally, Oklahoma statutes make it unprofessional conduct for a medical professional to willfully betray a professional secret to the detriment of the patient (*id.* tit. 59, § 509).

OREGON

Oregon Administrative Rules 333-70-055(18) (1986) requires medical record departments to maintain written policies on the release of medical record information, including patient access to medical records.

Oregon Revised Statutes § 433.045(3) (1986) states that no person shall disclose the identity of a person on whom a human immunodefiency virus (HIV)–related test was performed or the results of such a test in a manner that permits identification of the person unless he or she authorizes the disclosure or it is required by law.

Oregon Administrative Rules § 333-505-050(12) requires that healthcare providers take precautions to protect confidentiality of patient medical records. Further, Oregon Revised Statutes § 192.525 declares that the policy of the State of Oregon requires public and private healthcare providers to protect patients' rights of confidentiality of their medical records. Each provider must develop guidelines to ensure this protection (*id.* § 192.530).

Persons other than the patient who have received access to a patient's records may not disclose the contents to anyone without permission or as otherwise provided by law (*id.* § 179.505(12)).

Records of child abuse are confidential and not accessible for public inspection. Records may be disclosed as required for law enforcement, prevention of abuse, and as necessary to administer the services of the Child Welfare Division, if in the best interests of the affected child. Any record disclosed shall be kept confidential by the recipient (*id.* § 418.770).

The records of a patient at a drug or alcohol addiction treatment facility shall not be disclosed without the consent of the patient (*id.* § 426.460(5)).

PENNSYLVANIA

28 Pennsylvania Code § 115.27 (1991) requires hospitals to treat all medical records as confidential. Only authorized personnel shall have access to the records. The written authorization of the patient shall be presented and then maintained in the original record as authority for release of medical information outside the hospital. However, 42 Pennsylvania Consolidated Statutes § 6155 (1991) gives any patient whose medical charts or records are subpoenaed, any person acting on his or her behalf, and the healthcare facility having custody of the charts or records standing to apply to the court for a protective order denying, restricting, or otherwise limiting access to and use of the copies or records. Under 49 Pennsylvania Code § 16.61, revealing personally identifiable facts obtained as a result of the physician-patient rela-

tionship without the prior consent of the patient, except as authorized or required by statute, is unprofessional conduct.

28 Pennsylvania Code § 553.12 gives patients of ambulatory surgical facilities the right to have records pertaining to their medical care treated as confidential except as otherwise provided by law or third-party contractual arrangements.

Section 117.41(6)(8) requires emergency services to have the same policies on confidentiality of emergency room records as those that apply to other hospital medical records. The identity and general condition of the patient may be released to the public after the next of kin have been notified.

Ambulatory surgical facilities must also treat records as confidential, and only authorized personnel shall have access (*id.* § 563.9).

Long-term care nursing facilities must ensure confidentiality of medical records. Patients may approve or refuse the release of their personal and medical records to an individual outside the facility, except in case of a transfer to another healthcare institution or as required by statute or third-party payment contract (*id.* § 201.29). Subscribers of health maintenance organizations (HMOs) have the right to have all records pertaining to his medical care treated as confidential unless disclosure is necessary to interpret the application of the contract to care, or unless disclosure is otherwise provided for by law (*id.* § 9.77(a)(8)).

23 Pennsylvania Consolidated Statutes § 6340(A) and (B) make records of child abuse confidential and prevent disclosure except in limited circumstances.[32]

71 Pennsylvania Consolidated Statutes § 1690.108, discussed in Chapter 9, provides for confidentiality of records of alcohol and drug abuse patients.

RHODE ISLAND

Rhode Island General Laws § 5-37.3-3-2 ((9)(2) (1991), Confidentiality of Health Care Information Act, establishes "safeguards for maintaining the integrity of confidential health care information that relates to an individual." Section 5-37.3-3(c) defines "confidential health care information" as "all information relating to a patient's health care history, diagnosis, condition, treatment, or evaluation obtained from a health care provider who has treated the patient." The statute goes on to require that unless otherwise specifically provided by law, you may not release a patient's confidential healthcare information without the patient's consent or the consent of an authorized representative except

- To a physician, dentist, or other medical personnel who believes in good faith that the information is necessary to diagnose or treat the individual in a medical or dental emergency

- To medical peer review committees or the state board of medical review

---

32. *See* Chapter 8.

- To qualified researchers or auditors, provided they do not identify any individual patient in any report, audit, or evaluation or otherwise disclose patient identities

- To law enforcement personnel if someone is in danger from the patient, the patient tries to get narcotics from the healthcare provider illegally, in child abuse cases, and in gunshot wound cases

- For coordinating healthcare services and to educate and train within the same healthcare facility

- To insurers to adjudicate health insurance claims

- To malpractice insurance carriers or lawyers if the healthcare provider anticipates a medical liability action

- To a court or lawyer or medical liability insurance carrier if a patient brings a medical liability action against the provider

- To public health authorities in order to carry out their functions

- To the state medical examiner in the event of a fatality that comes under his jurisdiction

- Concerning information directly related to a claim for workers' compensation

- To the attorneys for a healthcare provider when release is necessary to receive adequate legal representation

- To school authorities of disease, health screening, or immunization information required by the school, or when a school-age child transfers from one school or school district to another

- To a law enforcement agency to protect the legal interests of an insurance institution agent or insurance support organization in preventing and prosecuting the perpetration of fraud upon them

- To a grand jury or court pursuant to a subpoena when the information is required for the investigation or prosecution of criminal wrongdoing by a healthcare provider and the information is unavailable from any other source

- To the state board of elections pursuant to a subpoena when required to determine the eligibility of a person to vote by mail due to illness or disability

- To certify the nature of permanency of a person's illness or disability, the date when the patient was last examined, and that it would be an undue hardship for the person to vote at the polls so he or she may obtain a mail ballot

- To the central cancer registry

- To the Medicaid fraud control unit of the attorney general's office for the investigation or prosecution of criminal or civil wrongdoing by a healthcare provider in connection with provision of medical care to Medicaid recipients. However, any information so obtained may not be used in any criminal proceeding against the patient on whom the information is obtained (*id.* § 5-37.3-4(b)).

A hospital may release the fact of a patient's admission and a general description of his or her condition to relatives, friends, and the news media.

The statute also provides that third parties receiving a patient's confidential healthcare information must establish security procedures including limiting access to those who have a "need to know"; identifying those who have responsibility for maintaining security procedures for such information; providing a written statement to each employee about the necessity of maintaining the confidentiality of the information and the penalties for unauthorized disclosure; and not taking disciplinary action against anyone who reports a violation of these rules (*id.* § 5-37.3-5(c)).

Section 5-37.3-5(a) establishes requirements for situations in which a patient is denied insurance, benefits, employment, and so forth, and requests amendment or expungement of erroneous information or addition of relevant information.

SOUTH CAROLINA

South Carolina Code § 44-52-190 (Law. Co-op. 1990) makes records of alcohol and drug abuse commitment confidential, as does § 44-20-340 for records of mentally retarded or developmentally disabled patients. Similarly, § 44-23-1090 reiterates confidentiality of patients who are mentally ill or retarded, as does § 44-36-30 for information, biomedical research, or medical data submitted to the Statewide Alzheimer's Disease and Related Disorders Registry.

Sexually transmitted disease records are confidential (*id.* § 44-29-135).[33]

The Bill of Rights for Residents of Long-Term Care Facilities provides for confidential treatment of personal and medical records. It specifies that residents may approve or disapprove release of their personal and medical records to any individual outside the facility, except they may not refuse in the case of transfer to another healthcare institution or when disclosure is required by law or third-party payment contract (*id.* § 44-81-40).

Section 38-33-260 makes health records in the custody of health maintenance organizations (HMOs) confidential.

Records of utilization reviews are also confidential (*id.* § 38-70-20).

---

33. *See* Chapter 10.

The identity of a veteran who may have been exposed to Agent Orange is confidential under the Agent Orange Information and Assistance Program (*id.* § 44-40-5(B)).

South Carolina Department for Health and Environmental Control Regulation for Minimum Standards for Licensing of Hospitals and Institutional General Infirmaries states that medical records will be treated as confidential.[34] Regulation 61-13, § 501 of the South Carolina Code states that medical records of residents of intermediate care facilities for the mentally retarded are confidential.

SOUTH DAKOTA

Administrative Rules of South Dakota 44:04:09:04 (1991) state that hospitals and nursing homes must have written policies and procedures pertaining to the confidentiality and safeguarding of medical records. South Dakota Codified Laws Annotated § 34-20A-91 (1992) requires information used for research into the causes and treatment of alcohol abuse to be kept confidential and not published in a way that discloses patients' names or other identifying information. Section 34-14-1 makes information procured in the course of a medical study strictly confidential and specifies that it may only be used for medical research.

TENNESSEE

Tennessee Code Annotated § 68-11-304 (1991) specifies that hospital records, except as otherwise provided by law, are not public records. Nothing in the medical record statutes should be considered to impair any privilege of confidentiality conferred by law on patients, their personal representatives, or their heirs.

Section 10-7-504 provides that the medical records of patients in state hospitals and medical facilities and those of persons receiving medical treatment, at any expense to the state, are confidential and are not open for public inspection. Any records containing the source of body parts for transplantation or any information concerning persons donating body parts is likewise confidential.

All records and information held by the Department of Health and Environment or a local health department relating to known or suspected cases of sexually transmitted disease are confidential and may only be released in limited circumstances (*id.* § 68-10-113).

The law concerning the rights of nursing home residents and patients states that every nursing home resident has the right to have records kept confidential and private (*id.* § 68-11-901).

---

34. South Carolina Code of Regulations 61-16, § 601.7 (1992).

Under § 68-1-108, the insurance commission may release health insurance entities' report of UB82 claims data for reporting inpatient services, but must keep any individual medical information confidential.

Finally, information furnished to medical review committees is privileged and confidential (*id.* § 63-6-219).

TEXAS

Texas Health and Safety Code Annotated § 81.046 (West 1992) provides for confidentiality of reports, records, and information relating to communicable diseases. For human immunodeficiency virus (HIV) test results, § 81.103(j) adds a criminal penalty for breach of such confidentiality.

Section 161.022 requires confidentiality of information used in medical research and education.

Similarly, §§ 533.010 and 595.001 provide for confidentiality of records of the identity, diagnosis, evaluation, or treatment of any person maintained in connection with the performance of any program or activity relating to mental retardation.

Communications between a patient or client and his or her physician for the purpose of diagnosis, evaluation, or treatment of any mental or emotional disorder are confidential. Also confidential are communications involving the treatment of sex offenders[35] and alcoholism and drug abuse.[36] Such communications will not be disclosed except in the limited circumstances listed in Chapter 9.

Texas Family Code § 34.08 (West 1992) makes reports of child abuse confidential.

Texas Department of Health, Hospital Licensing Standard ch. 12 § 8.7.3.1 (1991), covering special care facilities, states that such a facility shall protect medical records against loss, damage, destruction, and unauthorized use by safeguarding the confidentiality of medical record information and allowing access or release only under court order; by written authorization of the resident unless the physician has documented in the record that to do so would be harmful to the physical, mental, or emotional health of the resident; as allowed by state licensing agency law and rules for licensure inspection purposes and reporting of communicable disease information; or as specifically allowed by federal or state laws relating to facilities caring for residents with acquired immune deficiency syndrome (AIDS) or related disorders.

Under Texas Insurance Code art. 20A.17(c)(2) (West 1992), medical, hospital, and health records of enrollees and records of physicians and providers providing service under an independent contract with a health maintenance organization (HMO) are only subject to such examination as is necessary for an ongoing quality of health assurance program concerning

---

35. Texas Revised Civil Statute art. 4413(51) (West 1992).
36. Texas Code of Criminal Procedure art. 38.101 (West 1992).

healthcare procedures and outcome, in accordance with an approved plan. The plan shall provide for adequate protection of confidentiality of medical information.

UTAH

Utah Code Annotated § 26-25-1(3) (1992) only allows healthcare providers to release confidential information to state agencies, such as the Department of Human Services or the Utah State Medical Association, for efficiency, quality control, and research purposes. Section 26-25-2 places restrictions on the use of such data to ensure confidentiality. Section 26-25-3 provides that all information, including information required for the medical and health section of birth certificates, interviews, reports, statements, memoranda, or other data provided under the Health Code, and any findings or conclusions resulting from medical studies, are privileged communications. Section 26-25-4 adds that all such information must be held in strict confidence and any use, release, or publication resulting therefrom must preclude identification of any person or persons studied. Violation of these statutes is a misdemeanor, and the violator may be civilly liable (*id.* § 26-25-5).

Under § 58-12-43, information relating to the adequacy of quality of medical care provided to state or hospital boards is confidential.

Section 26-25a-101 provides for confidentiality of information regarding communicable or reportable diseases, as does § 62A-4-513 with regard to child abuse reports.

All hospital medical records must be kept confidential. Only authorized personnel may have access to medical records. The patient or his legal representative must give written consent to release medical information to unauthorized persons (Utah Administrative Rules 432-100-7.404 (1990)). Rule 432-100-7.414 requires hospitals to have written policies approved by the medical staff relating to release of information including child abuse records, psychiatric records, and drug and alcohol abuse records and for confidentiality of medical records. Mental retardation facilities shall keep confidential all information contained in clients' records as well as protect records against access by unauthorized individuals (*id.* at 432-152-4.201 and 432-15-4.203). Small healthcare facilities shall protect records against unauthorized access (*id.* at 432-200-6.102) and keep records confidential (*id.* at 432-200-6.103). Rules 432-201-4.201 and 432-201-4.203 establish similar rules for mental retardation facilities, as do rules 432-500-6.104 and 432-500-6.105 for freestanding ambulatory surgical centers and rules 432-600-6.104 and 432-600-6.105 for abortion clinics. Rules 432-550-8 and 432-650-3.206 provide that birthing centers and end-stage renal disease facilities, respectively, shall guard medical records against unauthorized access.

Home health agencies must develop policies that address confidentiality of medical records (*id.* at 432-700-3.701 and 432-700-3.704). In addition, Rule 432-700-3.602 gives home health agency patients the right to be assured confidential treatment of personal and medical records, and to approve or refuse their release to any individual outside the agency, except in the case of transfer to another agency or health facility, or as provided by law or third-party payment contract.

Medical records and audits of health maintenance organizations (HMOs) are confidential,[37] as is information involved in audits of HMOs.[38]

Under the Medical Benefits Recovery Act, medical billing information is confidential.[39] Finally, § 31A-22-617 provides for confidentiality of information in medical records of patients during audits of preferred provider organizations.

VERMONT

Vermont's Bill of Rights for Hospital Patients is contained in Vermont Statutes Annotated tit. 18, § 1852 (1991), which states that patients have the right to expect that all communications and records pertaining to their care shall be treated as confidential. Only medical personnel, individuals directly treating the patient under the supervision of medical personnel, or those persons monitoring the quality of that treatment or researching the effectiveness of that treatment shall have access to the patient's medical records. Others may have access to those records only with the patient's written authorization. Vermont's physician-patient privilege amplifies patients' rights to confidentiality by precluding disclosure of confidential information acquired by a healthcare practitioner in a professional capacity (*id.* tit. 12, § 1612).

Similarly, § 7301, the Nursing Home Residents' Bill of Rights, requires the staff of any facility to ensure that each person admitted to the facility is assured confidential treatment of his or her personal and medical records. Residents may approve or refuse the release of their records to any individual outside the facility, except in case of the resident's transfer to another healthcare institution or as required by law or third-party payment contract (*id.* tit. 33, § 7301).

Title 33, § 7506, specifies that in the absence of either written consent by a complainant or resident of a long-term care facility, or his or her guardian or legal representative, or court order, neither the state ombudsman nor any ombudsman shall disclose the identity of such person.

Vermont law also makes child abuse and neglect reports (*id.* tit. 33, § 4013), tuberculosis reports (*id.* tit. 18, § 1041), and venereal disease reports confidential (*id.* tit. 18, § 1099).

Title 33, § 7112, provides for confidentiality of information received by the licensing agency through filed reports, inspection, or as otherwise specified. It shall not disclose such information publicly in such manner as to identify individuals or facilities.

---

37. Utah Code Annotated § 31A-8-405.
38. *Id.* § 31A-8-404.
39. *Id.* § 26-19-18.

Title 12, § 1705(a), governing human immunodeficiency virus (HIV)–related testing information, provides that Vermont state courts shall not issue any orders requiring the disclosure of individually identifiable HIV-related testing or counseling information unless such court finds that the person seeking the information has demonstrated a compelling need for it that cannot be accommodated by other means. In assessing compelling need the court shall weigh the need for disclosure against the privacy interest of the test subject and the public interest that may be disserved by disclosure that deters future testing or that may lead to discrimination.

Before granting any such limited order to disclose HIV-related testing information, the court shall provide the individual whose test information is in question with notice and a reasonable opportunity to participate in the proceedings if he or she is not already a party (*id.* tit. 12, § 1705(c)).

Court proceedings as to disclosure of counseling and testing information shall be conducted *in camera*, unless the subject of the test agrees to a hearing in open court or unless the court determines that a public hearing is necessary to the public interest and the proper administration of justice (*id.* tit. 12, § 1705(d)).

Upon issuance of an order to disclose test results, the court shall impose appropriate safeguards against unauthorized disclosure, which shall specify the persons who may have access to the information, the purposes for which the information shall be used, and appropriate prohibitions on future disclosure (*id.* tit. 12, § 1705(e)).

Any party issuing pleadings pertaining to disclosure of HIV-related testing or counseling information shall substitute a pseudonym for the true name of the subject of the test. The subject's true name shall be communicated confidentially to the court and those parties who have a compelling need to know the subject's true name. All documents filed with the court that identify the subject's true name shall not be disclosed to any person other than those parties who have a compelling need to know the subject's true name and the subject of the test. All such documents shall be sealed upon the conclusion of proceedings (*id.* tit. 12, § 1705(b)).

In addition, title 18, § 7103(a) specifies that all certificates, applications, records, and reports (other than an order of a court made for the purposes of this part of this title), which directly or indirectly identify a patient, former patient, or an individual whose hospitalization or care has been sought, together with any clinical information relating to such persons, shall be kept confidential and shall not be disclosed by any person except insofar as

- The individual identified or his or her legal guardian, if any (or, if he or she is a minor, the parent or legal guardian), shall consent in writing

- Disclosure may be necessary to carry out any of the provisions of this part

- A court may direct on its determination that disclosure is necessary for the conduct of proceedings before it and that failure to make disclosure would be contrary to the public interest

Nothing in this section shall preclude disclosure, on proper inquiry, of information concerning the medical condition to the members of the family of a patient or to his or her clergyman, physician, attorney, or an interested party (*id.* tit. 18, § 7103(b)). Further, any person violating this section shall be fined not more than $500.00 or imprisoned for not more than one year, or both (*id.* tit. 18, § 7103(c)).

VIRGINIA

Several provisions of the Virginia Code address confidentiality of medical record information. For example, Virginia Annotated Code § 32.1-36.1 (Michie 1991) provides for confidentiality of test results for human immunodeficiency virus (HIV).

Under § 32.1-138, patients in nursing homes are assured confidential treatment of personal and medical records and may approve or refuse their release to any individual outside the facility, except in case of transfer to another healthcare institution or as required by law or third-party payment contract.

Section 32.1-74.4 makes information released to the Commissioner of Health concerning Alzheimer's disease and related disorders confidential. No publication of information, biomedical research, or medical data shall be made that identifies the patients.

Private review agents must ensure that patient-specific medical records and information are kept strictly confidential except as authorized by the patient or by regulations (*id.* § 38.2-5302).

Investigative information acquired by the Department of Health Professions medical complaint investigative committee or the Board of Medicine in connection with possible disciplinary proceedings is confidential (*id.* § 54.1-2910).

Department of Health, Rules and Regulations for the Licensure of Hospitals in Virginia Part III, § 208.6 (1982), specifies that medical records shall be kept confidential, that only authorized personnel shall have access to the records, and that the hospital shall release copies thereof only with the written consent of the patient, his legal representative, or to duly authorized state or federal health authorities or others authorized by the Virginia Code or federal statutes. If the patient is a minor, his parent, guardian, or legal representative must provide the consent. Under § 208.6.3, the hospital's permanent record may be removed from the hospital's jurisdiction only in accordance with a court order, subpoena, or statute. The same rules apply to nursing homes.[40]

WASHINGTON

A number of sections of the Revised Code of Washington make patient records confidential. For example, § 71.05.630 (1991) provides that treatment records of mental illness patients are confidential and may only be released as de-

---

40. Department of Health, Rules and Regulations for the Licensure of Nursing Homes in Virginia Part III, §§ 24.3 and 24.3.3 (1991).

tailed in Chapter 8. Similarly, §§ 42.48.020 and 42.48.040 provide for the confidentiality of records used for research purposes, while § 70.168.090 provides for confidentiality of patient care quality assurance proceedings, records, and reports. Records of human immunodeficiency virus (HIV) antibody testing and testing or treatment records of sexually transmitted disease patients (*id.* § 70.24.105), as well as records of alcoholics and intoxicated persons, are confidential (*id.* § 70.96A.150). Further, § 70.127.140 provides for patients' rights to have their records treated confidentially by home health, hospice, and home care agencies.

Hospitals must establish policies and procedures that govern access to and release of data in patients' individual medical records and other medical data, taking into consideration the confidential nature of these records.[41] These records and other personal or medical data on patients must be handled and stored so they are not accessible to unauthorized persons.

WEST VIRGINIA

A number of West Virginia Code sections and regulations provide for confidentiality. For example, West Virginia Legislature, Title 64 West Virginia Legislative Rule 16-5C Department of the Board of Health, series 13, § 9.7 (1987), covers nursing home patients' rights to confidentiality. The rule states that patients are assured confidential treatment of their personal and healthcare records and condition. Such information shall not be discussed, without the patient's consent, with persons not treating or caring for the patient. A patient has the right to refuse release of his or her personal or healthcare records to any individual outside the facility, except as required by law or third-party payment contracts. A specific release signed by the patient is required for all other releases. A prior-executed, blanket release is not acceptable.

Similarly, West Virginia Code § 27-3-1 (1992) provides for confidentiality of communications and treatment of mentally ill patients, including the fact that a person is or has been a client or patient, and provides limited circumstances under which confidential information may be disclosed.

Section 16-3C-3 makes the identity of a person on whom a human immunodeficiency virus (HIV)–related test is performed or the results of such a test confidential, with disclosure permitted only in the circumstances detailed in Chapter 10.

Section 33-25A-26 makes confidential any data or information pertaining to the diagnosis, treatment, or health of any enrollee or applicant, that a health maintenance organization (HMO) obtains from the person or a healthcare provider. The information may not be disclosed except

- As necessary to facilitate an assessment of the quality of care or to review the complaint system

---

41. Washington Administrative Code § 248-18-440 (1986).

- On the express written consent of the enrollee or legally authorized representative

- Pursuant to statute or court order

- In the event of a claim or litigation between such person and the HMO in which such data or information is pertinent

Further, the HMO may claim any privileges against disclosure that a provider could claim (*id.*).

Section 16-4A-3 makes laboratory reports of blood tests for syphilis of pregnant women confidential. Similarly, information received by the State Department of Health to enforce its rules and regulations is confidential.

WISCONSIN

Under Wisconsin law, all healthcare records are confidential and may only be released on informed consent or to those listed in Wisconsin Statutes § 146.82 (1990).[42]

In addition, records concerning individuals who have received services for mental illness, developmental disabilities, alcoholism, or drug dependence are confidential and may be released only pursuant to informed consent or as provided for by the statute (*id.* 51.30(2)). Similarly, § 51.45 provides for confidentiality of registration and treatment records of alcoholism treatment programs and facilities. Section 254.07 makes reports, examinations, inspections, and all records concerning sexually transmitted diseases confidential.

Finally, Wisconsin Administrative Code § HSS 92.03 (June 1986) establishes further rights to privacy for patients who received treatment for mental illness, developmental disability, and alcohol and drug abuse, except those provided by individual practitioners. Under § HSS 92.03 such records that in any way identify a patient are confidential and may be released only on informed consent by the patient or

- For management audits, financial audits, or program monitoring and evaluation

- For billing or collection

- For research

- By court order

- For progress determination and to determine adequacy of treatment

- Within the department

---

42. See also Chapters 8 through 12.

- In medical emergencies

- To facilities receiving an involuntarily committed person

- To correctional facilities or probation and parole agencies

- To counsel, guardians *ad litem,* counsel for the interest of the public, and court-appointed examiners

- To correctional officers of a change in status

- Between a social services department and a 51 Board

- Between subunits of a human services department and between the human services department and contracted service providers

- To law enforcement officers when necessary to return a patient on unauthorized absence from the facility

WYOMING

Wyoming Statutes § 35-2-609 (1991) provides that hospitals may not disclose any healthcare information about a patient to any other person without the patient's written authorization, except as authorized under § 35-2-606 (relating to disclosure to other providers who are providing care, for research, and so forth). Section 35-2-606(c), providing for such disclosure, requires that the receiver use reasonable care to protect the confidentiality of the information.

CHAPTER 8

Disclosure on Request

Introduction

Most states have statutes or administrative regulations that provide for patients and others to have access to medical records on request. Some are quite detailed, such as California's.[1] Others say little more than that patients are to have access to their records. If your state does not have a detailed procedure in its statutes or regulations or your licensing body does not have a detailed procedure in its rules, you should carefully consider a procedure and adopt one in your bylaws in order to allow for authorized access while maintaining confidentiality.[2]

Federal Laws

The Freedom of Information Act does not apply to private facilities, but rather to federal agencies. And medical information is not covered by the Act.[3]

The Occupational Safety and Health Administration (OSHA) requires that employers provide employees access to required medical records of employees exposed to toxic substances and harmful physical agents. On receiving a request from an employee or his designated representative, the employer must provide a copy of the record within 15 days.[4]

The Social Security Administration (SSA) and the Department of Health and Human Services (HHS) note that an individual can request medical records held by the SSA if the requesting person names a representative. Failure to name a representative may result in denial of request.[5]

45 C.F.R. § 5b.6 (1991) contains regulations and procedures relating to a person's access to medical and psychological records held by HHS.

1. California Civil Code §§ 56.10 and 56.105 (Deering 1992); California Evidence Code § 1158 (Deering 1992); California Code of Regulations tit. 22, § 70751(a) (1991).
2. *See* the discussion on security in Chapter 5 and privacy in Chapter 7.
3. 5 U.S.C. § 552 (1992).
4. 29 C.F.R. § 1910.20 (1991).
5. 20 C.F.R. § 401.410 (1991).

State Laws

ALABAMA

After noting that medical records are confidential, Alabama Administrative Code r. 420-5-7.07 (1990), concerning the Rules of the Alabama State Board of Health Division of Licensure and Certification, specifies that access to medical records shall be determined by the hospital governing board.

ALASKA

Alaska Statutes § 18.23.065 (1991) provides that patients are entitled to inspect and copy any record.

ARIZONA

Arizona's Compilation of Administrative Rules and Regulations 9-10-221 (1982), concerning healthcare institution licensure rules, specifies that medical record information shall be released only with the written consent of the patient, the legal guardian, or in accordance with law.

ARKANSAS

Arkansas' rules simply state that written consent of the patient or legal guardian shall be presented as authority for the release of medical information.[6]

However, Arkansas law, which permits patients' access to their medical records, requires healthcare providers to furnish copies of such records and limits the amount that a provider may charge for copying the records.[7] For example, in contemplation of preparation for, or use in, any legal proceeding, any current or former patient of a doctor, hospital, or other medical institution is entitled to obtain access, personally or through his or her attorney, to the information in the patient's medical records, on request and with written patient authorization. The doctor, hospital, or other medical institution must furnish copies of all medical records on the patient's tender of the cost of the copies.[8]

CALIFORNIA

California Health and Safety Code § 1795.12(b) and (c) (Deering 1992) provides access for patients or their representatives to their medical records in licensed health facilities on payment of reasonable clerical costs. The facility must provide for patient inspection within five working days and provide copies within 15 working days of the request and payment of fees. The

---

6. Arkansas Register 0601 U.
7. Arkansas Code Annotated § 16-46-106 (Michie 1992).
8. *Id.* § 16-46-106(a)(1).

facility may not refuse access to any person because such person has an unpaid bill for healthcare services (*id.* § 1795.12(g)). Further, a healthcare provider will not be liable to the patient or any other person for any consequences resulting from disclosure of patient records as required by this provision. However, a healthcare provider may not discriminate against classes or categories of providers in the transmittal of x rays or other patient records (*id.* § 1795.12(e)). Minors may only inspect their records if the records cover care to which a minor is lawfully able to consent (*id.*).

In lieu of granting full access to a patient's record, § 1795.20 allows healthcare providers to prepare a summary of the record. The healthcare provider must first confer with the patient in an attempt to clarify the patient's purpose and goal in obtaining his or her record. If as a consequence the patient requests information about only certain injuries, illnesses, or episodes, the provider is not required to prepare the summary for other than the injuries, illnesses, or episodes.

The summary shall contain for each injury, illness, or episode requested any information included in the record relative to the following:

- Chief complaint or complaints including pertinent history

- Findings from consultations and referrals to other healthcare providers

- Diagnosis, where determined

- Treatment plan and regimen including medications prescribed

- Progress of the treatment

- Prognosis including significant continuing problems or conditions

- Pertinent reports of diagnostic procedures and tests and all discharge summaries

- Objective findings from the most recent physical examination, such as blood pressure, weight, and actual values from routine laboratory tests

California's Confidentiality of Medical Information Act, California Civil Code § 56.10(c)(1)–(11) (Deering 1992), provides for disclosure of medical records on request to

- Providers of health care or other healthcare professionals or facilities for purposes of diagnosis or treatment

- An insurer, employer, healthcare service plan, hospital service plan, employee benefit plan, governmental authority, or any other entity responsible for paying for healthcare services rendered to the patient, as needed to determine responsibility for payment and for payment to be made

- Persons or entities that provide billing, claims management, medical data processing, or other administrative services for providers

- Organized committees and agents of professional societies or medical staffs or professional standards review organizations or to those insuring, responsible for, or defending professional liability that a provider may incur if such recipients are engaged in reviewing the competence or qualifications of healthcare professionals or reviewing healthcare services with respect to medical necessity, level of care, quality of care, or justification of charges

- Those responsible for licensing or accrediting

- The county coroner in the course of an investigation by his office

- Public agencies, clinical investigators, healthcare research organizations, and accredited public or private nonprofit educational or healthcare institutions for bona fide research purposes so long as no further disclosure by the recipient identifies the patient

- A provider of health care that has created medical information as a result of employment-related healthcare services to an employee (conducted at the specific prior written request and expense of the employer) may disclose to the employer that part of the information relevant in a lawsuit, arbitration, grievance, or other claim or challenge to which the employer and employee are parties and in which the patient has placed in issue his or her medical history, condition, or treatment and that describes functional limitations of the patient that may entitle him or her to leave from work for medical reasons or limit fitness to perform his or her employment.

- Unless informed in writing of an agreement to the contrary, to a sponsor, insurer, or administrator of a plan or policy under which the patient seeks coverage or benefits

- A group practice prepayment healthcare service plan

- An insurance institution, agent, or support organization that has complied with the requirements of the Insurance Code

Patients demanding settlement of actions against healthcare providers must authorize the providers to disclose medical information requested by persons or organizations insuring, responsible for, or defending professional liability actions. Such parties requesting disclosure must furnish notice of the request to the patient or his or her legal representative (*id.* § 56.105).

California Evidence Code § 1158 (Deering 1992) also requires healthcare providers to disclose a patient's records for inspection and copying on presentation of that patient's written authorization. The patient authorizing the disclosure is liable for reasonable costs of such inspection and copying.

California Code of Regulations tit. 22, § 70751(a) (1991) requires hospitals to maintain patient health records in such form as to be legible and readily available on the request of the admitting physician; the nonphysician granted privileges; the hospital or its medical staff, or any authorized officer, agent, or employee of either; authorized representatives of the Health Department; and any other person authorized by law to make such a request.

In addition to general acute care hospitals, Title 22 regulations specify that the following other types of facilities must maintain patient records available at the request of various authorized parties:

- Acute psychiatric hospitals (*id.* § 71551(a))

- Skilled nursing facilities (*id.* § 72543(a))

- Intermediate care facilities (*id.* § 73543(a))

- Home health agencies (*id.* § 74731(b))

- Primary care clinics (*id.* § 75055(a))

- Psychology clinics (*id.* § 75343(a))

- Psychiatric health facilities (*id.* § 77143(a))

- Adult day health facilities (*id.* § 78435(b))

- Chemical dependency recovery hospitals (*id.* § 79351(a))

COLORADO

Colorado Revised Statute § 25-1-801(1) (1991) allows patients in healthcare facilities or their designated representatives to inspect their records, other than those relating to psychiatric or psychological problems or those that an independent third-party psychiatrist believes would have a significant negative impact on the patient, at reasonable times and on reasonable notice. The patient or his representative is also entitled to a summary of his psychiatric or psychological problems following termination of the treatment program. Following the patient's discharge, he is entitled, on submission of a written authorization/request for records, and payment of reasonable costs, to have copies of his records, including x rays.

This statute does not require a person responsible for the diagnosis or treatment of venereal diseases or addiction to or use of drugs, in the case of minors, to release records of such diagnosis or treatment to a parent, guardian, or anyone other than the minor or a designated representative.

The attending healthcare provider or a designated representative shall note all requests by patients for inspection of their medical records made under this section with the time and date of the patient's request and the time and date of inspection. The patient shall acknowledge inspection by dating and signing the record file (*id.* § 25-1-801(2)).

Section 25-1-802 contains virtually identical language covering patient records in the custody of individual healthcare providers.

CONNECTICUT

Connecticut General Statutes § 20-7c (1990) requires healthcare providers to supply a patient, upon his or her request, complete and current information possessed by that provider concerning any diagnosis, treatment, and prognosis of the patient. Upon written request, the provider, except as provided in § 4-194, shall furnish the patient with a copy of his or her health record at a cost of not more than 25 cents per page plus postage. If the provider reasonably determines that the information is detrimental to the health of the patient or could cause harm to the patient or another, the provider may withhold the information from the patient. The provider, however, may supply the records to another provider or an appropriate third party. Further, the patient may, in writing, request that the provider furnish a copy of the medical records to another provider (*id.* § 20-7d).

Under § 17a-630, medical treatment facilities shall not disclose the fact that a minor sought treatment or rehabilitation for alcohol or drug abuse to the parents or legal guardian without his or her consent.

DELAWARE

Delaware Code Annotated tit. 16, § 1121(b) (1991), governing the rights of patients in sanatoria, rest homes, nursing homes, boarding homes, and related institutions, specifies that such facilities shall treat personal and medical records confidentially and not make them public without the consent of the patient or resident.

Section 1203 permits disclosure of human immunodeficiency virus (HIV)–related test information to the subject of the test or a legal guardian.[9] Further, the code defines "release of test results" as "written authorization for disclosure of HIV-related test results which is signed, dated and which specifies to whom disclosure is authorized and the time period during which the release is to be effective." (*id.* § 1201).

Delaware Code tit. 25, § 4306 gives any person who is legally liable, or against whom someone has asserted a claim for compensation for injuries, permission to examine the records of any association, corporation, or other institution or body maintaining a hospital in reference to the treatment, care, and maintenance of the injured person.

DISTRICT OF COLUMBIA

District of Columbia Code Annotated § 14-307(a) (1991) provides that a physician or surgeon may disclose confidential information acquired in the course of treating a patient only with the patient's consent. The statute has been construed to apply to hospital records, also.

---

9. *See also* Chapters 10 through 12.

FLORIDA

Florida Statutes ch. 395.017(1) (1991) requires that any licensed facility shall, on request, and only after discharge of the patient, furnish to any person previously admitted for care and treatment, to that person's guardian, curator, or personal representative, or to anyone designated by such person in writing a true and correct copy of all of that patient's records, including x rays, in possession of the licensed facility. However, healthcare providers do not have to furnish progress notes and consultation report sections of a psychiatric nature concerning the care and treatment performed by the licensed facility.

The person requesting such records must agree to pay a reasonable charge for copying the records. Licensed facilities shall further allow any such person to examine the original records, microfilms, or other suitable reproductions of the records in the facility's possession on such reasonable terms as shall be imposed to ensure that the records will not be damaged, destroyed, or altered.[10]

Florida Statutes ch. 455.241 requires the same access on request to records of psychiatric patients as does chapter 400.145 for records of nursing home residents.

Chapter 766.204(1) requires that copies of any medical record relevant to any litigation of a medical negligence claim or defense shall be provided to a claimant or a defendant, or to the attorney thereof, at a reasonable charge within 10 business days of a request for copies.

Florida Administrative Code r. 10D-29.118(10) provides that nursing homes, unless expressly prohibited by a legally competent resident, shall furnish to the spouse, guardian, or responsible party of a current or former resident, within 10 days of receipt of a written request, a copy of that resident's records that are in possession of the facility. Such records shall include medical and psychiatric records and any records concerning the care and treatment of the resident performed in the facility, except progress notes and consultation report sections of a psychiatric nature. Copies of such records are not part of a deceased resident's estate and may be made available prior to the administration of an estate. The facility may charge a reasonable fee for the copying of resident records. No persons may obtain copies of resident's records more often than once per month, except that physician reports in the resident's records may be obtained as often as necessary to effectively monitor the resident's condition. The facility shall allow any such spouse, guardian, or responsible party to reasonably examine original records in its possession (or microfilm or other suitable reproductions of the record) to help ensure that the records are not damaged, destroyed, or altered.

Rule 21D-17.0055 requires chiropractors to release copies of patient medical records on request of the patient or his legal representative.

---

10. Florida Administrative Code r. 10D-28.158(5) (1991).

GEORGIA

Official Code of Georgia Annotated § 31-33-2 (Michie 1991) governs instances when healthcare providers must furnish medical records on request. (Psychiatric, psychological, or other mental health records, however, are governed by § 31-33-4.) On receipt of a written request from the patient, you shall furnish a complete and current copy of the records to the patient, to any designated healthcare provider, or to any other person the patient designates unless disclosure would be detrimental to the physical or mental health of the patient. In such cases, you need not provide the record except to healthcare providers designated by the patient (*id.* § 31-33-2). The requester is responsible for paying the costs of copying and mailing the records unless they are records requested to apply for a disability benefit. You may require payment before you provide the records. Under § 33-33-5, if you provide records in good faith, you are not civilly or criminally liable for such release. Otherwise, however, the records remain confidential (*id.* § 31-33-6).

HAWAII

Under Hawaii Revised Statute § 622-57 (1991), if a healthcare provider's patient requests copies of his or her medical records, the facility shall make them available unless in the opinion of the provider obtaining such records would be detrimental to the patient's health. In such case, the provider shall advise the patient that it will make copies of the records available to the patient's attorney on presentation of a proper authorization signed by the patient.

If a patient's attorney requests copies of the patient's medical records and presents proper authorization from the patient, the facility must provide complete and accurate copies within 10 working days. The requester must pay reasonable costs for making copies of the records.

As a note, § 321-267 provides authority for the attorney general to represent a class of veterans or exposed residents, who may have been injured by Agent Orange or other agents, to obtain individual medical records.

IDAHO

Idaho law does not specify any particular requirements for release of medical records on request.[11]

ILLINOIS

Illinois Revised Statutes, ch. 110, ¶ 8-2001 (1985), requires every hospital to permit any patient it has treated and discharged, or the patient's attorney, to examine and copy the patient's records on request. The request must be in

---

11. *See* Chapters 7 and 9 through 12 for the confidentiality requirements and disclosure rules.

writing and be delivered to the hospital administrator. The hospital must comply within 60 days of receipt of the request.

Paragraph 8-2003 also requires physicians to permit patients' attorneys access to patient records and the right to copy them.

Records of clinical psychologists may not be examined or copied by patients, unless ordered by a court for good cause shown (*id.* ¶ 8-2004).

Under ch. 91 ½, ¶ 805, release of records relating to the care and treatment of patients with mental health problems or developmental disabilities may only be made on the written consent of the patient or a person authorized to consent for the patient.

Chapter 111 ½, ¶ 6358-2, provides that records of patients treated for alcohol or drug abuse may be disclosed with the prior written consent of the patient, but only under such circumstances as prescribed by the Department of Alcoholism and Substance Abuse. Illinois Administrative Code tit. 77, § 2058.318(a) (1991), by referring to 42 C.F.R. § 2.31(a) (1991), specifies that a written release must contain the

- Specific name or general designation of the program or person permitted to make the disclosure

- Name or title of the individual or name of the organization to which disclosure is to be made

- Name of patient

- Identification of the specific information to be released

- Reason for the release or disclosure

- Date on which the consent is signed

- Signature of the patient or patient's representative if patient is a minor (*id., referring to* 42 C.F.R § 2.14 (1991)) or incompetent (*id., referring to* 42 C.F.R § 2.15 (1991))

- A statement that the consent is subject to revocation at any time, except to the extent that the program or person who is to make the disclosure has already acted in reliance on the consent

- Date, event, or condition on which the consent will expire, if not revoked

The Illinois Administrative Code only recommends that hospitals issue definite policies and procedures pertaining to the use of medical records and the release of medical record information (*id.* § 250.1510(b)(5)).

INDIANA

Indiana Code 16-4-8-2(a) and (b), concerning access to health records, states that a provider shall furnish to the patient or the patient's designee the health records possessed by that provider concerning the patient. The provider shall furnish the records on written request at reasonable notice and may charge its total actual costs for the service. The provider may comply by supplying either

- A copy of the patient's health record, used in assessing the patient's health condition, or

- At the option of the patient, the pertinent portion of patient's health record relating to a specific condition, as requested by the patient

However, information concerning contact lenses may be given in general terms.

A request made under this section is valid for 60 days after the date the request is made (*id.* § 16-4-8-2(c)). On the patient's written request, under § 16-4-8-2.1, the provider shall provide the patient, or his or her designee, access to or a copy of the patient's x rays on payment of actual costs.

However, information may be withheld if a provider, as a healthcare professional, reasonably determines that the information requested is detrimental to the physical or mental health of the patient, or is likely to cause the patient to harm himself or another (*id.* § 16-4-8-6).

Section 16-4-8-3 specifies that healthcare records may be requested by a competent patient if the patient is emancipated and less than 18 years old, or if the patient is at least 18 years of age. However, if the patient is mentally incompetent, the request may be made by parent, guardian, or custodian of the patient.

Healthcare records of a deceased patient may be requested by the personal representative of the patient's estate. If the deceased does not have a personal representative, the spouse of the deceased patient may make a request, or, if no spouse exists, a child of the deceased patient (or the parent, guardian, or custodian of the child if the child is mentally incompetent) may make a request.

However, § 16-4-8-7 does not authorize a patient to obtain a copy of his health records while he is an inpatient of a hospital, health facility, or facility licensed under §§ 16-14-1 or 16-16-1. Notwithstanding this, during this time, if the patient is

- Unemancipated and less than 18 years old, then a parent, guardian, or next of kin (if the patient does not have a parent or guardian) is entitled to obtain a copy of the healthcare records

- Incompetent to request his own health records, then a spouse, parent, guardian, or next of kin (if the patient does not have a parent, spouse, or guardian) is entitled to obtain a copy of the healthcare records

- Competent, then a spouse, parent, or next of kin (if the patient does not have a parent or spouse) is entitled to obtain a copy of the healthcare records, if the inpatient requests that the records be released

Section 16-4-8-4 specifies that request for healthcare records must contain the name and address of the patient and provider, the person or organization to which disclosure is to be made, a statement that the request may be revoked by the patient, the specific information requested, the date of the request, and the signature of the patient.

Hospitals must keep their hospital medical records in such a manner that the information may be made readily available in written or printed form to authorized persons only (*id.* § 34-3-15.4). "Authorized persons" include

- The patient

- A person authorized by the patient to request the records, if the authorization was made in writing not more than 60 days before the date of the request for the records

- Physicians or other professionals within the hospital

- A person entitled to request health records, as discussed above in § 16-4-8-3

- A coroner who is investigating a death under § 36-2-14-6

- Any other person designated by order of a court of competent jurisdiction

Insurance companies may also obtain health records or medical information with a written consent (*id.* § 16-4-8-5).

IOWA

Iowa Code § 229.25 (1991), providing for confidentiality of medical records of mentally ill persons, specifies that the records maintained by a hospital or other facility, relating to the examination, custody, care, and treatment of any person in the facility, may be released to the person who is hospitalized once that person signs an informed consent to release the information. If the patient is a minor or not competent to sign an informed consent, the patient's guardian may sign instead. Each signed consent shall designate specifically the person or agency to whom the information is to be sent, and the facility may only send the information to that person or agency. The facility may also release such information to a licensed physician, attorney, or advocate who provides the chief medical officer with a written waiver signed by the person about whom the information is sought.

The subject of a human immunodeficiency virus (HIV)–related test or his or her guardian may execute a written release of the test results under § 141.23(1)(a) and (b), subject to the provisions of § 141.22(2) (governing disclosure of positive HIV-related tests of minors).

Section 249D.42(7) gives the long-term care resident's advocate access to residents' personal and medical records and access to other records maintained by the facilities or governmental agencies pertaining only to the person on whose behalf a complaint is being investigated.

Iowa Administrative Code r. 481-81.13(5)(e) (1990) specifies that residents of nursing facilities may approve or refuse the release of personal and clinical records to any person outside the facility. This right of refusal does not apply when the facility transfers the resident to another healthcare institution or when record release is required by law or third-party payment contract.

Rule 481-63.38(135C) notes that facilities for the mentally retarded shall require written consent for release of confidential information to persons not otherwise authorized by law to receive it. Only personnel concerned with the financial affairs of the resident may have access to financial records. The resident, or his or her responsible party, shall be entitled to examine all information contained in the resident's record and shall have the right to secure full copies of the record at reasonable cost on request, unless the physician determines that disclosure is contraindicated, in which case the facility will delete this information prior to making the record available. The facility must document the determination and the reasons for it in the record. Rule 481-57.40(135C) has identical provisions governing records of residential care facilities, as does Rule 481-59.49(135C) for skilled nursing facilities and Rule 481-58.44(135C) for intermediate care facilities.

KANSAS

Kansas Statutes Annotated § 59-2931(a)(1) (1990) provides the conditions under which medical treatment records of mentally ill patients or former patients may be disclosed:

- On the written consent of the patient or former patient if that person is an adult who has no guardian; the patient's or former patient's guardian, if any; or a parent, if the patient or former patient is less than 18 years old, except that a patient or former patient who is 14 or more years of age and who requested voluntary admission shall have capacity to consent to release of the records without parental consent. The head of any treatment facility, other than an adult care home, who has the records may refuse to disclose portions of such records if that person states in writing that such disclosure will be injurious to the welfare of the patient or former patient.

- On the sole consent of the head of the treatment facility who has the records after a written statement by that person that such disclosure is necessary for the treatment of the patient or former patient. The head may make such disclosure to the patient or any former patient, the former patient's next of kin, any state or national accreditation agency or scholarly investigator without making such determination. But the head of the treatment facility shall require, before such disclosure is made, a pledge from any state or national accreditation agency or scholarly investigator that such agency or investigator will not disclose the name of any patient or former patient to any person not authorized by law to receive such information (*id.* § 59-2931(a)(2)).

- On the order of any court of record after a determination by the court issuing the order that such records are necessary for the conduct of proceedings before it and are otherwise admissible as evidence (*id.* § 59-2931(a)(3))

- In proceedings under this act, on oral or written request of any attorney representing the patient, former patient, or applicant (*id.* § 59-2931(a)(4))

- To appropriate administrative or professional staff of the Department of Corrections whenever patients have been administratively transferred to the state security hospital or other state psychiatric institutions (*id.* § 59-2931(a)(4))

Similarly, disclosure may be made without the patient's consent for records of the treatment of drug abusers (*id.* § 65-5225(a)(2)(A)) and the treatment of alcohol abusers (*id.* § 65-4050).[12]

KENTUCKY

Patient information shall be released only on authorization of the patient, the patient's guardian, or the executor of his estate.[13]

LOUISIANA

Louisiana Revised Statutes Annotated § 40:2144(B)–(D) (West 1991) states that the information contained in a patient's hospital records is subject to reasonable access by that patient or an authorized representative. On written request, signed by the patient or authorized representatives, the hospital shall furnish the records as soon as practicable and on payment of reasonable costs. The only exception to this procedure is if good cause is shown, for example, if release of the patient's records is medically contraindicated. The hospital and its employees, acting in good faith, are justified in relying on the reasonable representations of the requester and may not be held liable for damages for complying or inability to comply with the request.

Section 40:1299.96(A)(1), concerning healthcare information and records, states that each healthcare provider shall furnish each patient, on request of the patient, a copy of any information related in any way to the patient that the healthcare provider has transmitted to any company, or any public or private agency, or any person.

Section 40:1299.96(A)(2)(b) states that a patient or his legal representative, or in the case of a deceased patient, the executor of the will, the admin-

---

12. *See* Chapter 9 for details.
13. 902 Kentucky Administrative Regulations 20:016 § 3(11)(c) (1991).

istrator of the estate, the surviving spouse, the parents, or the children of the deceased patient, seeking any medical, hospital, or other record relating to the patient's medical treatment, history, or condition, either personally or through an attorney, shall have a right to obtain a copy of such record on furnishing a signed authorization and on payment of a reasonable copying charge. This charge is not to exceed $1 per page for the first 25 pages, 50 cents per page thereafter, a handling charge not to exceed $10 for hospitals and $5 for other healthcare providers, and actual postage. The individuals named herein shall also have the right to obtain copies of patient x rays on payment of reasonable reproduction costs. In the event a hospital record is not complete, the copy of the records furnished hereunder may indicate, by use of a stamp, cover sheet, or otherwise, that the record is incomplete.

Section 40:1299.96(A)(2)(c), further states that if a copy of the record is not provided within a reasonable time, not to exceed 15 days following the receipt of the request and written authorization, and production of the record is obtained through a court order or subpoena *duces tecum,* the healthcare provider shall be liable for reasonable attorney fees and expenses incurred in obtaining the court order or subpoena *duces tecum.* Such sanctions shall not be imposed unless the person requesting the copy of the record has by certified mail notified the healthcare provider of his failure to comply with the original request, by referring to the sanctions available, and the healthcare provider fails to furnish the requested copies within five days from the receipt of such notice. Except for their own gross negligence, such healthcare providers shall not otherwise be held liable in damages by reason of their compliance with such request or their inability to fulfill the request.

A healthcare provider may deny access to a record if the healthcare provider reasonably concludes that knowledge of the information contained in the record would be injurious to the health or welfare of the patient or could reasonably be expected to endanger the life or safety of any other person (*id.* § 40:1299.96(A)(2)(d)).

Section 44:7(B), concerning public records, provides that the governing authority of each public hospital, adult or juvenile correctional institution, public mental health center, or public state school for the mentally deficient may make and enforce rules under which these charts, records, reports, documents, or other memoranda may be exhibited, or copied by or for persons legitimately and properly interested in the disease, physical or mental, or in the condition of patients.

Section 40:2013.3 requires superintendents of all hospitals caring for mentally ill patients that are administered by the Department of Health and Human Resources to furnish, on written request of a coroner of the parish from which the patient was committed, a report on patient's condition that specifies

- Diagnosis

- Laboratory findings

- Treatment prescribed

- Prognosis

On the written request of the attorney of the patient or a near relative, the hospital superintendent shall make the patient's medical record available for inspection by such attorney or relative at such time as may be fixed by the superintendent.

Section 23:1127(A), concerning worker's compensation records, provides that in any claim for compensation, a healthcare provider who has at any time treated the employee shall release any requested medical information and records relative to the employee's injury to the employee, employer, or its worker's compensation insurer or the agent or representative of the employee, employer, or the worker's compensation insurer. Any information relative to any other treatment or condition shall be available to the employer or the worker's compensation insurer by subpoena or through a written release by the claimant.

Any medical information released pursuant to this section shall be released in writing, and a copy shall be furnished to the employee at no cost simultaneously with its provision to the employer or its insurer. Such records or information furnished to the employer or insurer shall be held confidential by them, and the employer or insurer shall be liable to the employee for any actual damages sustained by him or her as a result of a breach of this confidence up to a maximum of $1,000, plus all reasonable attorney fees necessary to recover such damages. An exception to this breach of confidentiality shall be any introduction or use of such information in a court of law, or before the Office of Worker's Compensation Administration or the Louisiana Worker's Compensation Second Injury Board (*id.* § 23:1127(B)).

MAINE

Maine Revised Statutes Annotated tit. 22, § 1711 (West 1991), provides for patient access to hospital medical records, if the patient makes a written request. On such a request, the hospital shall make copies available within a reasonable time unless, in the opinion of the hospital, it would be detrimental to the health of the patient to obtain the records. In that event, the hospital shall advise the patient that it will make copies available to the patient's representative on presentation of a proper authorization signed by the patient. If a patient's authorized representative requests, in writing, a copy of the patient's records and presents a proper authorization from the patient, the hospital will provide copies within a reasonable time.

The hospital may require the requester to pay reasonable costs prior to responding to the request.

State of Maine, Regulations Governing Licensure and Functioning of General and Specialty Hospitals, ch. XII, § (A)(2) (1972), states that hospitals may require the requester to pay reasonable costs prior to responding to the request. However, the written consent of the patient is authority for release of medical information.

The state's law on release of human immunodeficiency virus (HIV) infection status is more specific, requiring that the patient elect, in writing, whether to authorize release of that portion of the record containing the HIV infection status information at or near the time the entry is made.[14]

MARYLAND

Maryland Health–General Code § 4-301(a) (1991), effective July 1, 1991, provides definitions relating to disclosure of medical records. It defines "person in interest" as

- An adult on whom a healthcare provider maintains a medical record

- A person authorized to consent to health care for an adult consistent with the authority granted

- A duly appointed personal representative of a deceased person

- A minor, if the medical record concerns treatment to which the minor has the right to consent and has consented

- A parent, guardian, custodian, or a representative of the minor designated by a court, in the discretion of the attending physician who provided the treatment to the minor

- A parent of the minor, except if the parent's authority to consent to health care for the minor has been specifically limited by a court order or a valid separation agreement entered into by the parents of the minor

- A person authorized to consent to health care for the minor consistent with the authority granted

- An attorney appointed in writing by a person previously listed (*id.* § 4-301(k)).

Section 4-306(a) permits facilities to disclose records to the following persons, without the authorization of the person in interest

- A unit of the state or local government, or a member of a multidisciplinary team assisting the unit, for purposes of investigation or treatment of suspected abuse or neglect of a child or an adult, subject to certain limitations

- Licensing and disciplinary boards, subject to limitations

- A healthcare provider or the provider's insurer or legal counsel. They may have access to all information in a medical record relating to a

---

14. Maine Revised Statutes Annotated tit. 5 § 19203-D(1). *See also* Chapter 10.

patient or recipient's health or treatment that forms the basis for the issues of a claim in a civil action initiated by the patient, recipient, or person in interest.

- A medical or dental review committee

- Another healthcare provider

- In accordance with compulsory process, a stipulation by a person in interest, or a discovery request permitted by law to be made to a court, an administrative tribunal, or a party to a civil court, administrative, or health claims arbitration proceeding

When a party seeks disclosure, the facility must place a written request for disclosure or written confirmation of an oral request that justifies the need for disclosure in the medical record (*id.* § 4-306(b)).

Section 8-601(c) notes that the disclosure and use of records of individuals served by alcohol abuse and drug abuse treatment centers are governed by federal regulations.

MASSACHUSETTS

Massachusetts General Laws ch. 111, § 70 (1992), provides that patients, or their attorneys when authorized in writing, may inspect medical records kept by the hospital or clinic, except a hospital or clinic under the control of the Department of Mental Health, and receive a copy on request and payment of a reasonable fee.

MICHIGAN

Under Michigan Compiled Laws § 333.5131 (1991), an individual tested or treated for serious communicable diseases or human immunodeficiency virus (HIV) infections or acquired immune deficiency syndrome (AIDS) may expressly authorize disclosure if the written authorization is specific to HIV infection, AIDS, or AIDS-related complex (ARC). If the individual is a minor or incapacitated, a parent or legal guardian may execute the authorization.

Section 333.6112(a) provides for disclosure of records involving substance abuse. The subject of such a record may consent in writing to the disclosure of the content of the record to

- Health professionals for the purpose of diagnosis or treatment of the individual

- Governmental personnel for the purpose of obtaining benefits to which the individual is entitled

- Any other person specifically authorized by the individual

The individual may revoke authorization for disclosure at any time, unless expressly prohibited by federal legislation on the confidentiality of alcohol and drug abuse patient records, by giving written notice to the licensee of the substance abuse service.[15]

MINNESOTA

Minnesota Statutes § 144.335(2)(a)–(b) (1991) states that on a patient's written request and payment of reasonable costs, a healthcare provider shall furnish the patient copies of his or her record or the pertinent part thereof or a summary. The provider may exclude written speculations about the patient's condition, except that all information necessary for informed consent must be provided. If the information is detrimental to the physical or mental health of the patient or is likely to cause him to harm himself or others, the provider may withhold information and may supply it to an appropriate third party or other provider, who may release it to the patient. The patient may consent to release to another healthcare provider (*id.* § 144.335(2)(c)–(d)).

Section 144.651(1) specifies that patients and residents of healthcare facilities may approve or refuse release of their personal and medical records to any individual outside the facility. Residents shall be notified when their records are requested, and may select someone to accompany them when the records or information are the subject of a personal interview. This section does not apply to complaint investigation and inspections by the Department of Health, where required by third-party payment contracts, or where otherwise provided by law.

Home care hospice program patients have the right to access to records and written information from records (*id.* § 144.335(2)).

Minnesota statutes make failing to comply with a patient's request for medical records a ground for disciplinary action (e.g., *id.* §§ 147.091 [physicians, surgeons, osteopaths] and 148.261 [registered and licensed practical nurses]).

Under § 145B.04(b), a proxy who is authorized to make healthcare decisions has the same rights as the declarant to receive information regarding proposed health care, to receive and review medical records, and to consent to the disclosure of medical records as does the declarant unless the declarant specifies otherwise (*id.* § 145B.08).

No applicant is eligible for state catastrophic health expense assistance unless he has authorized the commissioner of human services, in writing, to examine all personal medical records developed while the applicant received the medical care for which state assistance is sought.

MISSISSIPPI

Mississippi Code Annotated § 41-9-65 (1991) provides that hospital records are the property of the hospital subject to reasonable access on good cause

---

15. *See also* Chapter 9, for other reasons a healthcare provider may disclose such information.

shown by the patient, his personal representative or heirs, his attending medical personnel, and his duly authorized nominees, on payment of any reasonable charges for such access.

Sections 41-21-97(d) and 41-21-102(7) give mentally ill and mentally retarded persons the right of access to their medical records, unless disclosure is detrimental to their physical or mental health and the provider makes such a notation in their records. Civilly committed patients also have certain rights to access hospital records (*id.* § 13-1-21 notes *referring* to § 41-21-97(a) and (d)).

MISSOURI

Under Missouri Revised Statute § 334.100(2)(k) (1990), failure to furnish details of a patient's medical records to other treating physicians or hospitals on proper request, or failing to comply with any other law relating to medical records, is a ground for denial, revocation, or suspension of license.

Convalescent, nursing, and boarding homes must have written policies governing access to, duplication of, and dissemination of information from the resident's records (*id.* § 198.088(1)(5)). Written consent is required for release of information to persons not otherwise authorized under law to receive it.

Under § 191.317, before a facility may release confidential test results and personal information of those tested under genetic and metabolic disease programs, the facility must fully inform the individual, or his or parent or guardian, of the scope of the information to be released, the risks, benefits, and purpose of such release, and the identity of those to whom the information will be released.

Written consent of the patient or the patient's legal representative is required for access to or release of information, copies, or excerpts from hospital medical records to persons not otherwise authorized to receive them.[16]

Under Missouri Revised Statute § 630.110, mental health patients have the right to have access to their mental and physical records.

Information held by the Missouri Department of Social Services on convalescent, nursing, and boarding home residents may only be disclosed to

- The Department or any person or agency designated by the Department

- The attorney general

- The Department of Mental Health, for residents placed through that department

- Any appropriate law enforcement agency; the resident, his or her guardian, or any other person designated by the resident

- Appropriate committees of the general assembly

---

16. Missouri Code of Regulations tit. 13, § 50-20.021(D)(5) (1982).

- The state auditor, but only to the extent of required financial records (*id.* § 198.032(1))

Inspection reports and written reports of investigations of complaints, including reports of abuse and neglect and relating to the quality of care of residents, are accessible to the public, provided that they do not identify the complainant or any particular resident (*id.* § 198.032(2)).

The law permits the Missouri Department of Social Services to obtain medical insurance information from health maintenance organizations (HMOs) and others. A request for data must include sufficient information to identify each person named in the request in a form that is compatible with the record-keeping methods of the entity. Failure to provide the requested information within 60 days subjects the entity to civil penalties (*id.* § 208.217(2) and (4)).

MONTANA

Montana Code § 50-16-541(1)(a) through (e) (1992) specifies requirements for patient's examination and copying. On receipt of a written request from a patient to examine or copy all or part of his or her recorded healthcare information, a healthcare provider shall take the following steps as promptly as required under the circumstances but no later than 10 days after receiving the request:

- Make the information available to the patient for examination during regular business hours or provide a copy, if requested, to the patient.

- Inform the patient if the information does not exist or cannot be found.

- Inform the patient and provide the name and address, if known, of the healthcare provider who maintains the record, if the contacted healthcare provider does not maintain a record of the information.

- Deny the request in whole or in part under section 50-16-542, discussed below, and inform the patient.

On request, the healthcare provider shall provide an explanation of any code or abbreviation used in the healthcare information. If a record of the particular healthcare information requested is not maintained by the healthcare provider in the requested form, the provider is not required to create a new record or reformulate an existing record to make the information available in the requested form. The healthcare provider may charge a reasonable fee, not to exceed actual cost, for providing the healthcare information, and is not required to permit examination or copying until the fee is paid (*id.* § 50-16-541(2)).

Under § 50-16-542(1)(a) through (g), a healthcare provider may deny access to healthcare information by a patient if the provider reasonably concludes that

- Knowledge of the healthcare information would be injurious to the health of the patient.

- Knowledge of the healthcare information could reasonably be expected to lead to the patient's identification of an individual who provided the information in confidence and under circumstances in which confidentiality was appropriate.

- Knowledge of the healthcare information could reasonably be expected to cause danger to the life or safety of any individual.

- The healthcare information was compiled and is used solely for litigation, quality assurance, peer review, or administrative purposes.

- The healthcare information might disclose birth out of wedlock or provide information from which knowledge of birth out of wedlock might be obtained, which information is protected from disclosure pursuant to § 50-15-206.

- The healthcare provider obtained the information from a person other than the patient.

- Access to the healthcare information is otherwise prohibited by law.

Under the same statute, a healthcare provider may deny access to healthcare information by a patient who is a minor if

- The patient is committed to a mental health facility.

- The patient's parents or guardian have not authorized the healthcare provider to disclose the patient's healthcare information (*id.* § 50-16-542(2)).

However, this provision does not apply if the minor is authorized to consent to health care, under § 50-16-521.

Section 50-16-529 permits disclosure without patient authorization based on need to know. For example, such disclosure is permissible

- To a person who is providing health care to the patient

- To any other person who requires healthcare information for healthcare education; to provide planning, quality assurance, peer review, or administrative, legal, financial, or actuarial services to the healthcare provider; for assisting the provider in the delivery of health care; or to a third-party payer who requires healthcare information and if the provider reasonably believes that the person will

  - Not use or disclose the healthcare information for any other purpose

  - Take appropriate steps to protect the healthcare information

- To any other healthcare provider who has previously provided health care to the patient, to the extent necessary to provide health care to that patient, unless the patient has instructed the provider not to make the disclosure

- To immediate family members of the patient or other individuals with whom the patient is known to have a close personal relationship, if made in accordance with the laws of the state and good medical or other professional practice, unless the patient has instructed the provider not to make the disclosure

- To a healthcare provider who is a successor in interest to the healthcare provider maintaining the healthcare information

- For use in a research project[17]

- To a person who obtains information for purposes of an audit

- To an official of a penal or other custodial institution in which the patient is detained

NEBRASKA

Under Nebraska Revised Statutes § 44-32,172 (1990), data and information pertaining to the diagnosis, treatment, or health of any enrollee or applicant of a health maintenance organization (HMO) may be disclosed, on the express consent of the enrollee or applicant, pursuant to statute or court order for the production of evidence, or in the event of claim or litigation between such person and the HMO wherein such data or information is pertinent.

Nebraska statutes, providing for confidentiality of contagious disease information, specify that such information may be released if the patient consents (*id.* § 71-511(2)).

NEVADA

Each healthcare provider must make patient healthcare records available for physical inspection by the patient or a representative if the latter has written authorization from the patient. The healthcare provider must make copies available to such persons on request and payment of copying costs, not to exceed 60 cents per page for photocopies and a reasonable cost for copies of x rays and other records produced by similar processes.[18]

Each healthcare provider shall make available, on request of a law enforcement agency, the healthcare records of a patient that relate to a test of his or her blood, breath, or urine, if the patient is suspected of driving under the influence of alcohol or the records will aid in a related investigation.[19]

---

17. *See* Chapter 12.
18. Nevada Revised Statutes § 629.061(1) (1991).
19. *Id.* § 629.065.

NEW HAMPSHIRE

New Hampshire Revised Statutes Annotated 332-I:1 (1991) specifies that patients are entitled to copies of medical records in the possession of any licensed or registered medical provider on request and for a reasonable cost. Section 151:21(IX), concerning the Health Facilities Licensing Laws and Patient's Bill of Rights, specifies that patients are entitled to a copy of their personal and clinical records, on request, for a reasonable cost.

New Hampshire Code of Administrative Rules Department of Health and Human Services Regulations He-P 806.10(f) (1986) requires outpatient clinics to provide for written release of information of patient/client clinical records.

NEW JERSEY

Hospitals must require written consent by the patient for release of medical information.[20] The facility must have policies and procedures approved by the Department of Health governing the availability, release, or provision of copies of the medical record to patients, the patient's authorized representative, or both. The policies must include

- A description of the procedures to protect medical information against loss, destruction, or unauthorized use

- A schedule of fees, as established by the facility, for obtaining copies of the medical record

- The business hours, as defined by the facility, during which the patient has access to his or her medical records

- A statement that in the event that a patient's access to his or her medical record is medically contraindicated (as documented by a physician in the patient's medical record), the medical record shall be made available to the patient's authorized representative

The facility must ensure that it provides a patient's medical record within 30 calendar days of the written request.[21]

The Administrative Code of the State Board of Medical Examiners of New Jersey notes that licensees shall provide access to professional treatment records to a patient or an authorized representative in accordance with the following:

- No later than 30 days from receipt of a request from a patient or an authorized representative, the licensee shall provide a copy of the professional treatment record, billing records, or both, as requested. The

---

20. New Jersey Administrative Code tit. 8, § 43B-7.1(c)(4) (West 1991) (Standards for Hospital Facilities).
21. *Id.* § 43B-7.4.

record shall include all pertinent objective data, including test results and x-ray results as applicable as well as subjective information.

- The licensee may elect to provide a summary of the record, so long as that summary adequately reflects the patient's history and treatment, unless otherwise required by law.

- If, in the exercise of professional judgment, a licensee has reason to believe that the patient may be harmed by release of the subjective information contained in the professional treatment record or a summary thereof, the licensee may refuse to provide such information. That record or the summary, with an accompanying notice setting forth the reasons for the original refusal, shall nevertheless be provided on request of and directly to

  - The patient's attorney

  - Another licensed healthcare professional

  - The patient's health insurance carrier

- The licensee may require a record request to be in writing and may charge a reasonable fee for the reproduction of records, which shall be no greater than an amount reasonably calculated to recoup the cost of copying or transcription.

- If the patient or a subsequent treating healthcare professional is unable to read the treatment record, either because it is illegible or prepared in a language other than English, the licensee shall provide a transcription at no cost to the patient.

- The licensee shall not refuse to provide a professional treatment record on the ground that the patient owes the licensee an unpaid balance if the record is needed by another healthcare professional for the purpose of rendering care.[22]

Title 45, § 14B-32, provides that a patient who is receiving or who has received treatment from a licensed practicing psychologist may be requested to authorize the psychologist to disclose certain confidential information to a third-party payer for the purpose of obtaining benefits from the third-party payer for psychological services. Such information is limited to

- Administrative information

- Diagnostic information

- The status of the patient (voluntary or involuntary, inpatient or outpatient)

---

22. *Id*. tit. 13, § 35-6.5.

- The reason for continuing psychological services, limited to an assessment of the patient's current level of functioning and level of distress (both described by the terms mild, moderate, severe, or extreme)

- A prognosis, limited to the estimated minimal time during which treatment might continue

New Jersey Revised Statutes §§ 26:5C-8, 26:5C-12, and 26:5C-13 specify conditions for consensual disclosure of acquired immune deficiency syndrome (AIDS) and human immunodeficiency virus (HIV) infection patient records, which are discussed in Chapter 10 in more detail.

NEW MEXICO

Facilities should use New Mexico Hospital Association Form 2, which authorizes the hospital to release information in patient's records to designated individuals and entities.[23] If others request access to or copies of records, the hospital should require that the patient sign NMHA Form 14, Consent to Access Hospital Records and Release Medical Information. The hospital and the physician may decide whether disclosure is in the patient's best interest. If not, after advising the patient and the individual requesting the records of its decision, the hospital may withhold the record unless the patient obtains a court order for release thereof.

New Mexico Statute Annotated § 43-1-19 (Michie 1992) provides more details with regard to disclosure of confidential information of patients with mental health or developmental disabilities. It provides that no authorization for the transmission or disclosure of confidential information shall be effective unless it

- Is in writing and signed

- Contains a statement of the client's right to examine and copy the information to be disclosed, the name or title of the proposed recipient of the information, and a description of the use that may be made of the information

The statute adds that the client has a right of access to confidential information about himself and has the right to make copies of any information and to submit clarifying or correcting statements and other documentation of reasonable length for inclusion with the confidential information. If, however, a physician or other mental health or development disabilities professional believes and notes in the client's medical records that such disclosure would not be in the best interest of the client, the client may petition the court for an order granting access.

---

23. Healthcare Financial Management Association, *New Mexico Hospital Association Legal Handbook,* ch. V, § C, ¶ 1 at V-8 (rev. ed. 1991).

If the client is incapable of giving or withholding valid consent and does not have a court-appointed guardian or treatment guardian, the person seeking authorization shall petition the court to appoint a guardian to make a substitute decision for the client. If, however, the client is less than 14 years of age, the client's parent or guardian is authorized to consent on behalf of the client.

Section 14-6-1 provides for release of confidential health information on request to a governmental agency or its agent, a state educational institution, a duly organized state or county association of licensed physicians or dentists, a licensed health facility, or staff committees of such facilities without incurring liability for libel or slander.

NEW YORK

New York Public Health Law § 17 (McKinney 1992) specifies that on the written request of any competent patient, parent or guardian of an infant, committee for an incompetent, or conservator of a conservatee, a physician or hospital must release and deliver, exclusive of personal notes of the said physician or hospital, copies of all x rays, medical records, and test records including all laboratory tests regarding that patient to any other designated physician or hospital. However, records concerning the treatment of an infant patient for venereal disease or the performance of an abortion operation upon a minor patient shall not be released or in any manner be made available to the parent or guardian of such infant.

New York Compilation of Codes, Rules and Regulations tit. 10, § 405.10(a)(6) (1988) (Department of Health, Health Facilities Series H-40), notes that hospitals shall allow patients and other qualified persons to obtain access to their medical records. Section 505.5 adds that, other than to patients, hospitals may only release records to hospital staffs involved in treating the patient and individuals permitted by federal and state law.

Disclosure of human immunodeficiency virus (HIV) and acquired immune deficiency syndrome (AIDS)–related information is governed by New York Public Health Division § 2782.[24]

New York Mental Hygiene Law § 33.16 (McKinney 1992) contains detailed guidance on the release of clinical records of clients of facilities licensed by the Office of Mental Retardation and Developmental Disabilities. With the exceptions detailed below, facilities must provide an opportunity, on the written request of any patient or client, for such individual to inspect their clinical records. Similarly, the parent or a guardian of an infant has a right of access to such records unless the treating practitioner determines that access to the information requested by the parent or guardian would have a detrimental effect on the practitioner's relationship with the infant, or on the treatment of the infant or on the infant's relationship with his or her parents

---

24. *See also* Chapter 10.

or guardians. On the written request of any qualified person, the facility shall furnish a copy of the record if the person is entitled to inspect it.

However, on the receipt of any request to inspect or copy the record, the facility shall notify the treating practitioner. If he or he determines that the requested review can reasonably be expected to cause substantial and identifiable harm to the patient, client, or others, which would outweigh the qualified person's right to access, the facility may deny review. The requester must be notified of such denial and has a right to review of the decision by a clinical record access review committee and to judicial review of the determination.

Patient ombudsmen have a right to access to patient records if the patient gives consent.[25]

NORTH CAROLINA

North Carolina General Statutes § 8-53 (1991), dealing with the state's physician–patient privilege, states that confidential information in medical records shall be furnished only on the authorization of the patient or, if deceased, his or her executor, administrator, or next of kin or if ordered by a judge.

The Mental Health, Developmental Disabilities, and Substance Abuse Act specifies that facilities, physicians, or other individuals responsible for the evaluation, management, supervision, or treatment of respondents examined or committed for treatment may request, receive, and disclose confidential information

- To the extent necessary to enable them to fulfill their responsibilities

- To the Department of Correction in certain circumstances

- When a responsible professional opines that imminent danger exists to the health or safety of the client or another individual, or the commission of a felony or violent misdemeanor is likely

- To another healthcare provider who is providing emergency medical services to a client

- To the Department for the purpose of maintaining an index of clients

- To a provider of support services, when the facility has entered into a written agreement with a person to provide support services and the agreement includes a provision in which the provider of support services acknowledges in writing that he or she will safeguard and not further disclose the information

- Whenever reason exists to believe that the client is eligible for financial benefits through a governmental agency, a facility may disclose confi-

---

25. New York Public Health Law § 2803-c(3)(m).

dential information to state or federal agencies to the extent necessary to establish financial benefits.

- Within a facility, to employees, consultants, or volunteers involved in the care, treatment, or habilitation of a client as needed to carry out their responsibilities in serving the client

- On specific request, to a physician or psychologist who referred the client (*id.* in § 122C-55)

Nursing home licensure regulations require nursing homes to make provision for a patient or a resident or his or her legal guardian to have access to the information contained in the medical record unless otherwise ordered by his or her physician. As part of the patient's medical records, the facility must keep signed authorizations concerning approval or disapproval of medical information for licensure inspections.[26]

The Insurance Information and Privacy Protection Act specifies that if any individual, after proper identification, submits a written request to an insurance institution, agent, or insurance-support organization, the entity will provide specified information to the individual. The insurance entity will forward medical record information from the appropriate medical-care institution or medical professional together with the name of the professional or the institution to the individual or a medical organization designated by the individual, whichever the entity prefers. If the entity discloses the information to a medical professional, it will so notify the individual.

NORTH DAKOTA

North Dakota Administrative Code § 33-07-01-16.2(a) through (c) (1980), concerning hospital licensing rules, requires that hospitals keep medical records confidential. Only authorized persons shall have access to the record, and written consent of the patient must be presented as authority for the release of medical information.

North Dakota Century Code § 23-06.5-08 (1991), providing for durable powers of attorney, gives the agent in such a power of attorney the right to request, review, and receive any information regarding the principal's physical or mental health, including medical and hospital records; to execute any releases or other documents that may be required to obtain such information; and to consent to the disclosure of such medical information.

OHIO

According to Ohio Revised Code § 3701.74(C) (Baldwin 1992), a patient who wants to examine or obtain a copy of his or her medical records must submit to the hospital a signed, written request dated not more than 60 days before

---

26. North Carolina Administrative code tit. 10, 3H.0300 and 3H.0315 (Jan. 1991).

the date on which it is submitted and indicate whether the hospital is to send the copy to his residence or hold it at the hospital. The hospital shall permit inspection or provide the copy within a reasonable time, unless a physician determines for clearly stated treatment reasons that disclosure is likely to have an adverse effect on the patient. In that event, the hospital shall provide the record to a physician designated by the patient.

Ohio Administrative Code 5122-14-24 (1991) requires psychiatric hospitals and units to provide information regarding the facility's policy and procedures for patient access to their medical records to the patients. Section 5122:2-1-02 provides for disclosure of information on those hospitalized for mental illness. Such information may be disclosed to the person identified, or a legal guardian, if any, or if the person is a minor, if his or her parent or legal guardian consents, and if such disclosure is in the best interests of the person, as may be determined by the court for judicial records and the chief clinical officer for medical records. A patient shall have access to his or her own psychiatric and medical records unless access is restricted in the patient's treatment plan for clear treatment reasons.

Section 4121-17-30 notes that no employer, physician, healthcare professional, hospital, or laboratory that contracts with the employer to provide medical information pertaining to employees shall refuse, under a written request from the employee, to furnish the employee or former employee or an authorized representative a copy of such medical information. The employee shall provide a current signed release if requested by the employer.

Section 3701-55-15 notes that confidential records of patients of alcoholism inpatient/emergency care facilities shall be disclosed only to authorized persons. Confidential records of drug treatment programs may be disclosed when the patient gives consent in the form of a signed written release if the release

- Specifically identifies the person, official, or entity to whom the information is to be provided

- Describes with reasonable specificity the record, records, or information to be disclosed

- Describes with reasonable specificity the purposes of the disclosure and the intended use of the disclosed information

Ohio Revised Code § 5123.89 (Baldwin 1992) governs disclosure of records of the Department of Mental Retardation and Developmental Disabilities. Disclosure is permitted only if, in the judgment of the court for judicial records and the managing officer for institution records, that disclosure is in the best interest of the person and the person or his or her guardian, or, in the case of a minor, if the parent or guardian consents and as otherwise provided by law. Section 5123.61 makes information in reports of abuse of mentally retarded or developmentally disabled adults available to the adult who is the subject of the report, his legal counsel, and to agencies authorized to receive the report or to a county board of mental retardation and developmental disabilities.

Residential care facility residents have the right to confidential treatment of all information in their personal and medical records.[27]

Medical records of persons covered by health maintenance organizations (HMOs) are confidential and shall not be released without the written consent of the covered person or a responsible party.[28]

Ohio Revised Code § 3701.248 permits an emergency medical services worker who believes he or she has suffered significant exposure to a contagious or infectious disease through contact with a patient, to submit to the healthcare facility or coroner that received the patient a written request to be notified of the results of any test performed on the patient to determine the presence of a contagious or infectious disease. The request shall include

- The name, address, and telephone number of the emergency medical services worker submitting the request

- The name of the emergency medical services worker's employer, or the entity where he or she is a volunteer, and the supervisor's name

- The date, time, location, and manner of the exposure

The facility that receives a written request shall give an oral notification of the presence of a contagious or infectious disease, or of a confirmed positive test result, if known, within two days with a written notification to follow within three days. The notification shall include the name of the disease, its signs and symptoms, the date of exposure, the incubation period, the mode of transmission of the disease, the medical precautions necessary to prevent transmission to other persons, and the appropriate prophylaxis, treatment, and counseling for the disease. The notification shall not include the name of the patient or deceased person.

OKLAHOMA

Any patient is entitled, under Oklahoma Statutes tit. 76, § 19(A) (1991), to obtain access to the information in his or her medical records and to receive copies on payment of the costs of the copies, not to exceed 10 cents per page. Access to psychiatric records, however, requires a court order on a finding that access is in the best interest of the patient.

Title 43A, § 1-109(A)(1) (1991), provides that privileged or confidential medical information may not be released to anyone not involved in patient treatment programs without a written release by the patient (or, if the patient is a minor or if a guardian has been appointed for the patient, the guardian of the patient) or a court order.

Mental health or drug and alcohol abuse patients are not entitled to personal access to the information in their psychiatric or psychological records

---

27. Ohio Administrative Code 5123:2-3-18.
28. *Id.* § 5105:3-26-07.

or to copies unless the treating physician consents or a court orders access (*id*. tit. 43, § 3-422).

OREGON

Medical record departments must maintain a current written policy on the release of medical record information including patient access to his or her medical record.[29]

Patients or their legal guardians may request public healthcare providers to release the content of any record by means of a written, voluntary, informed consent, which includes the following:

- Name of provider directed to make disclosure

- Name of persons or organizations to which the information is to be disclosed, or released to the public

- Name of the patient

- Extent or nature of the information to be disclosed

- Statement that consent is revocable at any time[30]

The provider must release such information to the patient within five working days. Patients have the right to immediate inspection of any written record.[31]

PENNSYLVANIA

28 Pennsylvania Code §§ 103.22(b)(15) and 115.29 (1991) permit patients of general and special hospitals and their patient designees to have access to or a copy of their medical records unless access thereto is specifically restricted by the attending physician for medical purposes. On the death of a patient, the hospital shall provide the executor or next of kin, on request, access to all medical records of the deceased patient. The facility may charge the reasonable costs of making copies of the record (*id*. § 115.29). Section 115.28 adds that copies of medical records may be made available for appropriate purposes such as insurance claims and physician review, consistent with their confidential nature.

The hospital shall maintain the written authorization of the patient in the original record as authority for release of medical information outside the hospital (*id*. § 115.27). 49 Pennsylvania Code § 16.61 makes failing to make medical records available to a patient or another designated healthcare practitioner, upon a patient's written request, unprofessional conduct.

---

29. Oregon Administrative Rules § 333-505-050(18) (1990).
30. Oklahoma Revised Statute § 179.505(3) (1991).
31. *Id*. § 179.505(7).

Under 28 Pennsylvania Code § 563.11, patients of ambulatory surgical facilities or their designees have the same rights of access as detailed above. The written authorization of the patient shall be presented and then maintained in the original record as authority for release of medical information outside the facility (*id.* § 563.9).

Long-term care nursing facility patients may approve or refuse the release of their personal and medical records to an individual outside the facility, except in case of a transfer to another healthcare institution or as required by statute or third-party payment contract.[32] On request, the facility shall provide the patient or the patient designee access to information contained in the patient's medical records unless medically contraindicated. If the patient or designee wants a copy, the facility shall provide the copy and may charge a reasonable fee for reproducing copies. If requested, after the death of a patient, the facility shall make the patient's medical record available to the deceased person's executor or administrator of the decedent's estate or to the person responsible for the disposition of the body.[33]

Subscribers of health maintenance organizations (HMOs) have the right to all information contained in their medical records unless the attending physician specifically restricts access for medical reasons.[34]

Patients of birth centers have a right to review, or obtain, a copy of the mother's medical records.[35] Such patients have control over the release of health record information. Except in an emergency, a written release, signed by the mother, is required to release health record information except as otherwise provided by law or by third-party contractual arrangements.

RHODE ISLAND

Rhode Island General Laws § 5.37.3-4(a) (1991) states that healthcare providers may release confidential healthcare information on written consent of the patient or his authorized representative. The consent form must contain a statement of the need for and proposed uses of the information; a statement that all information is to be released or clearly indicating the extent of that to be released; and a statement that the consent may be withdrawn at any time and is subject to revocation, except where used in an application for a life or health insurance policy, in which case the authorization expires two years from the issue of the policy. Authorizations in connection with a claim for insurance benefits are valid during the pendency of the claim. Any revocations of consent must be in writing.

---

32. 28 Pennsylvania Code § 201.29(n).
33. *Id.* § 211.5(d) and (e).
34. *Id.* § 9.77(3) and (8).
35. *Id.* § 501.46(b)(7).

SOUTH CAROLINA

Under South Carolina Annotated § 44-52-170 (Law Co-op. 1990), patients of alcohol and drug abuse treatment facilities have access to their medical records. The Bill of Rights for Residents of Long-Term Care Facilities specifies that they may approve release of their personal and medical records to any individual outside the facility (*id.* § 44-81-40).

With regard to mentally retarded or developmentally disabled patients, § 44-20-340 provides that the South Carolina Department of Mental Retardation may release otherwise confidential records on written request of the client, the client's or applicant's parent with legal custody, legal guardian, the spouse with the written permission of the client or applicant, or under subpoena.

The records of mentally ill and mentally retarded patients are confidential (*id.* § 44-23-1090). Section 44-23-1090 provides that such records may not be disclosed except insofar as

- The individual identified or legal guardian, if any, or, if he or she is a minor, his parent or legal guardian shall consent

- Disclosure may be necessary to carry out the purposes of the laws related to mental health.

- A court may direct, on its determination that disclosure is necessary for the conduct of proceedings before it and that failure to make disclosure would be contrary to the public interest

- Disclosure is necessary in cooperating with state and federal agencies or subdivisions thereof in furthering the welfare of the patient or his family.

- Disclosure is necessary in cooperating with law-enforcement agencies.

- Public safety is involved; provided, when disclosure is so authorized, it may be made to such person as the Commissioner of Mental Health may in his or her discretion determine.

Violation of this section is a misdemeanor.

Section 38-33-260, governing health records of health maintenance organizations (HMOs), permits enrollees or applicants to consent to disclosure of data or information pertaining to their diagnosis, treatment, or health.

Under § 43-38-20, the ombudsman of the governor's office is authorized to investigate any complaint on behalf of any health facility and may have access to pertinent medical records, but may not further disclose such records unless

- Such complainant or resident, or his legal representative, consents in writing.

- Such disclosure is required by court order.

SOUTH DAKOTA

South Dakota Codified Laws Annotated § 34-12-15 (1992) specifies that hospitals or other institutions to which persons resort for treatment of disease shall provide copies of all medical records, reports, and x rays to a discharged patient or designee on receipt of a written request signed by the patient. The facility may require that the patient pay reproduction and mailing expenses. Section 36-2-16 contains a similar requirement for practitioners of the healing arts in general. Further, § 36-2-17 specifies that licensees who act in good faith within the requirements of § 36-2-16 are immune from any injury or damage caused by complying with that section.

TENNESSEE

Under both Tennessee statutory and administrative law, hospitals shall provide reasonable access to the information contained in health records on good cause shown by the patient, his or her personal representative or heirs, or attending medical personnel, and on payment of any reasonable charge for such service.[36]

In the case of children where only one parent has custody, the Tennessee Child Custody Act provides that the treating physician or hospital may release a copy of the child's medical records on written request by the noncustodial parent; in the case of joint custody, the parent with whom the child is not residing; or in the case of a child in the custody of a legal guardian, either parent.[37] Costs must be paid by the requesting party.[38]

Under Tennessee Code Annotated § 68-11-901(13), residents of nursing homes have the right to keep their records confidential and private. The home must obtain written consent of the resident before it can release any information, except for persons authorized under the law. If the resident is mentally incompetent, the facility must obtain written consent from his or her legal representative. Nursing homes must have a written policy governing access to and duplication of patient records, and copies of the policy shall be available to residents and their families on request.

TEXAS

Texas Revised Civil Statutes art. 4495b, § 5.08(j) (West 1992), governing the physician–patient privilege, specifies that consent for release of confidential information must be in writing and signed by the patient, or a parent or legal guardian if the patient is a minor, or a legal guardian if the patient has been

---

36. Tennessee Code Annotated § 68-11-304 (1991); Tennessee Administrative Rules and Regulations tit. 1200, ch. 8-4-.03(1)(b)(ii) (1986) (Rules of the Board for Licensing Healthcare Facilities).
37. Tennessee Code Annotated § 36-6-103(4).
38. *Id.*

adjudicated incompetent to manage his or her legal affairs, or an attorney *ad litem* (for the lawsuit) appointed for the patient, or a personal representative if the patient is deceased. The written consent must specify

- The information or medical records to be covered by the release

- The reasons or purposes for the release

- The person to whom the information is to be released

The patient, or other person authorized to consent, has the right to withdraw consent.

Article 4495, § 5.08(k), also provides that a physician shall furnish copies of medical records requested, or a summary or narrative of the records, pursuant to a written consent as above, unless the physician determines that access to the information would be harmful to the physical, mental, or emotional health of the patient. The physician shall furnish the information within a reasonable time; however, the patient may be required to pay reasonable fees.

Texas Health and Safety Code § 81.046 (West 1992) provides that reports, records, and information furnished to a health authority or to the department that relate to cases or suspected cases of diseases or health conditions may be released with the consent of each person identified in the information.

Sections 595.001 and 533.010(c) through (d) note that records maintained for any program or activity relating to mental retardation must maintain confidentiality regarding patient identity, diagnosis, evaluation, or treatment. Such records, however, may be disclosed with the written consent of the patient, or parent if such person is a minor, or guardian if such person has been adjudicated incompetent. If, however, a qualified professional responsible for supervising the patient's habilitation states, in writing, that it would not be in the best interest of the person, the disclosure should not be made to that person but only to the parent of a minor or a guardian. If the patient is deceased and does not have an executor or administrator, his or her spouse or a person related within the first degree of family relationship may consent to the release of the records.

Providers may disclose such information, without the patient's consent, to

- Medical personnel to the extent necessary to meet a bona fide emergency

- Qualified personnel for management audits, financial audits, program evaluation, or research approved by the Department of Health. However, such personnel may not identify, directly or indirectly, any individual receiving services in any report or otherwise disclose identities.

- Parties authorized access by a court order on a showing of good cause

- Personnel authorized to conduct investigations concerning abuse or denial of rights of retarded persons

Texas Department of Health, Hospital Licensing Standards ch. 12, § 8.7.3.1 (1991), states that special care facilities may allow access or release by written authorization of the resident unless the physician has documented in the record that to do so would be harmful to the physical, mental, or emotional health of the resident.

Texas Human Resources Code § 101.058(a) (West 1992) gives the state long-term care ombudsman access to patient care records of elderly residents of long-term care facilities, but does not provide such access to certified volunteer ombudsmen.

Under Texas Health and Safety Code Annotated § 81.103, a person tested for acquired immune deficiency syndrome (AIDS), human immunodeficiency virus (HIV), or other communicable disease, or a person legally authorized to consent to such test on the patient's behalf, may voluntarily release or disclose that person's test results to any other person, and may authorize the release or disclosure of the test results. Such authorization must be in writing and signed by the person tested or the person legally authorized to consent to the test on the person's behalf. The authorization must state the person or class of persons to whom the test results may be released or disclosed.

UTAH

Utah Administrative Rules 432-100-7.404 (1990), concerning health facility licensure rules, states that hospital medical records shall be readily available to "other persons authorized by consent forms." The rule adds that the patient or his legal representative must give written consent to release medical information to unauthorized persons.

Rules 432-152-4.201 and 432-201-6.103, respectively, require mental retardation and small healthcare facilities to develop and implement policies and procedures governing the release of any client information, including consents necessary from the client, parents, if the client is a minor, or legal guardian. In addition, small healthcare facilities may only disclose such information to authorized persons in accordance with federal, state, and local laws (*id.* r. 432-200-6.103). If the patient is judged incompetent, requests for information requiring the patient's signature shall be fulfilled on the written consent of the patient or guardian. Authorized representatives of the Department of Health may review records to determine compliance with licensure rules and standards.

Rules 432-500-5.401 and 432-600-6.105 contain the same language with regard to freestanding ambulatory surgical centers and abortion clinics, respectively. Home health agencies must have written procedures for the use and removal of medical records. Release of information requires written consent of the patient, but authorized representatives of the Department of Health are allowed to review records to determine compliance with licensure rules and standards. Even when a patient is referred to another agency or facility, the home health agency may release information only with the written consent of the patient (*id.* r. 432-700-4).

Utah Code Annotated § 78-25-25 (1992) requires practitioners and hospitals to make patient medical records available for inspection and copying to a patient's attorney if he or she presents a written authorization signed by the patient and notarized, or by the parent or guardian of a minor, or by the personal representative or an heir of a deceased patient. The attorney shall pay for the costs of the copies, and the practitioner or facility may retain possession of the actual record.

VERMONT

Vermont's Bill of Rights for Hospital Patients, contained in Vermont Statutes Annotated tit. 18, § 1852 (1991), states that a patient has the right to expect that all communications and records pertaining to his or her care shall be treated as confidential. Only medical personnel, or individuals under the supervision of medical personnel and directly treating the patient, or those persons monitoring the quality of that treatment, or researching the effectiveness of that treatment, shall have access to the patient's medical records. Others may have access to those records only with the patient's written authorization.

Title 14, § 3458, governing durable powers of attorney for health care, specifies that an agent may, for the purpose of making healthcare decisions, do the following:

- Request, review, and receive any information, oral or written, regarding the principal's physical or mental health, including, but not limited to, medical and hospital records

- Execute any releases or other documents that may be required in order to obtain such medical information

- Consent to the disclosure of such medical information

VIRGINIA

Hospitals may release copies of a patient's medical record if the patient or a legal representative consents in writing. In the case of a minor, the parent, guardian, or legal representative may consent.[39] The same rules apply to nursing homes.[40]

---

39. Division of Medical and Nursing Facilities Services, Rules and Regulations for the Licensure of Hospitals in Virginia, part III, § 208.6.2 (1982).
40. Division of Medical and Nursing Facilities Services, Rules and Regulations for the Licensure of Nursing Homes, § 24.3.2 (1991).

WASHINGTON

Revised Code of Washington § 71.05.630(1) (1991) specifies the conditions under which mental illness treatment records may be released. Of course, the provider may release such records pursuant to an informed written consent. Without an informed written consent, the provider may release such records

- To an individual, organization, or agency as necessary for management or financial audits, or program monitoring and evaluation. Information obtained for these purposes shall remain confidential and may not be used in a manner that discloses the name or other identifying information about the individual whose records are being released.

- To the department, the director of regional support networks, or a qualified staff member designated by the director only when necessary to be used for billing or collection purposes. The information shall remain confidential.

- For purposes of research

- Pursuant to lawful order of a court

- To qualified staff members of the department, to the director of regional support networks, to resource management services responsible for serving a patient, or to service providers designated by resource management services, as necessary to determine the progress and adequacy of treatment and to determine whether the person should be transferred to a less restrictive or more appropriate treatment modality or facility

- Within the treatment facility where the patient is receiving treatment, confidential treatment may be disclosed to individuals employed, serving in bona fide training programs, or participating in supervised volunteer programs at the facility when necessary to perform their duties.

- Within the department as necessary to coordinate treatment for mental illness, developmental difficulties, alcoholism, or drug abuse of individuals who are under the supervision of the department

- To a licensed physician who has determined that the life or health of the individual is in danger and that treatment without the information contained in the treatment records could be injurious to the patient's health. Disclosure shall be limited to the portions of the records necessary to meet the medical emergency.

- To a facility that is to receive an individual who is involuntarily committed under Chapter 71.05, or on transfer of the individual from one treatment facility to another. The release shall be limited to the treatment records required by law, a record or summary of all somatic treatments, and a discharge summary.

- To a correctional facility or officer under certain conditions

- To the individual's counsel or guardian *ad litem* to prepare for involuntary commitment or recommitment proceedings, reexaminations, appeals, or other actions relating to detention, admission, commitment, or patient's rights

- To a corrections officer of the department who has custody of or is responsible for the supervision of an individual who is transferred or discharged from a treatment facility

- To staff members of the protection and advocacy agency or to staff members of a private, nonprofit corporation, for the purpose of protecting and advocating the rights of persons with mental illness or developmental disabilities with certain specified limitations

Whenever federal law or regulations restrict the release of such information concerning patients who receive treatment for alcoholism or drug dependency, the release should be restricted to comply therewith (*id.* § 71.05.630(2)).

Section 70.96A.150, discussed in Chapter 9, specifies the conditions under which a facility may disclose records of alcoholics and intoxicated persons.

The state long-term care ombudsman has access to patient records (*id.* § 43.190.030), as do researchers (*id.* § 42.48.020; *see also* Chapter 12).

WEST VIRGINIA

West Virginia Code § 16-29-1 (1992) provides that any licensed healthcare provider shall, on the patient's written request, provide the patient, authorized agent, or representative with a copy or summary of the patient's records within a reasonable time. Furnishing a copy or summary of reports of x-ray examinations is sufficient to comply with this section, and the patient shall reimburse the provider for all reasonable expenses incurred in complying with this statute.

However, under § 16-29-1(b), healthcare providers responsible for diagnosing, treating, or administering healthcare services in the case of drug rehabilitation or related services may not release patient records of such diagnosis, treatment, or provision of health care to a parent or guardian without prior written consent from the patient. This general rule has the two exceptions described below, which are discussed in Chapter 9:

- In the case of a patient receiving treatment for psychiatric or psychological problems, a summary shall be made available to the patient, an authorized agent, or authorized representative following termination of the program (*id.* § 16-29-1 (a)).

- Under § 16-30A-12, except to the extent the right is limited by a medical power of attorney, a representative designated to make healthcare decisions under a medical power of attorney has the same legal right as the principal to receive information, including information requiring a special release, to receive and review medical records, and to consent to the disclosure of medical records.

A provider may disclose confidential identities of those tested for human immunodeficiency virus (HIV) or the results to the subject of the test or a person who secures a specific release executed by the subject (*id.* § 16-3C-3(a)). "Release of test results" is defined in § 16-3C-1(k) as signed and dated written authorization for disclosure of HIV-related test results that specifies to whom disclosure is authorized and the time period during which the release is to be effective. Section 16-3C-4(a) adds if the person whose consent is necessary for disclosure of HIV-related test results is unable to give such authorization because of mental incapacity or incompetency, the authorization shall be obtained from another person in the following order of preference:

- A person holding a durable power of attorney for healthcare decisions

- The person's duly appointed legal guardian

- The person's next of kin in the following order of preference: spouse, parent, adult child, sibling, uncle or aunt, and grandparent

Healthcare providers treating minors for birth control, prenatal care, drug rehabilitation, or venereal disease need not, under the above rule, release such patient records to a parent or guardian without the prior written consent of the patient (*id.* § 16-29-1 (b)).

Long-term care ombudsmen have access to residents' records, including medical records, under the following conditions:

- If the resident is competent and has the ability to write, access may only be obtained by the written consent of the resident.

- If the resident is competent but unable to write, oral consent may be given in the presence of a third party who shall witness the resident's consent in writing.

- If the resident is under a guardianship committee or has granted a medical power of attorney which is in effect, or granted any other power of attorney which is in effect, access may only be obtained by the written consent of the guardian or attorney in fact, unless the existence of the guardianship, medical power of attorney, or attorney in fact is unknown to the long-term care ombudsman on investigation and to the long-term care facility, or unless the guardian or attorney in fact cannot be reached through normal communications within five working days.

- If the resident is unable to express written or oral consent and does not have a guardian or attorney in fact, or the notification of the guardian or attorney in fact is not achieved for the above reasons, the ombudsman may inspect the records (*id.* § 16-5L-12).

WISCONSIN

Under Wisconsin Statutes § 146.83(1)(a) through (c) (1990), patients may inspect or receive a copy of their healthcare records on submitting a statement of informed consent and paying reasonable costs. "Informed consent for disclosure" means consent, in writing on an informed consent form, to disclosure to another specified person of the results of a test administered to the person consenting (*id.* § 146.025(1)(d)).

Written consent of the patient or the patient's legally authorized representative shall be presented as authority for release of medical information to persons not otherwise authorized to receive such information.[41]

Wisconsin Statutes § 51.30(4) (1990) requires informed consent for disclosure of information and records of individuals who are receiving or have received treatment for mental illness, developmental disabilities, alcoholism, or drug dependence from court or treatment records to an individual, agency, or organization. Such consent must contain

- The name of the individual, agency, or organization to which the disclosure is to be made

- The name of the subject individual whose treatment record is being disclosed; the purpose or need for the disclosure

- The specific type of information to be disclosed

- The time during which the consent is effective

- The date on which the consent is signed

- The signature of the individual or person legally authorized to give consent for the individual (*id.* § 51.30(2))

Without the patient's informed consent, providers may release such records

- To healthcare facility staff committees, or accreditation or healthcare services review organizations for the purposes of conducting management and financial audits, program evaluation, healthcare service reviews, or accreditation

- To healthcare providers to the extent their duties require access

- To the extent that the records are needed for billing, collection, or payment of claims

- Under lawful order of a court[42]

---

41. Wisconsin Administrative Code § HSS 124.14(2)(b) (July 1988).
42. *See* Chapter 11.

- In response to a written request of any federal or state governmental agency to perform a legally authorized function

- For research[43]

- To a county agency designated, under § 46.09(2), to receive reports of elder abuse

- To the Department of Health, under § 46.73, relating to cancer reporting

- To staff members of the protection and advocacy agency to protect the rights of persons with developmental disabilities or mental illness

- To persons, as provided under § 655.17(7)(b), relating to filing malpractice claims if the patient files a submission of controversy

- To a county department or law enforcement agency to investigate child abuse

- To school district employees when they have responsibility for health records or when access is necessary for them to comply with federal or state law

- To persons and entities, under § 940.22, relating to reporting sexual exploitation by a therapist (*id.* § 146.82(2)(2)–(12)

The director of the facility may restrict patient access to records during treatment. Following discharge, the patient has a right to a complete record of all medications and somatic treatments and to a copy of the discharge summary. He or she shall also have a right, on request, to have access to and to receive a photostatic copy of any or all treatment records (*id.* § 51.30(4)(b)). Parents, guardians, or persons in place of a parent of a minor, or the guardian of an incompetent adult, may consent to the release of confidential information and have access to treatment records, except in the case of a minor aged 14 or older who files a written objection. A minor aged 14 or older may consent to disclosure. The statute also contains detailed guidelines concerning to whom the facility may release such information without informed consent (*id.* § 51.30(5)). The facility may also release treatment records to the following without the consent of the patient:

- To individuals, organizations, or entities designated by the Department of Health and Social Services for the purposes of management audits, financial audits, or program monitoring and evaluation

- To the department or county department or qualified staff member for billing or collection purposes

---

43. *See* Chapter 12.

- For research, if the department has approved the project and the researcher has provided assurances that the information will be used only for the purpose for which it was provided, that it will not be released to anyone not connected with the research, and the final product will not identify the individual

- Pursuant to a lawful court order

- To staff members of the department or the director of the county department to determine adequacy of treatment, whether the person should be transferred, and so forth

- Within the treatment facility when and to the extent that the individuals employed, serving in bona fide training programs, or participating in supervised volunteer programs need access in the performance of their duties

- Within the department to the extent necessary to coordinate treatment

- To a licensed physician who has determined that the life or health of the individual is in danger and treatment without the information could be injurious to the patient's health

- To a facility that is to receive an individual who is involuntarily committed

- To the subject individual's counsel or guardian *ad litem* to prepare for involuntary commitment or recommitment proceedings, reexaminations, appeals, or other actions relating to detention, admission, commitment, or patients' rights (*id.* § 51.30(4)(b) 1–8, 9, and 11)

Wisconsin Administrative Code § HSS 92.05 (June 1986), relating to records of patients treated for mental illness, developmental disabilities, or alcohol or drug abuse, provides that patients have access to their treatment records during treatment unless the director has reason to believe that the benefits of allowing access to a patient are outweighed by the disadvantages. After discharge, a patient is allowed access, on one working day's notice, and may have a copy of his or her records, subject to payment of a uniform and reasonable fee.

Wisconsin Statutes 146.025 provides that results of a test for the presence of human immunodeficiency virus (HIV) or an HIV antibody may not be disclosed, without the subject's informed consent, except as detailed in Chapter 10. No person to whom such test results have been disclosed may disclose them except under the same rules.

WYOMING

Under Wyoming Statute § 35-2-607(a) (1991), a patient may authorize a hospital to disclose his or her healthcare information. To be valid, the authorization shall

- Be in writing and dated and signed by the patient

- Identify the nature of the information to be disclosed

- Identify the person to whom the information is to be disclosed

A patient may revoke an authorization to disclose healthcare information at any time, unless disclosure is required to effectuate payments for health care that has been provided. However, the revocation is not effective unless the healthcare provider has notice of the revocation, if the healthcare provider made the disclosure in good faith based on reliance on an authorization (*id.* § 35-2-608).

Except for authorizations to provide information to third-party healthcare payers, authorizations shall not permit the release of healthcare information relating to future care that the patient receives more than 12 months after he or she signs the authorization. All authorizations are invalid after the expiration date, which shall not exceed 48 months. If the authorization does not contain an expiration date, it expires 12 months after it is signed. The hospital shall retain each authorization or revocation of an authorization in conjunction with any healthcare information from which disclosures are made. Section 35-2-608 provides for patient's revocation of authorization for disclosure.

Section 35-2-606(b) requires hospitals to maintain a record of each person who has received or examined the recorded healthcare information of a patient during the preceding three years; however, no such recording is required for disclosures made to other healthcare providers providing care, to successor healthcare facilities, to researchers, or to peer review or quality assurance committees under § 35-2-609(a)(i) through (iii).

CHAPTER 9

Disclosure of Drug
and Alcohol Abuse Records

Introduction

Generally, as discussed in Chapter 7, states require healthcare providers to maintain the confidentiality of patients who receive voluntary or involuntary drug or alcohol abuse treatment. However, under certain circumstances healthcare providers may disclose this information.

Federal Laws

Federal statutes establish standards for disclosure of medical records of drug abusers. Violating patients' confidentiality may result in a criminal penalty. Under federal law, written consent must include the date, the name of the patient and the facility, the name of the party to whom the information may be disclosed, the purpose of the disclosure, the precise nature of the information to be disclosed, and the length of time the authorization is valid.[1] A similar provision affects the Veterans Administration.[2]

Any program relating to alcohol or drug abuse education, treatment, rehabilitation, or research that receives federal assistance, directly or indirectly, and that maintains records of the identity, diagnosis, or prognosis of any patient in connection with such programs must keep such records confidential.[3]

Information on participants in an alcohol or drug program can be disclosed if the patient consents in writing, if there is an emergency situation where medical history is necessary, for scientific research or other studies where the individual will not be identified, or by court order.

Federal regulations require public, nonprofit, and for-profit private entities conducting, regulating, or assisting alcohol or drug abuse programs to maintain records showing patient consent to disclosure and documenting

---

1. 42 U.S.C. § 242(a) (1992) (the Comprehensive Alcohol Abuse and Alcoholism Prevention, Treatment, and Rehabilitation Act of 1970); 42 U.S.C. § 290ee-2 (1992); 21 U.S.C. § 872(e) (1992) (as amended); 42 U.S.C. § 290ee-3 (1992) (transferred from 21 U.S.C. § 1175(b)(2)(c) (1992)).
2. 38 U.S.C. § 7333 (1992).
3. 42 U.S.C. § 290dd-3 (1992).

any disclosure from confidential records to medical personnel in a medical emergency.[4] The regulation does not specify a retention period.

The federal regulations also require alcohol, drug abuse, and mental health researchers to maintain confidentiality certificates showing that the Secretary of Health and Human Services has authorized the researcher to withhold the identity of research subjects in the face of any legal proceedings to compel the disclosure of the identity of research subjects, again without specifying a retention period.[5]

State Laws

ALABAMA

Alabama has no additional requirements over and above the federal confidentiality and disclosure requirements for drug and alcohol abuse records.

ALASKA

Alaska has no additional requirements over and above the federal confidentiality and disclosure requirements for drug and alcohol abuse records.

ARIZONA

Medical records of patients of substance abuse units are confidential and may not be released.[6]

Persons registered to manufacture, distribute, or dispense controlled substances must keep records and maintain inventories in conformance with federal and state law. These records and inventories are open to inspection by peace officers in the performance of their duties.[7] Pharmacists must maintain a bound record book for dispensing of controlled substances that shall contain the name and address of the purchaser, the name and quantity of the controlled substance purchased, the date of each purchase, and the name or initials of the pharmacist or pharmacy intern who dispensed the substance.[8]

ARKANSAS

A patient has the privilege of refusing to disclose and preventing others from disclosing confidential communications made for the purpose of diagnosis or treatment of his or her physical, mental, or emotional condition, including alcohol or drug addiction.[9]

---

4. 42 C.F.R. § 2.31-2.35 and 2.51-2.53 (1991).
5. *Id.* § 2a-3–2a-8.
6. Arizona Compilation Administration Rules and Regulations 9-10-221 (1982).
7. *Id.* § 36-2523B
8. *Id.* §§ 36-2525F.4 and 36-2523 (for specific record-keeping requirements).
9. Arkansas Code Annotated § 16-41-101, art. V, r. 503(b) (1991).

CALIFORNIA

The California Penal Code requires mandatory release of medical information if there is reason to believe that a crime was committed by or to a patient, presumably including drug abuse.[10] The California Health and Safety Code states that the division may not require a healthcare provider to permit inspection or provide copies of alcohol and drug abuse records where, or in a manner, prohibited by the federal drug laws or regulations.[11]

COLORADO

Registration and other records of alcoholics' and intoxicated persons' treatment facilities are confidential and privileged to the patient. However, the director may make available information from such records for purposes of research into the causes and treatment of alcoholism, but such information may not be published in a way that discloses patients' names or other identifying information.

Colorado revised statutes, which provide for patient access to medical records, specify that persons responsible for the diagnosis or treatment of drug addiction are not required, in the case of minors, to release patient records of such diagnosis or treatment to a parent, guardian, or person other than the minor or a designated representative.[12]

CONNECTICUT

Under Connecticut General Statute § 17-630(b) (1990), medical treatment facilities must promptly furnish a record of all applicants for enrollment and all enrolled patients in a program for drug-dependent persons to the commissioner of mental health. However, no hospital may report or disclose to the public the name of a person who requests treatment and rehabilitation for drug dependence (*id.* § 17a-630(c)). If the patient is a minor, the minor's request for treatment or the treatment itself may not be disclosed to his or her parents or guardian without the minor's consent (*id.* § 17a-630(d)).

DELAWARE

Delaware Code Annotated tit. 16, § 5161 (1991) specifies that no information reported to the Division of Public Health and no clinical records maintained with respect to patients are public records. Such information may not be disclosed outside the Division, except pursuant to court order, to attorneys representing the patient, with the consent of the patient or one authorized to

---

10. California Penal Code § 1543 (Deering 1992).
11. California Health and Safety Code § 1795.18 (Deering 1992). *See also* 42 U.S.C. §§ 290aa-1–290ee-3, 1101-1102, 1115, 1171, 177-79, 1181, 4577, 4591-4594 (1988).
12. Colorado Revised Statute § 25-1-802 (2) (1991).

act on the patient's behalf, or where the patient has been transferred to an institution outside the Division.

DISTRICT OF COLUMBIA

The District of Columbia has no additional requirements over and above the federal confidentiality and disclosure requirements for drug and alcohol abuse records.

FLORIDA

Notwithstanding confidentiality of medical records, hospitals may release evidence relating to the alcoholic content of the blood or the presence of chemical substances to a court, prosecuting attorney, defense attorney, or law enforcement official.[13] Records of alcohol testing should not be released without a written request from the state assuring that it is pursuing a drinking violation.

GEORGIA

Georgia provides that the records and name of any drug-dependent person who seeks or obtains treatment, therapeutic advice, or counsel from any drug abuse treatment and education program licensed under Georgia law is confidential and will not be revealed except to the extent authorized in writing by the drug-dependent person affected.[14] Likewise, any communication by such person to an authorized employee of such a program is confidential.[15] However, the records of such person and information about such person may be produced in response to a valid court order after a show-cause hearing and in response to a Department of Human Resources request for access for licensing purposes when accompanied by a written statement that no record of patient identifying information will be made.[16] Allowing unauthorized access to juvenile drug use records is a misdemeanor.[17]

HAWAII

Hawaii has no additional requirements over and above the federal confidentiality and disclosure requirements for drug and alcohol abuse records.

IDAHO

Idaho provides for confidentiality regarding records of alcoholics or intoxicated or addicted persons. The registration and other records of treatment

---

13. Florida Statute Annotated ch. 316.1933 (1991).
14. Georgia Code Annotated § 26-5-17 (Michie 1991).
15. *Id.*
16. *Id.*
17. *Id.* § 49-5-45.

facilities are confidential and privileged to the patient.[18] However, the director may make available information from patient records for purposes of research into the causes and treatment of alcoholism or drug addiction. Such information, however, may not be published in a way that discloses patients' names or other identifying information.

No physician or person acting under a physician's supervision may report or disclose the names of persons who request treatment or rehabilitation for addiction or dependency on any drug.[19]

ILLINOIS

Illinois requires those who treat patients for alcohol or drug abuse to keep patient records strictly confidential.[20] Records may be disclosed with the prior written consent of the patient, but only under such circumstances and for such purposes as prescribed by the Department of Alcoholism and Substance Abuse. The Illinois administrative code specifies that release must comport with the federal guidelines implementing the Drug Abuse Prevention, Treatment and Rehabilitation Act.[21]

INDIANA

Indiana has no additional requirements over and above the federal confidentiality and disclosure requirements for drug and alcohol abuse records.

IOWA

Records of the identity, diagnosis, prognosis, or treatment of a person maintained in connection with the provision of substance abuse treatment services are confidential (Iowa Code § 125.93 (1991)), and the Iowa code requires employers to protect the confidentiality of the results of any drug tests on employees (*id.* § 730.5(8)).

KANSAS

Under Kansas Statute Annotated § 65-5225 (1990), a healthcare provider commits a misdemeanor when it discloses records showing treatment of a drug abuser, unless the patient or former patient consents in writing. If the patient or former patient is less than 16 years of age, consent in writing must be provided by a parent of the patient or former patient, or if the patient or former patient has a guardian, by the guardian. However, the head of the treatment facility or state institution, or the head of the other facility for care or treatment who has the records, may refuse to disclose such records if he

---

18. Idaho Code § 39-308 (1991).
19. *Id.* § 37-3105.
20. Illinois Revised Statute ch. 111 ½, ¶ 6358-2 (1988).
21. Illinois Administration Code tit. 77, § 200.602 (1991).

or she has stated in writing that such disclosure will be injurious to the welfare of the patient or former patient (*id.* § 65-5225(a)(2)(A)).

Further, in a bona fide medical emergency (*id.* § 65-5225(a)(2)(B)), on court order (*id.* § 65-5225(a)(2)(D)), or for research purposes (*id.* § 65-5225(a)(2)(C)), disclosure may be made without the consent of the patient or former patient.

Similar rules exist with regard to records of alcoholism and intoxication treatment (*id.* § 65-4050).

KENTUCKY

Kentucky has no additional requirements over and above the federal confidentiality and disclosure requirements for drug and alcohol abuse records.

LOUISIANA

Louisiana has no additional requirements over and above the federal confidentiality and disclosure requirements for drug and alcohol abuse records.

MAINE

Registration and other records of alcohol and drug abuse treatment facilities are confidential and are privileged to the patient.[22] However, the Director of the Office of Alcoholism and Drug Abuse Prevention may make available information from patients' records for purposes of research, so long as it does not disclose patients' names or other identifying information.[23]

MARYLAND

Maryland's general medical record confidentiality and disclosure statute, Maryland Health–General Code § 4-302(a) (1991), does not apply to information governed by the federal confidential alcohol and drug abuse patient records regulations (*id.* § 8-601).[24]

Oral or written statements of a person who seeks counseling, treatment, or therapy for any form of drug or alcohol abuse, made to a physician, psychologist, hospital, or person certified to provide counseling or treatment for such abuse, are privileged, as are observations and conclusions that the practitioner makes. Such information is not admissible in any proceeding against the individual except parole, probation, or conditional release proceedings and commitment proceedings.[25] The disclosure and use of records of individuals served by alcohol and drug abuse treatment programs are

---

22. Maine Revised Statute Annotated tit. 5, § 20047(1) (West 1991).
23. *Id.* § 20047(2).
24. *See also* 42 C.F.R. §§ 2.31–2.35 and 2.51.
25. Maryland Health–General Code § 8-601 (1991).

governed by federal regulations on the confidentiality of alcohol and drug abuse patient records.[26]

Each person authorized to administer, use professionally, or dispense drugs must release to the Alcohol and Drug Addiction Administration, on request, information that deals with drug and alcohol abuse and dependency.[27] Such reports should include the name of the person with the drug or alcohol problem, subject to regulations governing confidentiality.[28]

MASSACHUSETTS

Massachusetts has no additional requirements over and above the federal confidentiality and disclosure requirements for drug and alcohol abuse records.

MICHIGAN

As discussed in Chapter 7, records of the identity, diagnosis, prognosis, and treatment of an individual for substance abuse are confidential, but the statute provides for disclosure of the record with the patient's consent.[29] The statute also permits disclosure of such records without the patient's consent, but only as follows:

- To medical personnel to the extent necessary to meet a bona fide medical emergency

- To qualified personnel for the purpose of conducting scientific statistical research, financial audits, or program evaluation. However, the personnel shall not directly or indirectly identify an individual in a report of the research, audit, or evaluation or otherwise disclose an identity in any manner.

- On application to a court of competent jurisdiction and a ruling by such court ordering disclosure concerning whether a specific individual is under treatment by an agency. In all other respects the confidentiality is the same as the physician-patient relationship.

- On application to a court of competent jurisdiction and a ruling by such court ordering disclosure of a record for the purpose of a hearing to determine whether substance abuse treatment and rehabilitation is necessary in the case of a minor and for review of a minor's treatment plans[30]

---

26. *Id.* § 8-601(c).
27. *Id.* § 8-205(b) (1990).
28. *Id.*
29. Michigan Compiled Laws § 333.6112 (1991).
30. *Id.* § 333.6113 (discussing §§ 333.6124 and 333.6126).

MINNESOTA

Minnesota requires the Department of Human Services to ensure confidentiality to individuals who are the subject of research by the state authority or are recipients of alcohol or drug abuse information, assessment, or treatment from a licensed or approved program.[31] The commissioner of the Department of Human Services must withhold from all persons not connected with the conduct of research the names or other identifying characteristics of a subject of research, unless the subject gives written permission for release. Persons authorized to protect the privacy of a subject of research may not be compelled to reveal the identity or disclose confidential information about the individuals. Before a court may order release, it must determine that the information is relevant and weigh the public interest and the need for disclosure against the injury to the patient, to the treatment relationship, and the harm to the ability of programs to attract and retain patients if disclosure occurs.

MISSISSIPPI

Mississippi has no additional requirements over and above the federal confidentiality and disclosure requirements for drug and alcohol abuse records.

MISSOURI

Missouri has no additional requirements over and above the federal confidentiality and disclosure requirements for drug and alcohol abuse records.

MONTANA

Montana has no additional requirements over and above the federal confidentiality and disclosure requirements for drug and alcohol abuse records.

NEBRASKA

The Nebraska Department of Health/Healthcare Facilities Regulations note that such centers must maintain confidential case records for residents and that confidential information concerning a resident should not be released to any person or agency, except an authorized representative of the department, without prior written consent of the resident.[32]

Nebraska's only statutory reference to records of alcohol and drug abuse treatment states that the director of the Department of Health may obtain a warrant to examine the books and accounts of a facility providing treatment for alcoholism under circumstances listed in the statute.[33]

---

31. Minnesota Statutes § 245A.09 (Supp. 1991).
32. Nebraska Administration Rules and Regulations 175-1-005.19 (1974) (Regulations and Standards Governing Treatment Centers for Persons with Alcohol Problems or the Chemically Dependent).
33. Nebraska Revised Statute § 71-5037 (1991).

NEVADA

Nevada has no additional requirements over and above the federal confidentiality and disclosure requirements for drug and alcohol abuse records, except that healthcare providers may disclose communications made to a physician in an attempt to unlawfully obtain controlled substances. No physician–patient privilege exists for such communications.[34] Otherwise, the records of facilities for the treatment of alcohol and drug abuse are confidential.[35]

NEW HAMPSHIRE

So as not to breach the confidentiality of patient records, healthcare practitioners must keep separate records to show the receipt and disposition of all controlled drugs. Such records are confidential and open to inspection only by law enforcement officers and officers, agents, inspectors, representatives of the board of pharmacy, the attorney general, and all county attorneys whose duty involves enforcing controlled drug laws.[36]

NEW JERSEY

New Jersey has no additional requirements over and above the federal confidentiality and disclosure requirements for drug and alcohol abuse records.

NEW MEXICO

The *New Mexico Hospital Association Legal Handbook* notes that before a program may release a patient's record relating to drug or alcohol treatment, the provider must obtain the written consent of the patient.[37] The consent must

- Specify the name of the program to make the disclosure
- Specify the person or organization to whom disclosure will be made
- Specify the name of the patient
- Specify the purpose of the disclosure
- Specify the information to be disclosed
- Specify that consent may be withdrawn at any time
- Specify a determinable expiration date
- Specify the date on which the consent is signed

---

34. Nevada Revised Statute § 49.245 (1991).
35. *Id.* §§ 458.055 and 458.280.
36. New Hampshire Revised Statute Annotated § 318-B:12(1) (1991).
37. Healthcare Financial Management Association, *New Mexico Hospital Association Legal Handbook* ch. 3, ¶ E(4) at 56 (rev. ed. 1991).

- Be signed by the patient or his or her authorized representative[38]

The *Handbook* also notes that providers should use NMHA Form 12, rather than NMHA Form 11 (the general consent form).[39]

NEW YORK

New York Mental Hygiene Law § 23.05 (McKinney 1992) specifies that all records of identity, diagnosis, prognosis, or treatment in connection with a person's receipt of substance abuse services must be confidential and must be released only in accordance with applicable provisions of the public health law, any other state law, federal law, and court orders.

Section 19.07 gives the Division of Alcoholism and Drug Abuse the authority to obtain information from anyone licensed or permitted to dispense, administer, or conduct research with respect to a controlled substance, consistent with the law as to confidentiality.

NORTH CAROLINA

The North Carolina general statute provides that confidential information acquired in attending or treating a client for mental health, developmental disabilities, or substance abuse is not a public record, is confidential, and may not be disclosed except with client consent, in child abuse reporting, and in court proceedings.[40] Unauthorized disclosure is a misdemeanor.[41] Further, state agencies may inspect such information regardless of any privilege or confidentiality.[42]

The law provides for confidentiality for subjects of research programs on the uses and effects of controlled substances.[43] A practitioner shall not disclose the name of any person who has requested treatment and rehabilitation for drug dependence from him or her to any law-enforcement agency.[44]

NORTH DAKOTA

The North Dakota code has established an addiction counselor–client privilege.[45] Under the code, a client has a privilege to disclose, and to prevent any other person from disclosing, confidential communications made for the purpose of diagnosis or treatment of the client's physical, mental, or emotional condition, including alcohol or drug addiction, among the client, the client's

---

38. *Id.*
39. *Id.* at 57 NMHA Form 12 is referred to as the Consent to Release of Records Concerning Drug or Alcohol Use.
40. North Carolina General Statute § 122C-52 (1991).
41. *Id.*
42. *Id.* §§ 122C-192, 131E-105, 131E-141, and 131E-150.
43. *Id.* § 90-113.3(e).
44. *Id.* § 90-109.1.
45. North Dakota Century Code §§ 31-01-06.3–31-01-06.5 (1991).

counselor, and persons who are participating in the diagnosis or treatment under the direction of the counselor, including members of the client's family.[46] Exceptions include

- Communication relevant to an issue in proceedings to hospitalize the client for mental illness, including alcohol and drug abuse

- When a court orders an examination of the client's physical, mental, or emotional condition

- When a client relies on his physical, mental, or emotional condition as an element of his claim or a defense.[47]

OHIO

Records or information pertaining to the identity, diagnosis, or treatment of drug treatment program patients are confidential and may only be disclosed on patient consent or to qualified personnel for research, management, audits, or program evaluation. However, such personnel may not identify any individual patient in any report or otherwise disclose a patient's identity.[48]

Disclosure may be made without the patient's consent for scientific research (*see* Chapter 8), management, financial audits, or program evaluation so long as the personnel to whom the records were disclosed do not identify any individual patient in any report. A court may also order disclosure in certain circumstances.[49]

Likewise, communications by a person seeking aid in good faith for drug dependence or danger of such dependence are confidential.[50]

OKLAHOMA

Oklahoma has established a confidentiality rule concerning treatments for alcohol and drug abuse.[51] All written communications relating to the treatment and rehabilitation of drug-dependent persons must be contained in folders clearly marked "Confidential," and may be used only by persons actively involved in treatment and rehabilitation. Those persons may not testify about information relating to drug possession or dependency nor may medical records compiled during treatment and rehabilitation be admitted into evidence. Information in the records is confidential and privileged to the patient, but the administrator of an approved facility may make information

---

46. *Id.*
47. *Id.* § 31-01-06.6.
48. Ohio Revised Code § 3793.13(A) and (B) (Baldwin 1992).
49. *Id.* § 3793.13(D) and (E).
50. *Id.* § 3793.12.
51. Oklahoma Statute Annotated tit. 43A, § 3-422 (West 1991).

from such records available for research into the causes and treatment of alcohol and drug abuse so long as the patient is not identified.[52]

OREGON

Oregon Administrative Rules § 426.460(5) provides that the records of a patient at a drug or alcohol addiction treatment facility shall not be disclosed without the consent of the patient.

PENNSYLVANIA

Information from the records of drug and alcohol abuse patients may be disclosed, but only with patients' consent.[53] Clients of hospitalization activities, outpatient activities, and shelter activities that are part of a healthcare facility have the right to inspect their own records.[54] The project director may temporarily remove portions of the record, prior to inspection by the client, if the director determines that the information may be detrimental if presented to the client, but the reasons must be documented.[55] The director must also develop a written procedure covering confidentiality of client identity and records, and staff access to records. Project directors must obtain an informed and voluntary consent from each client for disclosure of information. The disclosure must be in writing and must include the following:

- Name of the person, agency, or organization to whom disclosure is made

- Specific information disclosed

- Purpose of disclosure

- Dated signature of the client or guardian

- Signature of a witness

- Expiration date of the consent[56]

The facility should offer a copy of the consent to the client and keep a copy in the records. Where consent is not required, the project personnel must fully document the disclosure in the client records and inform the client, as quickly as possible, of the disclosure, its purposes, and to whom the disclosure was made.[57] Inpatient nonhospital activities—transitional living

---

52. *Id.* § 3-423.
53. 71 Pennsylvania Consolidated Statute § 1690.108(b) (1991).
54. 28 Pennsylvania Code §§ 711.83(b), 711.93(b), and 711.102(b) (1991).
55. *Id.*
56. 28 Pennsylvania Code §§ 711.83(c)(1) and (2), 711.93(c)(1) and (2), and 711.102(c)(1) and (2).
57. *Id.* §§ 711.83(c)(3), 711.93(c)(3), and 711.102(c)(3).

facilities,[58] intake evaluation and referral activities,[59] and inpatient nonhospital activities—short-term detoxification[60] have identical client access and confidentiality requirements.

RHODE ISLAND

Rhode Island law permits disclosure of otherwise confidential healthcare information to law enforcement personnel if a patient has or is attempting to obtain narcotic drugs from the healthcare provider illegally.[61]

Rhode Island law states that all providers of treatment for substance dependency and abuse shall maintain and make available to third-party insurers medical records attesting to the medical necessity of the treatment. In the absence of such information, insurers are not obliged to reimburse the healthcare facility for the care in question.[62]

SOUTH CAROLINA

All certificates, applications, records, and reports identifying patients hospitalized for alcohol or drug abuse are confidential and may not be disclosed except on consent; on court order; for research conducted or authorized by the State Department of Mental Health or the South Carolina Commission on Alcohol and Drug Abuse, as may be necessary to cooperate with law enforcement, health, welfare, and other state agencies; or as necessary to carry out the provisions of state law concerning such treatments.[63]

SOUTH DAKOTA

South Dakota requires alcohol and drug abuse facilities to protect client case records against loss, tampering, or unauthorized disclosure of information, and maintain confidentiality of client case records in accordance with federal regulations.[64] Each healthcare provider must have policies and procedures that govern client access to case records. South Dakota administrative rules require each healthcare provider to assure the timely closing of case records of inactive clients.[65] The maximum time a case record may be kept open without client contact may not exceed

* Detoxification records, not more than six months

---

58. *Id.* § 711.72.
59. *Id.* § 711.43.
60. *Id.* § 711.62.
61. Rhode Island General Law § 5-37.3-4(b)(4) (1991).
62. *Id.* § 27-38-2.
63. South Carolina Code Annotated § 44-52-190(4) (1991).
64. South Dakota Administration Rules 44:14:33:01 (1986); *see also* 42 C.F.R. § 2.23 (1991). Subsection (a) deals with patients' access to alcohol and drug abuse information, and subsection (b) concerns healthcare providers' and others' use of such information.
65. *Id.* at 44:14:33:03.

- Support service records, not more than six months

- Community counseling records, not more than three months

- Outpatient treatment records, not more than three months

- Residential treatment records, not more than one month

- Transitional care records, not more than one month

- Custodial care records, not more than one month[66]

The agency must arrange for safe storage and recall of client case records for at least six years.

TENNESSEE

Tennessee has no additional requirements over and above the federal confidentiality and disclosure requirements for drug and alcohol abuse records.

TEXAS

Communications between a patient or client and any healthcare provider for the purpose of diagnosing, evaluating, or treating a mental or emotional disorder, including alcoholism and drug abuse, are confidential and will not be disclosed except in limited circumstances listed below:

- In court proceedings

  - When the proceedings are brought by the patient against a professional, and in criminal or license revocation proceedings where disclosure is relevant to the claim or defense of a professional

  - When the patient waives his or her right in writing or other persons acting on his or her behalf do so

  - When the purpose of the proceeding is to collect on a claim for mental or emotional health services rendered to the patient

  - When a judge finds that the patient, after being previously informed that the communications would not be privileged, communicated to a professional in the course of a court-ordered examination relating to his mental or emotional condition or disorder

    - In criminal prosecution where the patient is a victim, witness, or defendant

- In other than court proceedings

---

66. *Id.*

- To governmental agencies where required or authorized by law

- To medical or law enforcement personnel where the professional determines that a probability of imminent physical injury by the patient or client to himself or herself or others, or a probability of immediate mental or emotional injury to the patient exists

- To qualified personnel for the purpose of management and financial audits, program evaluations, or research

- To a person bearing the written consent of the patient, or a parent or guardian if the patient is a minor or has been adjudicated incompetent, or to his personal representative if deceased

- To individuals, corporations, or governmental agencies involved in the payment or collection of fees for mental or emotional health services

- To other professionals and personnel under their direction who are participating in the diagnosis, evaluation, or treatment of the patient

- In official legislative inquiries[67]

A person aggrieved by a violation of this statute may sue for an injunction and for civil damages.[68]

UTAH

Utah has no additional requirements over and above the federal confidentiality and disclosure requirements for drug and alcohol abuse records.

VERMONT

Any information concerning drug test results held by an employer is confidential and may not be released to anyone except the employer, applicant, or employee, and may only be obtained by court order as provided in the statute.[69] Employers, laboratories, and their agents, who receive or have access to information about drug test results, must keep all information confidential. Release must be made solely pursuant to a written voluntary consent form signed by the tested person.[70] Should any information about such drug test be released contrary to the above provisions, such information will be inadmissible as evidence in most judicial or quasi-judicial proceedings.[71]

---

67. Texas Revised Civil Statute Annotated art. 4495b, § 5.08(j) (West 1992).
68. *Id.*
69. Vermont Statute Annotated tit. 21, § 516(a) (1991).
70. *Id.* § 516(b); § 518 (1991).
71. *Id.* § 516(c).

VIRGINIA

Virginia has no additional requirements over and above the federal confidentiality and disclosure requirements for drug and alcohol abuse records.

WASHINGTON

Washington law specifies the conditions under which a facility may disclose confidential records of alcoholics and intoxicated persons.[72] For example, records may be disclosed

- With the prior written consent of the patient

- If authorized by an appropriate order of a court of competent jurisdiction granted after application showing good cause

- To comply with state laws mandating the reporting of suspected child abuse or neglect

- When a patient commits a crime on program premises or against program personnel, or threatens to do so[73]

WEST VIRGINIA

As discussed in Chapter 8, healthcare providers responsible for the diagnosis, treatment, or provision of healthcare services in the case of drug rehabilitation or related services may not, with two exceptions, release patient records of such diagnosis, treatment, or provision of health care to a parent or guardian, without prior written consent from the patient.[74]

WISCONSIN

Wisconsin law establishes a drug dependence and drug abuse program that allows the department to collect data on drug abuse treatment from all treatment facilities.[75] Wisconsin also permits access to medical records of persons treated for mental illness, developmental disabilities, alcohol or drug abuse, without patient consent for authorized research.[76]

In addition, patients treated for mental illness, developmental disabilities, or alcohol or drug abuse may have access to their treatment records during treatment unless the director of the treatment facility has reason to believe that the benefits of allowing access to a patient are outweighed by the disadvantages.[77] After discharge, a patient is allowed access, on one working day's

---

72. Washington Revised Code § 70.96A.150(1) (1991).
73. *Id.*
74. West Virginia Code § 16-29-1(b) (1991).
75. Wisconsin Statutes § 140.81 (1990).
76. Wisconsin Administration Code § HSS 92.04(3) (June 1986).
77. *Id.* § HSS 92.05.

notice, and may have a copy of his or her records subject to payment of a uniform and reasonable fee.

WYOMING

A hospital may disclose healthcare information about a patient without the patient's authorization to the extent a recipient needs to know the information, if the disclosure is

- To an official of a penal or other custodial institution in which the patient is detained[78]

- To federal, state, or local public health authorities, to the extent the hospital is required by law to report healthcare information or when needed to protect the public health

- To federal, state, or local law enforcement authorities to the extent required by law[79]

---

78. Wyoming Statute § 35-2-609(a)(x) (1991).
79. *Id.* § 35-2-609(b)(i)-(iv).

CHAPTER 10

Disclosure of Communicable Disease Information

Introduction

As discussed in Chapter 7, patients have a right to privacy for healthcare records that contain information concerning communicable diseases. Thus, healthcare providers must be careful not to disclose information that would violate a patient's right of privacy. This chapter will discuss the instances in which a healthcare provider is authorized to release communicable disease information.

Federal Laws

Federal law does not provide specific requirements concerning disclosure of communicable disease information. Thus, a national healthcare organization must consider each state in which it has a facility to determine the law that applies.

State Laws

ALABAMA

Alabama does not provide specific requirements concerning disclosure of communicable disease information.

ALASKA

Alaska does not provide specific requirements concerning disclosure of communicable disease information.

ARIZONA

Communicable disease information is confidential.[1] Arizona provides detailed guidance concerning to whom a practitioner may release such information including

---

1. Arizona Revised Statute Annotated § 36-664 (1991).

- The protected person or, if the protected person lacks capacity to consent, a person authorized by law to consent

- Agents or employees of health facilities or providers, if the agents or employees are authorized to access medical records, if the facilities or providers are authorized to obtain such information, and if the agents or employees provide health care to the protected individual or maintain or possess medical records for billing or reimbursement

- Healthcare providers or facilities, if knowledge of the communicable disease–related information is necessary to provide appropriate care or treatment to the person or a child

- Health facilities or providers in relation to the procurement, processing, distributing, or use of a human body or a human body part, including fluids, for use in medical education, research, or therapy or for transport to another person

- A peer review, utilization review, or similar activity so long as the disclosure does not include information directly identifying the protected person

- Federal, state, county, or local health officers, if disclosure is mandated by law

- Government agencies authorized by law to receive the information

Information may also be released pursuant to a court order or a written release if any of the following conditions exist:

- Disclosure is authorized by law

- Disclosure is made to a contact of the protected person

- Disclosure is made pursuant to a release of confidential communicable disease information

- Disclosure is for the purpose of research[2]

Any disclosure made pursuant to a release must be accompanied by a statement in writing warning that the information is from confidential records and is protected by state law prohibiting further disclosure without the specific written consent of the person to whom it pertains or as otherwise permitted by law. The person making a disclosure must keep a record of all disclosures.

Under Arizona revised statutes, tuberculosis control officers may, with the consent of the attending physician, examine any and all records, reports, and other data pertaining to the tuberculosis condition of tuberculosis pa-

---

2. *Id.*

tients. However, information so obtained is confidential, privileged, and cannot be divulged so as to disclose the identity of the person to whom it relates.[3]

ARKANSAS

Arkansas does not provide specific requirements concerning disclosure of communicable disease information.

CALIFORNIA

California does not provide specific requirements concerning disclosure of communicable disease information.

COLORADO

Colorado does not provide specific requirements concerning disclosure of communicable disease information.

CONNECTICUT

Under Connecticut General Statute § 19a-583 (1991), no person may disclose human immunodeficiency virus (HIV)–related information except to the following:

- The protected individual or legal guardian

- Any person who secures a release of confidential HIV-related information

- Federal, state, or local health officers, when such disclosure is mandated or authorized by federal or state law.

- Healthcare providers or health facilities when knowledge of the HIV-related information is necessary to provide appropriate care or treatment to the protected individual or a child, or when confidential HIV-related information is already recorded in a medical chart or record and a healthcare provider has access to such record for the purpose of providing medical care to the protected individual

- Medical examiner to assist in determining the cause or circumstances of death

- Health facility staff committees or accreditation or oversight review organizations conducting program monitoring, program evaluation, or service reviews

- Healthcare provider or other person in cases where such person in the course of occupational duties has had significant exposure to HIV infection, provided detailed criteria are met

---

3. *Id.* § 36-714.

- Employees of hospitals for mental illness operated by the Department of Mental Health, if the infection control committee of the hospital determines that the behavior of the patient poses a significant risk of transmission to another patient and specific criteria are met

- Employees of facilities operated by the Department of Correction, if specific criteria are met

- By court order, which is issued in compliance with the following provisions:

  - The court finds a clear and imminent danger to the public health or the health of a person, and the person has demonstrated a compelling need for the test results that cannot be accommodated by other means.

  - Pleadings pertaining to disclosure of confidential HIV-related information substitute a pseudonym for the true name of the subject of the test.

  - Before granting any such order, the court provides the individual whose test result is in question with notice and a reasonable opportunity to participate in the proceedings.

  - The court proceedings are conducted *in camera* unless the subject of the test agrees to a hearing in open court or unless the court determines that a public hearing is necessary to the public interest and the proper administration of justice.

  - On issuance of an order to disclose test results, the court imposes appropriate safeguards against unauthorized disclosure, which must specify the persons who may have access to the information, the purposes for which the information must be used, and appropriate prohibitions on future disclosure.

- Life and health insurers, government payers, and healthcare centers and their affiliates, reinsurers, and contractors (except agents and brokers) in connection with underwriting and claim activity for life, health, and disability benefits

- Any healthcare provider specifically designated by the protected individual to receive such information received by a life or health insurer or healthcare center pursuant to an application for life, health, or disability insurance *(id.)*

Whenever confidential HIV-related information is disclosed, it must be accompanied by a statement in writing, whenever possible, that includes the following or substantially similar language:

This information has been disclosed to you from records whose confidentiality is protected by state law. State law prohibits you from making any further disclosure of it without the specific written consent of the person to whom it pertains, or as otherwise permitted by said law. A general authorization for the release of medical or other information is NOT sufficient for this purpose (*id.* § 19a-585).

A notation of all permitted disclosures should be placed in the medical record.

DELAWARE

Information and records held by the Division of Public Health relating to known or suspected sexually transmitted diseases, including human immunodeficiency virus (HIV) infection, are confidential and may only be released in the following limited circumstances:

- Release is made of medical or epidemiological information for statistical purposes so that no person can be identified.

- Release is made of medical or epidemiological information with the consent of all persons identified in the information released.

- Release is made of medical or epidemiological information to medical personnel, appropriate state agencies, or state courts to the extent required to enforce the provisions of the law and related rules and regulations concerning the control and treatment of sexually transmitted diseases, or as related to child abuse investigation.

- Release is made of medical or epidemiological information to medical personnel in a medical emergency to the extent necessary to protect the health or life of a named party.

- Release is made during the course of civil or criminal litigation to a person allowed access to said records by a court order issued in compliance with the detailed requirements of the law.[4]

Violations of these reporting requirements may result in a fine of between $100 and $1,000.[5] A violation of this law and the law concerning reporting of sexually transmitted diseases may result in a fine of $25 to $200.[6]

No person may disclose or be compelled to disclose the identity of any person on whom an HIV-related test is performed or the results of such test in a manner that permits identification of the subject of the test, except to the following persons[7]:

---

4. Delaware Code Annotated tit. 16, §§ 711–712 or 702 (1991).
5. *Id.* § 713(a). This section does not cover reporting of sexually transmitted diseases.
6. *Id.* §§ 713 and 702.
7. *Id.* § 1203.

- Subject of the test or subject's legal guardian

- Any person who secures a legally effective release of test results executed by the subject of the test or subject's legal guardian

- Authorized agent or employee of a healthcare facility or healthcare provider, if the facility or provider itself is authorized to obtain the test results, if the agent or employee provides patient care or handles or processes specimens of body fluids or tissues, and the agent or employee has a medical need to know such information to provide health care to the patient

- Healthcare providers giving medical care to the subject of the test, when knowledge of test results is necessary to provide appropriate medical care or treatment

- When part of an official report to the Division of Public Health, as may be required by regulation

- Health facility or healthcare provider that procures, processes, distributes, or uses

  - Blood

  - Human body part from a deceased person donated for a purpose specified under the Uniform Anatomical Gift Act

  - Semen provided prior to July 11, 1988, for the purpose of artificial insemination

- Health facility staff committees or accreditation or oversight review organizations conducting program monitoring, program evaluation, or service reviews

- For the investigation of child abuse.[8]

- For the control of sexually transmitted diseases.[9]

- Pursuant to a court order issued in compliance with the detailed requirements of the statute[10]

Anyone aggrieved by an improper disclosure of such information may recover damages of $1,000 or actual damages, whichever is greater, if the violation is negligent; damages of $5,000 or actual damages, if the violation is intentional or reckless; and reasonable attorney's fees and other relief, such as an injunction, that the court deems appropriate.[11]

---

8. *Id.* §§ 901–909.
9. *Id.* §§ 701–713.
10. *Id.* § 1203.
11. *Id.* § 1204(a).

DISTRICT OF COLUMBIA

Records related to cases of communicable disease or environmentally or occupationally related disease or medical conditions may be used for statistical and public health purposes only. Any identifying information in the records may be disclosed only when necessary to safeguard the physical health of others. No person is allowed to disclose or redisclose identifying information from such records unless the patient gives prior written permission or a court finds, on clear and convincing evidence, that the disclosure is necessary to safeguard another's health or to provide evidence probative of guilt or innocence in a criminal prosecution.[12]

The head of Preventive Health Services Administration, Commission on Public Health, Department of Human Services, is authorized to make any necessary investigation to determine the source of the infection and the nature of treatment. Hospitals, laboratories, and physicians are required to make medical records and histories available to the administrator to facilitate such investigations. The administrator, however, may not disclose the identity of an acquired immune deficiency syndrome (AIDS) patient without that person's written permission.

The provisions of the Preventive Health Services Amendments Act of 1985, pertaining to the confidentiality of medical records and information on persons with AIDS, apply to AIDS treatment.[13]

FLORIDA

Florida does not provide specific requirements concerning disclosure of communicable disease information.

GEORGIA

Georgia does not provide specific requirements concerning disclosure of communicable disease information.

HAWAII

Hawaii requires the director of health to ensure that the state hospital keeps medical records of every patient.[14]

Hawaii provides for confidentiality in such reports by prohibiting disclosures that would identify the persons to whom the records relate, except as necessary to safeguard the public health against those who disobey the rules relating to such diseases.[15] The confidentiality of human immunodeficiency virus (HIV) infection, AIDS-related complex (ARC), and acquired immune

---

12. District of Columbia Code Annotated § 6-117 (1991).
13. *Id.* § 6-2805.
14. Hawaii Revised Statute § 334-35 (1991).
15. *Id.* § 325-4.

deficiency syndrome (AIDS) records information is assured and may not be released or made public on subpoena or any other method of discovery.[16] However, release of this information is permitted under the following circumstances, if

- Release is made to the Department of Health in compliance with federal reporting requirements imposed on the state. The department must ensure that personal identifying information in these records is protected from public disclosure.

- Release is made of the records, or of specific medical or epidemiological information contained therein, with the prior written consent of the person or persons to whom the records pertain.

- Release is made to medical personnel in a medical emergency only to the extent necessary to protect the health, life, or well-being of the named party.

- Release to or by the Department of Health is necessary to protect the health and well-being of the general public, provided such release is made in such a way that no person can be identified, except as specified in law.

- Release is made by the Department of Health of medical or epidemiological information from the records to medical personnel, appropriate county and state agencies, blood banks, plasma centers, organ and tissue banks, schools, preschools, day care centers, or county or district courts to enforce this part and to enforce rules adopted by the Department of Health concerning the control and treatment of HIV infection, AIDS, and ARC, provided that release of information is only made by confidential communication to a designated individual.

- Release of a child's records is made to the Department of Human Services for the purpose of enforcing child abuse laws or suspect transmission of HIV.

- Release of a child's records is made within the Department of Human Services and to child protective services team consultants under contract to the Department of Human Services for the purpose of enforcing and administering the law on a need-to-know basis pursuant to a written protocol to be established and implemented, in consultation with the director of health, by the director of human services.

- Release of a child's records is made by employees of the Department of Human Services authorized to do so by the protocol established in the law to a natural parent of a child who is the subject of the case (when the

---

16. *Id.* § 325-101(a).

natural parent is a client in the case), to the guardian *ad litem* of the child, to the court, to each party to the court proceedings, and also to an adoptive or a prospective adoptive parent, to an individual or an agency with whom the child is placed for 24-hour residential care, and to medical personnel responsible for the care or treatment of the child. When a release is made to a natural parent of the child, it must be with appropriate counseling as required by the law.[17] In no event may proceedings be initiated against a child's natural parents for claims of child abuse or harm to a child or to affect parental rights solely on the basis of the HIV seropositivity of a child or of the child's natural parents.

- Release is made to the patient's healthcare insurer to obtain reimbursement for services rendered to the patient, provided that release will not be made if, after being informed that a claim will be made to an insurer, the patient is afforded the opportunity to make the reimbursement directly and actually makes the reimbursement.

- Release is made by the patient's healthcare provider to another healthcare provider for the purpose of continued care or treatment of the patient.

- Release is made pursuant to a court order, after an *in camera* review of the records, on a showing of good cause by the party seeking the release of the records.[18]

IDAHO

Confidential disease reports containing patient identification reported under the statute may be only used by public health officials who must conduct investigations, and may be disclosed only as provided by law. Any person who willfully or maliciously discloses the content of any of these confidential public health records is guilty of a misdemeanor.[19]

ILLINOIS

Reports of incidents of sexually transmitted diseases, including acquired immune deficiency syndrome (AIDS), to the Public Health Department are confidential, but may be disclosed

- With consent

- For statistical purposes and medical or epidemiologic information, if summarized so no one can be identified and no names are revealed

- When made to medical personnel, appropriate state agencies, or courts to enforce the statute

---

17. *Id.* § 325-101(b) (*see* § 325-16).
18. *Id.*
19. Idaho Code § 39-606 (1991) (effective July 1, 1993).

- When pursuant to a subpoena. In such cases, the information must be sealed by the court, except as necessary to reach a decision or as otherwise agreed by all parties; the proceedings must be *in camera* and the record sealed.[20]

- When authorized by the AIDS Confidentiality Act.[21]

- When made to a school principal[22]

- When authorized by the AIDS Registry System Regulations[23]

Insurance companies and health service corporations that require patients or applicants for new or continued coverage to be tested for AIDS must keep the results confidential.[24]

INDIANA

Communicable or other disease information is confidential, but disclosure is permitted for statistical purposes if done in a manner that does not identify any individual, with the individual's consent, or to the extent necessary to enforce public health laws or to protect the life or health of a third party.[25] The law also specifies the conditions under which a practitioner may notify a person at risk of a dangerous communicable disease of otherwise confidential information.[26]

IOWA

Reports on acquired immune deficiency syndrome (AIDS) are confidential, and information in such reports may not be released except under the following circumstances[27]:

- Medical or epidemiological information may be released for statistical purposes in a manner such that no individual person can be identified.

- Medical or epidemiological information may be released to the extent necessary to enforce the provisions of the statute and related rules concerning the treatment, control, and investigation of the human immunodeficiency virus (HIV) infection by public health officials.

---

20. Illinois Revised Statute ch. 111½, ¶ 7408(a)–(c) (1991).
21. Illinois Administrative Code tit. 77, § 693.100(b)(5) (1991). *See also* Illinois Revised Statute ch. 111½, ¶ 7315 (1991); Illinois Revised Statute ch. 23, ¶ 2055 (1991); Illinois Revised Statute ch. 37, ¶ 802-11 (1991).
22. Illinois Administrative Code tit. 77, § 693.100(b)(6) (1991); Illinois Revised Statute ch. 111½, ¶ 22.12(a) (1991).
23. Illinois Administrative Code tit. 77, § 693.100(b)(4) (1991).
24. Illinois Revised Statute ch. 111½, ¶ 5403(b) (1991).
25. Indiana Code § 16-1-9.5-7 (1979 and Supp. 1991).
26. *Id.* § 16-1-10.5-11.5.
27. Iowa Code § 141.10 (1991).

- Medical or epidemiological information may be released to medical personnel in a medical emergency to the extent necessary to protect the health or life of the named party.

- Test results concerning a patient may be released pursuant to procedures established under the Iowa code.[28]

Iowa permits disclosure of otherwise confidential HIV information to protect a third party from the direct risk of transmission after making a reasonable attempt to warn, in writing, the infected person of the nature of and reason for the disclosure, the date of disclosure, and the name of the party or parties to whom the disclosure is to be made.[29]

The State Department of Health, the Iowa Medical Society or any of its allied medical societies, the Iowa Society of Osteopathic Physicians and Surgeons, or any in-hospital staff committee may use or publish material from any morbidity or mortality studies only to advance medical research or education, except that a summary of such studies may be published. In all events, the identity of any patient will be confidential. Violation of such confidentiality is a misdemeanor.[30]

KANSAS

Information required to be reported and information obtained through laboratory tests conducted by the Department of Health and Environment relating to human immunodeficiency virus (HIV) or acquired immune deficiency syndrome (AIDS) and persons suffering from or infected with HIV or AIDS is confidential. This information may not be disclosed beyond what is necessary to comply with the law,[31] or the usual reporting of laboratory test results to persons specifically designated by the secretary as authorized to obtain such information. Such information may be disclosed, however, if

- No person can be identified in the information to be disclosed, and the disclosure is for statistical purposes.

- All persons who are identifiable in the information to be disclosed consent in writing to its disclosure.

- Disclosure is necessary, and is made only to the extent necessary to protect public health as specified by rules and regulations of the secretary.

- A medical emergency exists and disclosure is to medical personnel qualified to treat AIDS, but only to the extent necessary to protect the health or life of a named party.

---

28. *Id.*
29. *Id.* § 141.6(2)(d)(2).
30. *Id.* § 135.41.
31. Kansas Statute Annotated § 65-6003(a) (1991).

- Information to be disclosed is required in a court proceeding involving a minor, and the information is disclosed *in camera*.[32]

The secretary of Health and Environment may adopt and enforce rules and regulations for the prevention and control of AIDS and for such other measures as may be necessary to protect the public health.[33] Physicians are authorized to disclose that a patient has AIDS or has had a positive reaction to an AIDS test to other healthcare providers who will be placed in contact with bodily fluids of such patient during medical procedures. Such information is otherwise confidential.[34]

KENTUCKY

Kentucky does not provide specific requirements concerning disclosure of communicable disease information.

LOUISIANA

Louisiana does not provide specific requirements concerning disclosure of communicable disease information.

MAINE

Maine statutes provide confidentiality of human immunodeficiency virus (HIV) test results. Disclosure of the results of an HIV test to state agencies is permitted, however, including the Department of Corrections, Department of Human Services, and Department of Mental Health and Mental Retardation to the extent that these departments are responsible for the treatment or care of the subject.[35] Such agencies must promulgate rules covering disclosure of test results. The statute also provides for court-ordered disclosure and disclosure to the Bureau of Health.

MARYLAND

Maryland does not provide specific requirements concerning disclosure of communicable disease information.

MASSACHUSETTS

Massachusetts does not provide specific requirements concerning disclosure of communicable disease information.

---

32. *Id.* §§ 65-6002(c) and 65-6003(b).
33. *Id.* § 65-6003(a).
34. *Id.* § 65-6004(a).
35. Maine Revised Statute Annotated tit. 5, § 19203(7) (1991).

MICHIGAN

Any release of reports, records, and data pertaining to the testing, care, treatment, reporting, and research associated with serious communicable diseases or human immunodeficiency virus (HIV) infections, acquired immune deficiency syndrome (AIDS), and AIDS-related complex (ARC) to a legislative body shall not contain information that identifies a specific individual who was tested.[36] In addition, such information may be released to the Department of Public Health, a local health department, or other healthcare provider for one or more of the following reasons:

- To protect the health of an individual

- To prevent further transmission of HIV

- To diagnose and care for a patient[37]

Michigan law also provides for disclosure to an employee of a school district if necessary to prevent a reasonably foreseeable risk of transmission of HIV to pupils.[38] Further, an individual may expressly authorize disclosure if the written authorization is specific to HIV infection, AIDS, or ARC. If the individual is a minor or incapacitated, a parent or legal guardian may execute such an authorization.[39] A provider may also disclose such information under the child abuse reporting laws.[40]

Violation of this law is a misdemeanor and subjects the violator to actual damages or $1,000, whichever is greater, and costs and reasonable attorney fees.[41]

MINNESOTA

Minnesota does not provide specific requirements concerning disclosure of communicable disease information.

MISSISSIPPI

Mississippi does not provide specific requirements concerning disclosure of communicable disease information.

MISSOURI

All information and records held by healthcare providers or the state of

---

36. Michigan Compiled Laws Annotated § 333.5131(4) (1991).
37. *Id.* § 333.5131(5)(a).
38. *Id.* § 333.5131(5)(c).
39. *Id.* § 333.5131(5)(d).
40. *Id.* §§ 722.626(2)–722.636.
41. *Id.* § 333.5131(8).

Missouri are confidential, and such information and records may be disclosed to the following[42]:

- Public employees within the agency, department, or political subdivision who need to know to perform their public duties

- Public employees of other agencies, departments, or political subdivisions who need to know to perform their public duties

- Persons other than public employees who are entrusted with the regular care of those under the care and custody of a state agency, including but not limited to operators of day care facilities, group homes, residential care facilities, and adoptive and foster parents[43]

- The Department of Health

- Healthcare personnel working directly with the infected individual, who have a reasonable need to know the results for the purpose of providing direct patient health care

- The spouse of the subject of the test result or results

- The subject or legal guardian or custodian of the subject of the testing, if he or she is an unemancipated minor

- Pursuant to the written authorization of the subject of the test result or results[44]

MONTANA

Montana does not provide specific requirements concerning disclosure of communicable disease information.

NEBRASKA

Nebraska does not provide specific requirements concerning disclosure of communicable disease information.

NEVADA

Nevada does not provide specific requirements concerning disclosure of communicable disease information.

NEW HAMPSHIRE

The identity of the person tested for human immunodeficiency virus (HIV) may not be disclosed. Under New Hampshire law, all records and other

---

42. Missouri Revised Statute § 191.656 (1990).
43. *Id.* § 191.656(1)(1)(a)–(c).
44. *Id.* § 191.656(2)(1)(a)–(f).

information relating to persons testing for this virus shall be maintained as confidential and protected from inadvertent or unwarranted intrusion.[45] Such information may be released, however, on request if the patient has given written authorization or to other healthcare providers when necessary to protect the health of the patient tested. Anyone who purposely violates these confidentiality requirements and thereby discloses the identity of a person infected by HIV is both (1) liable for actual damages, court costs, and attorney's fees, plus a civil penalty of up to $5,000 for such disclosure,[46] and (2) guilty of a misdemeanor.[47]

A report provided to the director that identifies a specific individual as having a communicable disease may only be released to persons demonstrating a need essential to health-related research. Any release of information must be conditioned on individual identities remaining confidential. The physician–patient privilege does not apply to communicable disease information.[48]

Healthcare providers may not disclose the identity of an individual reported to the cancer registry as having cancer, except to persons demonstrating a need essential to health-related research. The release must be conditioned on the personal identities of these cancer patients remaining confidential. The physician–patient privilege does not apply to reports to the cancer registry.[49]

Similarly, reports of critical health problems or other data that disclose the identity of such person's problem may be made available only to persons who demonstrate a need for the material essential to health-related research. The physician–patient privilege does not apply to such reports.[50]

NEW JERSEY

Healthcare providers may disclose the content of records concerning diagnosed cases of acquired immune deficiency syndrome (AIDS) or human immunodeficiency virus (HIV) infections if the subject of the record has given prior written informed consent[51] or if the subject is deceased or legally incompetent.[52]

If the prior written consent of such person was not obtained, the person's records may be disclosed only under the following conditions:

- To qualified personnel for the purpose of conducting scientific research, but a record must be released for research only following review of the research protocol by an Institutional Review Board constituted pursuant

45. New Hampshire Revised Statute Annotated § 141-F:8(I) and (II) (1991).
46. *Id.* § 141-F:10.
47. *Id.* § 141-F:11.
48. *Id.* § 141-C:7.
49. *Id.* § 141-B:9.
50. *Id.* § 141-A:5.
51. New Jersey Revised Statute § 26:5C-8 (1991).
52. *Id.* § 26:5C-12.

to federal regulation.[53] The person who is the subject of the record may not be identified in any report, and research personnel may not disclose the patient's identity.

- To qualified personnel for the purpose of conducting management audits, financial audits, or program evaluation, but the personnel shall not identify the person who is the subject of the record in any report or otherwise disclose the person's identity. The facility shall not release identifying information to audit personnel unless it is vital to the audit or evaluation.

- To qualified personnel involved in medical education or in the diagnosis and treatment of the person who is the subject of the record. Disclosure is limited to only personnel directly involved in medical education or in the diagnosis or treatment of the person.

- To the Department of Health as required by state or federal law

- As permitted by rules and regulations adopted by the commissioner for the purposes of disease prevention and control

- In all other instances authorized by State or federal law[54]

While New Jersey law requires consent for disclosure of the records of a person who has or is suspected of having AIDS or HIV infection, if such person is deceased or legally incompetent, the facility may obtain the consent from the following:

- Executor or administrator of such person's estate

- Authorized representative of the legally incompetent or deceased person

- Such person's spouse or primary caretaking partner or, if none, by another member of the person's family

- Commissioner of Health in the event that a deceased person has neither an authorized representative nor next of kin[55]

Similarly, when disclosure involves a minor, the provider may obtain consent from the parent, guardian, or other individual authorized under state law to act in the minor's behalf.[56]

Healthcare providers and personnel may disclose AIDS or HIV information pursuant to a court order conditioned on a showing of good cause.[57] New Jersey law specifies that the limitations on disclosure in the law continue to apply to a person who has been a patient or participant in a program

53. *Id.* § 26:5C-12 *referring to* 45 C.F.R. § 46.101 *et seq.* (1991).
54. *Id.* § 26:5C-8.
55. *Id.* § 26:5C-12.
56. *Id.* § 26:5C-13.
57. *Id.* § 26:5C-9.

whether or not the person remains a patient or participant.[58] New Jersey law also states that the recipient of any record disclosed under the statute shall hold it as confidential and not release it unless the conditions of the statute are met.[59]

New Jersey provides sanctions for violation of the confidentiality provisions.[60] A person who has or is suspected of having AIDS or HIV infection who is aggrieved as a result of a violation of the statute may sue to obtain appropriate relief, including actual damages, equitable relief (such as an injunction), and reasonable attorney's fees and court costs. The court may award punitive damages when the violation was reckless or intentionally malicious.

NEW MEXICO

Under the Human Immunodeficiency Virus Test Act,[61] no one may disclose the identity of any person and the test results other than to

- The subject of the test, the subject's legally authorized guardian or custodian, and any person designated in a legally effective release executed by the subject

- An authorized agent or a credentialed or privileged physician or employee of a health facility or healthcare provider, if the facility or provider itself is authorized to obtain the test results; the agent or employee provides patient care or handles or processes specimens of bodily fluids or tissues; and the agent or employee has a need to know such information

- A health facility or healthcare provider that processes, procures, distributes, or uses

  - Human body parts from deceased persons with respect to medical information regarding that person

  - Semen provided prior to the effective date of the Human Immunodeficiency Virus Test Act for purposes of artificial insemination

  - Blood or blood products for transfusion or injection

  - Human body parts for transplant with respect to medical information regarding the donor recipient

- Health facility staff committees or accreditation or oversight review organizations conducting program monitoring, evaluation, or service (so long as any identity remains confidential)

---

58. *Id.* § 26:5C-10.
59. *Id.* § 26:5C-11.
60. *Id.* § 26:5C-14.
61. New Mexico Statute Annotated § 24-2B-6 (Michie 1992).

- For purposes of application or reapplication for insurance coverage, an insurer or reinsurer at whose request the test is performed.[62]

Disclosure under this Act must be accompanied by a written statement that includes the following or similar language:

> This information has been disclosed to you from records whose confidentiality is protected by state law. State law prohibits you from making any further disclosure of such information without the specific written consent of the person to whom such information pertains, or as otherwise permitted by state law.[63]

NEW YORK

Under New York public health law, reports of sexually transmissible diseases are confidential except as necessary to control such diseases.[64] Human immunodeficiency virus (HIV) and acquired immune deficiency syndrome (AIDS)–related information is confidential and may not be disclosed except to[65]

- Protected individuals, or when such individual lacks capacity to consent, a person authorized pursuant to law to consent to health care for the individual

- Any person to whom disclosure is authorized pursuant to a release of confidential HIV-related information

- Agents or employees of a health facility or healthcare provider if (1) the agent or employee is permitted to access medical records; (2) the health facility or healthcare provider itself is authorized to obtain the HIV-related information; and (3) the agent or employee provides health care to the protected individual, or maintains or processes medical records for billing or reimbursement

- Healthcare providers or health facilities, when knowledge of the HIV-related information is necessary to provide appropriate care or treatment to the protected individual or child of the individual

- Health facilities or healthcare providers, in relation to the procurement, processing, distributing, or use of a human body or body part including organs, tissues, eyes, bones, arteries, blood, semen, or other body fluids, for use in medical education, research, therapy, or for transplantation to individuals

- Federal, state, county, or local health officers when such disclosure is mandated by federal or state law

---

62. *Id.* § 24-2B-6(A)–(F), (H).
63. *Id.* § 24-2B-7; *see also* Healthcare Financial Management Association, *New Mexico Hospital Association Legal Handbook,* ch. 3, ¶ E (4) at 55–56 (rev. ed. 1991).
64. New York Public Health Law § 2306 (McKinney 1992).
65. *Id.* § 2782.

- Authorized agencies in connection with foster care or adoption of a child

- Insurance institutions or other third-party reimbursers or their agents to the extent necessary to reimburse healthcare providers for health services; provided that, where necessary, an otherwise appropriate authorization for such disclosure has been secured by the provider

- Any person to whom disclosure is ordered by a court of competent jurisdiction

- Employees or agents of the division of parole under certain circumstances

- Employees or agents of the division of probation under certain circumstances

- Medical directors of a local correctional facility under certain circumstances

- Employees or agents of commissions of correction under certain circumstances

- Law guardians, appointed to represent a minor pursuant to the social services law or the family court act, with respect to confidential HIV-related information relating to the minor and for the purpose of representing the minor. If the minor has capacity to consent, the law guardian may not redisclose the information without his or her permission. If the minor does not consent, the guardian may redisclose information for the sole purpose of representing the minor.[66]

No person to whom confidential HIV-related information has been disclosed may disclose it to another person except as authorized by this statute.[67]

A physician may disclose confidential HIV-related information under the following conditions:

- Disclosure is made to a contact or to a public health officer for the purpose of making the disclosure to said contact.

- The physician reasonably believes disclosure is medically appropriate and there is a significant risk of infection to the contact.

- The physician has counseled the protected individual regarding the need to notify the contact, and the physician reasonably believes the protected individual will not inform the contact.

- The physician has informed the protected individual of his or her intent to make such disclosure to a contact and has given the protected individual the opportunity to express a preference whether the physician should make the disclosure directly or to a public health officer.[68]

---

66. *Id.*
67. *Id.*
68. *Id.* § 2782(4)(a).

A physician may also, on the consent of a parent or guardian, disclose confidential HIV-related information to a health officer for the purpose of reviewing the medical history of a child to determine the fitness of the child to attend school.[69]

The physician may also disclose such information to a person authorized to consent to health care for a protected individual when the physician reasonably believes that (1) disclosure is medically necessary in order to provide timely care and treatment for the protected individual; and (2) after appropriate counseling as to the need for such disclosure, the protected individual will not inform a person authorized by law to consent to health care. However, the physician shall not make such a disclosure if it would not be in the best interest of the protected individual or he is authorized by law to consent to such care and treatment.[70]

Whenever anyone discloses confidential HIV-related information, except to the individual or the person authorized to consent to health care, the disclosure will be accompanied by a statement:

> This information has been disclosed to you from confidential records which are protected by state law. State law prohibits you from making any further disclosure of this information without the specific written consent of the person to whom it pertains, or as otherwise provided by law. Any unauthorized further disclosure in violation of state law may result in a fine or jail sentence or both. A general authorization for the release of medical or other information is NOT sufficient authorization for further disclosure.[71]

Hospitals must have an infection control officer who must maintain a log of occurrences of infections and communicable diseases and who must report increased incidence of infections, including nosocomial infections, to the appropriate area office of the Office of Health Systems Management.[72]

NORTH CAROLINA

North Carolina provides for confidentiality of records of communicable diseases.[73] All information and records that identify a person who has acquired immune deficiency syndrome (AIDS) virus infection or who has or may have a reportable disease or condition must be strictly confidential. This information shall not be released or made public except under the following circumstances, among others:

- Release is made of specific medical or epidemiological information for statistical purposes in a way that no person can be identified.

---

69. *Id.*
70. *Id.* § 2782(4)(e).
71. *Id.* § 2782(5)(a).
72. New York Compilation Codes Rules and Regulations tit. 405, §§ 8 and 11 (1988) (Department of Health Memorandum, Health Facilities Series H-40).
73. North Carolina General Statutes § 130A-143 (1991).

- Release is made of all or part of the medical record with the written consent of the person or persons identified or their guardian.

- Release is made to healthcare personnel providing medical care to the patient.

- Release is necessary to protect the public health and is made as provided by the Commission in its rules regarding control measures for communicable diseases and conditions.

- Release is made pursuant to other provisions of this Article.

- Release is made pursuant to subpoena or court order.[74]

NORTH DAKOTA

North Dakota requires healthcare providers, blood banks, blood centers, and plasma centers that obtain or test specimens of body fluids for human immunodeficiency virus (HIV) antibody to maintain records of consent to testing and the result of the tests.[75] Such information is confidential[76] and may only be released to

- The subject of the test, in the case of a minor the parent or legal guardian or custodian of the subject; in the case of an incapacitated person, the legal guardian of the subject. In the event the subject is in a foster home, or to be adopted, the parent, legal guardian, or custodian may disclose the results to the foster parents or potential adoptive parents.

- The test subject's healthcare provider, including those instances in which a healthcare provider provides emergency care to the subject

- An agent or employee of the test subject's healthcare provider who provides patient care or handles or processes specimens of body fluids or tissues

- A blood bank, blood center, or plasma center that subjects a person to a test for any of the following purposes:

  - Determining the medical acceptability of blood or plasma secured from the test subject

  - Notifying the test subject of the test results

  - Investigating HIV infections in blood or plasma

- A healthcare provider who procures, processes, distributes, or uses a donated human body part for the purpose of assuring the medical acceptability of the gift for the purpose intended

---

74. *Id.*
75. North Dakota Century Code § 23-07.5 (1991).
76. *Id.* § 23.07.5-05.

- The state health officer or his or her designee, for the purpose of providing epidemiologic surveillance or investigation or control of communicable disease

- An embalmer

- A healthcare facility staff committee or accreditation or healthcare service review organization, for the purposes of conducting program monitoring and evaluation and healthcare service reviews

- A person who conducts research if the researcher

  - Is affiliated with the test subject's healthcare provider

  - Has obtained permission from an institutional review board to perform the research

  - Provides written assurance to the person disclosing the test results that the information requested is only for the purpose of research, the information will not be released to a person not connected with the study, and the final research product will not reveal information that may identify the test subject unless the researcher has first received informed consent for disclosure from the test subject[77]

The test results may be disclosed under a lawful court order. In addition, the individual tested may authorize disclosure to any person.[78]

OHIO

Ohio does not provide specific requirements concerning disclosure of communicable disease information, except that any person or institution who provides care or treatment to an individual suffering from a communicable disease must permit the director of health or authorized representative to have access to the patient's medical record.[79]

OKLAHOMA

Reports concerning venereal and other statutorily designated diseases are confidential[80] and may be released only under the following circumstances:

- Release is made on court order.

- Release is made in writing, by or with the written consent of the person whose information is being kept confidential, or with the written consent of the legal guardian or legal custodian of such person, or if

77. *Id.*
78. *Id.*
79. Ohio Revised Code Annotated § 3701-3-08 (Baldwin 1992).
80. Oklahoma Statutes tit. 63, § 1-502.2(A) (1991).

such person is a minor, with the written consent of the parent or legal guardian of such minor.

- Release is necessary as determined by the State Department of Health to protect the health and well-being of the general public. Any such order for release by the Department and any review of such order shall be in accordance with the procedures specified by law. Only the initials of the person whose information is being kept confidential shall be on public record for such proceedings, unless the order by the Department specifies the release of the name of such person and such order is not appealed by such person or such order is upheld by the reviewing court.

- Release is made of medical or epidemiological information to those persons who have had risk exposure to communicable diseases.[81]

- Release is made of medical or epidemiological information to health professionals, appropriate state agencies, or district courts to enforce the Oklahoma law and related rules and regulations concerning the control and treatment of communicable or venereal diseases.

- Release is made of specific medical or epidemiological information for statistical purposes in such a way that no person can be identified.

- Release is made of medical information among healthcare providers within a therapeutic environment for the purpose of diagnosis and treatment of the person whose information is released. This exception shall not authorize the release of confidential information by a state agency to a healthcare provider unless such release is otherwise authorized by this section.[82]

Violation of the confidentiality requirements is a misdemeanor[83] and makes the offender liable for any civil damages caused by the disclosure.[84]

Reports concerning cancerous, precancerous, and tumorous disease information are confidential, but may be released for legitimate research activities if the identity of each patient is protected.[85]

OREGON

Oregon does not provide specific requirements concerning disclosure of communicable disease information.

---

81. *Id.* (*referring to* § 1-502.1).
82. *Id.*
83. *Id.* tit. 63, § 1-502.2(D).
84. *Id.* tit. 63, § 1-502.2(E).
85. *Id.* tit. 63, § 1-551.1.

PENNSYLVANIA

Pennsylvania does not provide specific requirements concerning disclosure of communicable disease information.

RHODE ISLAND

Rhode Island general laws provide that no person may disclose the results of another person's acquired immune deficiency syndrome (AIDS) test without the prior written consent of that individual, or, in the case of a minor, of the minor's parent, guardian, or agent, on a form that specifically states that the AIDS test result may be released.[86] However, a licensed laboratory or healthcare facility that performs AIDS tests may release the results to a physician and to the director of the Department of Health.

A physician may disclose the test results to other health professionals involved in the care of a person who tests positive for the AIDS virus, and to persons who are in close contact with, or exposed to bodily fluids of, a person who tests positive for AIDS if there is, in the physician's opinion, a clear and present danger of transmission of the virus to the third party.[87]

SOUTH CAROLINA

South Carolina does not provide specific requirements concerning disclosure of communicable disease information.

SOUTH DAKOTA

South Dakota does not provide specific requirements concerning disclosure of communicable disease information.

TENNESSEE

All records and information held by the Department of Health and Environment or a local health department relating to known or suspected cases of sexually transmitted disease shall be strictly confidential.[88] Such information shall not be released or made public on subpoena, court order, discovery, search warrant, or otherwise, except that release may be made under the following circumstances:

- Release is made of medical or epidemiological information to medical personnel, appropriate state agencies, or county and district courts to enforce the provisions of this chapter and related regulations governing the control and treatment of sexually transmitted diseases.

---

86. Rhode Island General Law § 23-6-17 (1991).
87. *Id.* § 23-6-17(a) and (b).
88. Tennessee Code Annotated § 68-10-113(1)–(6)(A) (1991).

- In a case involving a minor not more than 13 years of age, only the name, age, address, and sexually transmitted disease treated shall be reported to appropriate agents as required by the Tennessee Child Abuse Law. No other information shall be released. If the information to be disclosed is required in a court proceeding involving child abuse, the information shall be disclosed *in camera.*

- Release is made during a legal proceeding when ordered by a trial court judge, designated by § 16-2-502, through an order explicitly finding each of the following:

  - The information sought is material, relevant, and reasonably calculated to be admissible evidence during the legal proceeding.

  - The probative value of the evidence outweighs the individual's and the public's interest in maintaining its confidentiality.

  - The merits of the litigation cannot be fairly resolved without the disclosure.

  - The evidence is necessary to avoid substantial injustice to the party seeking it and either the disclosure will result in no significant harm to the person examined or treated or it would be substantially unfair as between the requesting party and the person examined or treated not to require the disclosure.[89]

However, before making such findings, the trial court judge may examine the information *in camera* and may order the information placed under seal.[90]

TEXAS

A test result for acquired immune deficiency syndrome (AIDS) and related disorders is confidential, and a person who knows of a test result may not disclose the test result except as provided under the statute.[91] The test result may be disclosed to the following:

- Department of Health

- Local health authority, if reporting is required by the law governing communicable diseases

- Centers for Disease Control if reporting is required by federal law or regulation

- Physician or other person authorized by law who ordered the test

---

89. *Id.*
90. *Id.* § 68-10-113(6)(B).
91. Texas Health and Safety Code Annotated § 81.103(a) (West 1992).

- Physicians, nurses, or other health personnel who have a legitimate need to know the test results in order to provide for their protection and to provide for the patient's health and welfare

- Persons tested or persons legally authorized to consent to the test on the patient's behalf

- Spouse of the person tested if the person tests positive for AIDS or human immunodeficiency virus (HIV) infection, antibodies to HIV, or infection with any other probable causative agent of AIDS and if the physician who ordered the test makes the notification

- Victims of sexual offenses[92]

- If the person tested allegedly committed the offense and the test was required under that article[93]

A blood bank may report positive blood test results to other blood banks, indicating the name of a donor with possible infectious disease, so long as the blood bank does not disclose the infectious disease the donor has or is suspected of having. It may report blood test results to hospitals where the blood was transfused, to the physician who transfused it, and to the recipient; it may also disclose the results for statistical purposes. Such a report may not disclose the name of the donor or the person tested or any information that could result in the disclosure of the donor's or person's name, including an address, social security number, a designated recipient, or replacement information.[94]

A healthcare facility employee whose job requires him or her to deal with permanent medical records may view test results in the performance of his or her duties under reasonable healthcare facility practices.[95] However, anyone who releases or discloses a test result in violation of this section commits a misdemeanor when he, with criminal negligence, releases or discloses a test result on AIDS or HIV status or allows such information to become known other than as authorized under this statute.[96]

Hospital licensing standards permit disclosure of medical record information maintained by special care facilities for reporting of communicable disease information.[97]

UTAH

Utah does not provide specific requirements concerning disclosure of communicable disease information.

---

92. Texas Code Criminal Procedure Annotated art. 21.31(a) (West 1992) (qualifying victims are listed in this article).
93. *Id.;* Texas Health and Safety Code Annotated § 81.103(b) (West 1992).
94. *Id.* § 81.103(g).
95. *Id.* § 81.103(i).
96. *Id.* § 81.103(j).
97. Texas Department of Health, Hospital Licensing Standards ch. 12, § 8.7.3.1 (1991).

VERMONT

Vermont does not provide specific requirements concerning disclosure of communicable disease information.

VIRGINIA

Virginia Code Annotated § 32.1-36.1(A) (1991) states that results of tests for human immunodeficiency virus (HIV) are confidential but may be released to the following, among others:

- Subject of the test or a legally authorized representative

- Any person designated in a release signed by the subject of the test or a legally authorized representative

- Department of Health

- Healthcare providers, for the purposes of consultation or providing care and treatment to the person who was the subject of the test

- Any facility that procures, processes, distributes, or uses blood, other body fluids, tissues, or organs

- Any person authorized by law to receive such information

- The parents of the subject of the test if the subject is a minor

- The spouse of the subject of the test

A willful or grossly negligent unauthorized disclosure subjects the offender to a $5,000 civil penalty as well as to payment of actual damages or $100, whichever is greater (*id.* § 32.1-36.1(B) and (C)).

WASHINGTON

No person may disclose or be compelled to disclose the identity of any person on whom a human immunodeficiency virus (HIV) antibody test is performed, or the results of such a test. Nor may any person disclose the result of a test for any other sexually transmitted disease when it is positive, or disclose any information relating to diagnosis of or treatment for HIV infection or any other confirmed sexually transmitted disease.[98] The following persons, however, may receive such information:

- The subject of the test or the subject's legal representative for healthcare decisions, with the exception of such a representative of a minor child more than 14 years of age and otherwise competent

- Any person who secures a specific release or test results, or information executed by the subject or the subject's legal representative for

---

98. Washington Revised Code § 70.24.105(1) (1991).

healthcare decisions, with the exception of such a representative of a minor child more than 14 years of age and otherwise competent

- The state public health officer, a local public health officer, or the Centers for Disease Control in accordance with reporting requirements for a diagnosed case of a sexually transmitted disease

- A health facility or healthcare provider that procures, processes, distributes, or uses

  - A human body part, tissue, or blood from a deceased person with respect to medical information regarding that person

  - Semen, including that provided prior to March 23, 1988, for the purpose of artificial insemination

  - Blood specimens

- Any state or local public health officer conducting an investigation to determine whether an infected person is engaging in conduct that endangers the public health, provided that such record was obtained by means of court-ordered HIV testing[99]

- A person allowed access to the record by a court order granted after application showing good cause

- Persons who, because of their behavioral interaction with the infected individual, have been placed at risk for acquisition of a sexually transmitted disease, if the health officer or authorized representative believes that the exposed person was unaware that a risk of disease exposure existed and that the disclosure of the identity of the infected person is necessary

- A law enforcement officer, firefighter, healthcare provider, healthcare facility staff person, or other persons as defined by the board of health, who has requested a test of a person whose bodily fluids he or she has been substantially exposed to, if a state or local public health officer performs the test

- Claims management personnel employed by or associated with an insurer, healthcare service contractor, health maintenance organization, self-funded health plan, state-administered healthcare claims payer, or any other payer of healthcare claims where such disclosure is to be used solely for the prompt and accurate evaluation and payment of medical or related claims. Information released under this subsection must be confidential and may not be released or available to persons who are not involved in handling or determining medical claims payment.

---

99. *Id.* § 70.24.105(2)(e) (*referring to* § 70.24.024).

- A Department of Social and Health Services worker, a child placing agency worker, or a guardian *ad litem* who is responsible for making or reviewing placement or case-planning decisions or recommendations to the court regarding a child who is less than 14 years of age, has a sexually transmitted disease, and is in the custody of the Department or a licensed child placing agency. This information may also be received by a person responsible for providing residential care for such a child when the Department or a licensed child placing agency determines that it is necessary for the provision of childcare services.[100]

No person to whom the results of a test for a sexually transmitted disease have been disclosed may disclose the results to another except as authorized above.[101] Whenever disclosure is made, except to the subject or a representative for healthcare decisions, or among healthcare providers in order to provide healthcare services, the disclosure must be accompanied by a written statement:

> This information has been disclosed to you from records whose confidentiality is protected by state law. State law prohibits you from making any further disclosure of it without the specific written consent of the person to whom it pertains, or as otherwise permitted by state law. A general authorization for the release of medical or other information is NOT sufficient for this purpose.[102]

If the disclosure is oral, the discloser will provide the written notice, above, within 10 days.[103]

WEST VIRGINIA

No person may disclose or be compelled to disclose the identity of any person on whom an human immunodeficiency virus (HIV)–related test is performed or the results of such a test in a manner that permits identification of the subject of the test,[104] except, among others, to

- Subject of the test

- Any person who secures a specific release of test results executed by the subject

- Funeral directors, authorized agents, or employees of a health facility or healthcare provider, if the funeral establishment, health facility, or provider itself is authorized to obtain the test results, if the agent or the employee provides patient care or handles or processes specimens of

---

100. *Id.* § 70.24.105(2).
101. *Id.* § 70.24.105(3).
102. *Id.* § 70.24.105(5).
103. *Id.*
104. West Virginia Code § 16-3C-3(a)(1)–(7) (1992).

body fluids or tissues, and if the agent or employee has a need to know such information. The recipient must maintain the confidentiality of the information.

- Licensed medical personnel or appropriate healthcare personnel providing care to the subject of the test, when knowledge of the test results is necessary or useful to provide appropriate care or treatment in an appropriate manner, provided that such personnel must maintain the confidentiality of such test results

- Department of Health or Centers for Disease Control in accordance with reporting requirements for a diagnosed case of acquired immune deficiency syndrome (AIDS), or a related condition

- Health facilities or healthcare providers that procure, process, distribute, or use

  - A human body part from a deceased person with respect to medical information regarding that person

  - Semen provided prior to September 1, 1988, for the purpose of artificial insemination

  - Blood or blood products for transfusion or injection

  - Human body parts for transplant with regard to medical information regarding the donor or recipient

- Health facility staff committees or accreditation or oversight review organizations that are conducting program monitoring, program evaluation, or service reviews so long as any identity remains anonymous[105]

The statute also permits disclosure to inform sex partners or contacts or persons who have shared needles that they may be at risk of having acquired the HIV infection, but the name or identity of the person whose test was positive is to remain confidential.[106]

Whenever anyone discloses information under this statute that does not fall within one of the exceptions listed above, that person must add a written statement:

> This information has been disclosed to you from records whose confidentiality is protected by state law. State law prohibits you from making any further disclosure of the information without the specific written consent of the person to whom it pertains, or as otherwise permitted by law. A general authorization for the release of medical or other information is NOT sufficient for this purpose.[107]

---

105. *Id.*
106. *Id.* § 16-3C-3(b).
107. *Id.* § 16-3C-3(c).

WISCONSIN

Results of tests for the presence of human immunodeficiency virus (HIV) or an HIV antibody may not be disclosed, without the subject's consent[108] except to the following, among others:

- Subject of the test

- Healthcare providers

- Blood banks

- State epidemiologist

- Funeral directors

- Healthcare facility staff committees or accreditation or healthcare service review organizations

- Under court order

- Researchers

- Persons who render aid to the victim of an accident if exposed thereby to the disease

- A coroner

- Sheriffs or jailkeepers

- Those who have had sexual contact with the subject or who shared intravenous drug use paraphernalia, if the person is deceased

No person to whom such test results have been disclosed may disclose the results except under the same rules.[109]

The healthcare provider, blood bank, or plasma center that obtains specimens to test for HIV must maintain a record of informed consent for testing or disclosure and maintain a record of the results.[110] Notwithstanding the confidentiality requirements, such persons may only report positive test results for HIV or an antibody to

- State epidemiologist for the purpose of providing epidemiologic surveillance or investigation or control of communicable disease

- Healthcare facilities staff committees or accreditation or healthcare service review organizations for the purposes of conducting program monitoring and evaluation and healthcare service reviews

- Researchers, if the researcher is affiliated with a healthcare provider, has obtained permission to perform the research from an institutional

---

108. Wisconsin Statute § 146.025(2)(a)(5m) (1990).
109. *Id.* § 146.025(5).
110. *Id.* § 146.025(4).

review board, and provides written assurance to the person disclosing the test results that use of the information is only for the purpose for which it is provided to the researcher, that the information will not be released to a person not connected with the study, and that the final research product will not reveal information that may identify the subject unless the researcher has first received informed consent for disclosure from the subject.[111]

The healthcare provider, blood bank, or plasma center that obtains specimens to test for HIV may report positive test results for HIV or an antibody, when required by law, to

- Sheriffs, jailers, or keepers of a prison, a jail, or a house of correction to permit the assigning of a private cell to a prisoner with a positive test result

- Coroners, medical examiners, or appointed assistants, if the possible HIV-infected status is relevant to the cause of a death under direct investigation, or if the coroner, medical examiners, or appointed assistants are significantly exposed to a person whose death is under direct investigation, or a physician certifies in writing that such individuals have been significantly exposed and the certification accompanies the request for disclosure[112]

Violations of this statute can result in civil liability of up to $5,000 or a criminal penalty.[113]

WYOMING

A hospital may disclose healthcare information about a patient without the patient's authorization to the extent a recipient needs to know the information, if the disclosure is

- To an official of a penal or other custodial institution in which the patient is detained[114]

- To federal, state, or local public health authorities, to the extent the hospital is required by law to report healthcare information or when needed to protect the public health

- To federal, state, or local law enforcement authorities to the extent required by law[115]

---

111. Wisconsin Statute § 146.025(5)(a), (8), and (10) (1991).
112. *Id.* § 146.025(5)(a)(12) and (13).
113. *Id.* § 146.025(8) and (9).
114. Wyoming Statute § 35-2-609(a)(x) (1991).
115. *Id.* § 35-2-609(b)(i)–(iv).

CHAPTER 11

Disclosure When a Court Orders You To

Introduction

A subpoena is a court order that commands someone to come to court. A subpoena *duces tecum* is a court order that commands one who has possession or custody of a record to bring it to court. If someone serves a subpoena on you, you should document its receipt in a log book and record every action you take with respect to the subpoena. Before producing any records, you should contact your legal advisor to ensure that such production is proper. You may also call the attorney who sent the subpoena to verify the information requested and ask if you can mail the records to the court instead of appearing with the records in person. You may also want to ask the attorney to notify you if it turns out that the record is not needed, for example, if the case is settled before trial.

Federal Laws

Rule 34 of the Federal Rules of Civil Procedure allows a party access to records held by another during pretrial discovery. Rule 34 also allows access to records held by nonparties to the suit.[1]

Further, Rule 45 of the Rules of Civil Procedure allows a party to subpoena documents from another person for admission at trial. Rule 45 has been rewritten to allow greater access to records at trial (*id*. Rule 45).

Although the federal rules apply to actions brought in federal court, issues of privilege, such as the physician–patient privilege, which may affect the availability of a subpoena for medical records, are controlled by state law in the trial.

For criminal proceedings in federal court, subpoenas are issued under 18 U.S.C. Federal Rule of Criminal Procedure 17 (1990).

---

1. 28 U.S.C. Federal Rules of Civil Procedure 34 (1989).

State Laws

ALABAMA

Code of Alabama § 12-21-5 (1991) provides that a copy of medical records is admissible in evidence when certified and affirmed by the custodian of the records if kept in the usual and regular course of business, so long as the records were made at the time that such acts, transactions, occurrences, or events therein referred to occurred or within a reasonable time thereafter. Section 12-21-6 provides that any litigant can obtain a copy of medical records by subpoena *duces tecum,* and provides that in such cases the custodian of the records shall prepare a copy and securely seal the same in an envelope or other container and date, fill out, and sign a certificate and place on, or securely fasten said certificate to the outside of, said envelope or container, and deliver the records to the clerk or register of the court hearing the case. The custodian need not appear at trial, and the records shall not be open to inspection or copying by other persons than the parties and their attorneys until the court orders them published at the time of trial.

Appendix B of Alabama Administrative Code r. 420-5-7, of the Rules of Alabama State Board of Health Division of Licensure and Certification, states that when records are removed by court order, they should be accompanied by a responsible hospital employee and returned to the hospital at the end of the hearing for which they were directed to be produced or at the direction of the court.

ALASKA

Alaska statutes do not contain any specific rules for subpoena of medical records. However, Alaska Administrative Code tit. 7, § 13.130 (April 1984), specifies that information regarding a patient may be released without the patient's consent to a person authorized by court order.

ARIZONA

Arizona Revised Statutes § 12-2282(4) (1991), concerning compliance with subpoena *duces tecum* for hospital records, states that except as provided in § 12-2285, when a subpoena *duces tecum* is served on the custodian of records or other qualified witness from a hospital in an action in which the hospital is not a party, and such subpoena requires the production of all or any part of the records of the hospital relating to the care or treatment of a patient in the hospital, compliance is sufficient if the following steps are taken: The custodian or other officer of the hospital must, within five days after the receipt of such subpoena, deliver by registered mail or in person a true and correct copy of all the records described in such subpoena to the clerk of the court or other tribunal or, if there is no clerk, then to the court or tribunal, together with the affidavit as described in § 12-2283, below.

The copy of the records shall be separately enclosed in an inner envelope or wrapper and sealed, with the title and number of the action, name of witness, and date of subpoena clearly inscribed thereon. The sealed envelope or wrapper shall then be enclosed in an outer envelope or wrapper, sealed and directed to the clerk of the court or tribunal, or if there is no clerk, then to the court or tribunal.

Section 12-2283 requires that the records must be accompanied by the affidavit of the custodian or other qualified witness, stating in substance each of the following:

- That the affiant is the duly authorized custodian of the records and has authority to certify the records

- That the copy is a true copy of all the records described in the subpoena

- That the records were prepared by the personnel of the healthcare institution or staff physicians, or persons acting under the control of either, in the ordinary course of healthcare institution business at or near the time of the act, condition, or event

If the healthcare institution has none of the records described, or only part thereof, the custodian shall so state in the affidavit, and deliver the affidavit and such records as are available in the manner provided in § 12-2282, above (*id.* § 12-2283(B)).

ARKANSAS

Title 16 of the Arkansas Code Annotated § 16-46-302 (Michie 1992) provides that when a subpoena *duces tecum* is served on a record custodian of any hospital licensed in the state, or in a proceeding in which the hospital is neither a party nor the place where any cause of action is alleged to have arisen, and such a subpoena requires the production of all or any part of the records of the hospital relating to the treatment of a patient in the hospital, then compliance is satisfied if the custodian delivers by hand or by registered mail to the court clerk or the officer, court reporter, body, or tribunal issuing the subpoena or conducting the hearing, a true and correct copy of all records described in the subpoena together with an affidavit.

Under *id.* § 16-46-305, the affidavit must state

- That the affiant is the duly authorized custodian of the records and has authority to certify the records

- That the copy is a true copy of all the records described in the subpoena

- That the records were prepared by personnel of the hospital, staff physicians, or persons acting under the control of either, in the ordinary course of the hospital's business at or near the time of the act, condition, or event reported therein

If the hospital has none of the records described, or only part of them, the custodian shall state so in the affidavit and file the affidavit and any records in the manner described in §§ 16-46-302 and 16-46-303 (*id.* 16-46-305(a)).

The custodian of the records may also enclose a statement of costs for copying the records, and that cost shall be borne by the party requesting the subpoena (*id.* § 16-46-305(c)).

Section 16-46-303 states that copies of the records shall be separately enclosed in an inner envelope or wrapper, sealed, with the title and number of the action, the name of the custodian, and the date of the subpoena clearly inscribed thereon. The sealed envelope or wrapper shall be enclosed in an outer envelope or wrapper, sealed and directed as follows:

- If the subpoena directs attendance in court, to the clerk or the judge of the court

- If the subpoena directs attendance at a deposition, to the officer before whom the deposition is to be taken, at the place designated in the subpoena for the taking of the deposition or at his place of business

- In other cases, to the officer, body, or tribunal conducting the hearing, at a like address

CALIFORNIA

A provider of health care may disclose medical information if the disclosure is compelled by a court order; by a board, commission, or administrative agency for purposes of adjudication pursuant to its lawful authority; by a party to a proceeding before a court or administrative agency pursuant to a subpoena *duces tecum,* notice to appear, or any provision authorizing discovery in a proceeding before a court or administrative agency; by a board, commission, or administrative agency pursuant to an investigative subpoena; by an arbitrator or arbitration panel when arbitration is lawfully requested, pursuant to a subpoena *duces tecum;* by a search warrant lawfully issued to a government law enforcement agency; or when otherwise specifically required by law.[2]

California Penal Code § 1543 (Deering 1992) requires healthcare facilities to disclose records of the identity, diagnosis, prognosis, or treatment of any patient that are not privileged records, or records required by law to be confidential, to law enforcement agencies if authorized by an appropriate order of a court of competent jurisdiction in the county where the records are located, granted after application showing good cause.

California Welfare and Institutions Code § 107 (Deering 1992) allows court-appointed special advocates on specific court order to inspect and copy any health records of a child involved in a juvenile court appointment proceeding without consent of the child's parents.

---

2. California Civil Code § 56.10 (Deering 1992).

COLORADO

While Colorado does not have any specific statutory requirements for subpoena of medical records, Colorado Revised Statutes §§ 13-90-111 and 13-90-112 (1991) govern subpoenas in general. In addition, several statutes, such as § 12-32-108.3, allow professional boards to subpoena patient records during investigations concerning disciplinary matters.

CONNECTICUT

According to Connecticut General Statute § 4-104 (1990), if any private hospital, public hospital, society, or corporation receiving state aid is served with a subpoena issued by a competent authority directing the production of any hospital record in connection with any proceedings in any court, the hospital, society, or corporation on which the subpoena is served may, except where such record pertains to a mentally ill patient, deliver such record or a copy thereof to the clerk of the court. Any such record or copy delivered to such clerk shall be sealed in an envelope that shall indicate the name of the patient, the name of the attorney subpoenaing the same, and the title of the case referred to in the subpoena. A subpoena for the production of hospital records shall be valid if notice of intent to subpoena is given not less than 24 hours nor more than two weeks prior to the time of production, and the subpoena itself is served not less than 24 hours before the time for production.

DELAWARE

The Delaware Code does not contain any specific requirements for subpoena of medical records. However, they can be subpoenaed, subject to confidentiality requirements.[3] Delaware Code Annotated tit. 16, § 711 (1991), provides a procedure for release of confidential records and information concerning sexually transmitted disease pursuant to court order, as does *id.* § 1202 for human immunodeficiency virus (HIV) tests.

DISTRICT OF COLUMBIA

See the federal rules, above.

FLORIDA

While Florida Administrative Code r. 10D-28.158(3) (1991) provides that patient records shall have a privileged and confidential status and shall not be disclosed without the consent of the person to whom they pertain, appropriate disclosure may be made without such consent in any civil or criminal action, unless otherwise prohibited by law, on the issuance of a subpoena

---

3. *See* Shipmark v. Division of Social Services, 442 A.2d 101 (1951).

from a court of competent jurisdiction, if proper notice is given by the party seeking such records to the patient or his or her legal representative.

Florida Statutes ch. 395.017(1) (1991) provides that on issuance of such a subpoena, a licensed facility shall release all patient records requested (including x rays), except progress notes and consultation report sections of a psychiatric nature concerning the care and treatment performed by the licensed facility.

Section 110.123(3) provides that patient medical records and medical claims records of state employees, former employees, and eligible dependents in the custody or control of the state group insurance program may be furnished in any civil or criminal action, unless otherwise prohibited by law, on issuance of a subpoena from a court of competent jurisdiction and proper notice to the employee or his or her legal representative by the party seeking such records.

Florida Administrative Code r. 10D-29.082(2)(c) (1991) provides that nursing homes shall release patient records on court order.

GEORGIA

According to Georgia Code Annotated § 24-10-72 (Michie 1991), an institution and its personnel shall be in compliance with a subpoena or order for production if the facility shows timely delivery of the medical records, or substitutes, and accompanying certificate to the clerk of the court or other authorized person by any means, including, but not limited to, certified or registered mail.

HAWAII

According to Hawaii Revised Statutes § 622-52 (1990), whenever a medical record custodian receives a subpoena *duces tecum* requiring production of medical records, he or she may comply by delivering by messenger or by certified or registered mail, within five days after receipt of the subpoena, a true and correct copy to the clerk of court or the clerk's deputy authorized to receive it, together with an affidavit certifying that he or she is the custodian, has authority to certify medical records, that the copy is a true copy, and that the records were prepared by medical facility personnel in the regular course of business at or near the time of the act, condition, or event. A notary public must notarize the certificate (*id.* §§ 622-52 and 622-53).

IDAHO

A copy of medical records, certified by the custodian of the originals and authorized to certify that they are true copies, may be used to satisfy a subpoena, provided that the hospital holds the originals available for inspection and comparison.[4] The hospital must file a certified copy of the resolution of

---

4. Idaho Code § 9-420(1) (1991).

the governing board authorizing and identifying such employee in order to avail itself of this procedure.

When such an employee receives a subpoena *duces tecum,* he or she may comply by promptly notifying the party causing service of the subpoena and all other parties of the hospital's election to proceed under this statute and of the expenses of reproducing such records. Upon payment, the employee must deliver, by mail or otherwise, a true, legible, and durable certified copy to the clerk of the court before which the proceeding is pending or to the officer, body, or tribunal, if the case is not before a court. The copies must be separately enclosed and sealed in an outer envelope or wrapper, with the title and number of the action, cause, or proceeding, the name of the hospital, and the employee's name. He or she must then place the sealed envelope in an outer envelope for delivery.[5]

Personal attendance of the custodian is required if the subpoena so states. Any patient whose records are thus copied and delivered, any person acting on his or her behalf, the hospital having custody, or any physician, nurse, or other person responsible for entries on such records, may apply to the court or other body for a protective order denying, restricting, or otherwise limiting access to and use of such records.[6]

ILLINOIS

Illinois has several statutes that permit various state agencies to subpoena medical records. For example, Illinois Revised Statute, ch. 111 ½, ¶ 148(c) (1991), permits the Director of Public Health or a hearing officer to issue a subpoena for hospital records in licensing proceedings. Others, however, must use the general subpoena statute, *id.* ch. 110, ¶ 2-1101.

A subpoena for records of sexually transmissible diseases, including acquired immune deficiency syndrome (AIDS), requires that the court seal the information, except as necessary to reach a decision or as otherwise agreed by all parties. The proceedings must be held *in camera* and the record of the proceeding sealed.[7]

INDIANA

According to Indiana Code § 34-3-15.5-6(a) (1991), when a subpoena or a subpoena coupled with a patient's written authorization or a court order requiring the production of a hospital medical record is served on any hospital employee, the hospital employee with the custody of the original medical record may elect, in lieu of personally appearing and producing the original hospital medical record, to furnish the requesting party or party's attorney

---

5. *Id.* § 9-420(2).
6. *Id.* § 9-420(3).
7. Illinois Administrative Code tit. 77, § 693.100(d) (1991).

with a photostatic copy of the hospital medical record, certified in accordance with § 34-3-15.5-6(c) as described below.

If the hospital elects to proceed as discussed above, the hospital employee with custody of the original hospital medical records shall, on receipt of payment for the reproduction of the hospital medical records, promptly deliver, by certified mail or personal delivery, copies of the records specified in the subpoena to the person specified in the subpoena (*id.* § 34-3-15.5-6(b)).

Section 34-3-15.5-6(c) requires the hospital employee's certification of the records to

- Be signed by the hospital employee with custody of the records

- Include

  - Full name of the patient

  - Patient's medical record number

  - Number of pages in the hospital medical record

  - Statement in substantially the following form

The copies of records for which this certification is made are true and complete reproductions of the original or microfilmed hospital medical records that are housed in _____ (name of hospital). The original records were made in the regular course of business and it was the regular course of _____ (name of hospital) to make the records at or near the time of the matter recorded. This certification is given pursuant to IC 34-3-15.5-6 by the custodian of the records in lieu of the custodian's personal appearance.

The hospital shall place the copies of the hospital medical records in an envelope or wrapper and write or type on the envelope or wrapper the words "Confidential Medical Records," the title and number of the action or proceeding, and the name and business telephone number of the hospital employee making the certification (*id.* § 34-3-15.5-6(d)).

However, if the hospital does not have the hospital medical records or has only part of the hospital medical records specified in the subpoena, the hospital employee with custody of the original hospital medical record shall

- Execute an affidavit, either notarized or by affirmation, stating that the hospital does not have or has only a part of the subpoenaed hospital medical records.

- Follow the procedures detailed above in delivering the part of the hospital medical records that are in the possession of the hospital (*id.* § 34-3-15.5-6(e)).

When records are confidential under 42 U.S.C. §§ 290dd-3 or 290ee-3 because they involve records of alcoholism patients, because they concern the treatment of mental illness, or under Indiana Code § 16-1-9.5-7 (1991) they concern dangerous or communicable diseases, the hospital employee having custody of the original medical records shall

- Execute a verified affidavit

    - Identifying the record or part of it that is confidential

    - Stating that the confidential record or part of the record will only be provided under the federal procedure for production of the record

- Comply with the requirements specified above in delivering the record or part of the record that is not confidential (*id.* § 34-3-15.5-6(f), (g), and (h)).

The hospital may charge a reasonable fee to cover the costs of reproducing the hospital medical records (*id.* § 34-3-15.5-6(i)).

IOWA

Iowa Code § 141.23(1)(g) (1991) provides for access to records of human immunodeficiency virus (HIV)–related tests by court order, which is issued in compliance with the following provisions:

- A court finding that the person seeking the test results has demonstrated a compelling need for the test results that cannot be accommodated by other means

- Pleadings pertaining to the disclosure of the test results shall substitute a pseudonym for the true name of the subject of the test. The disclosure to the parties of the subject's true name shall be communicated confidentially, in documents not filed with the court.

- Before granting an order, the court shall provide the person whose test results are in question with notice and a reasonable opportunity to participate in the proceedings if the person is not already a party.

- Court proceedings as to disclosure of test results shall be conducted *in camera* unless the subject of the test agrees to a hearing in open court or unless the court determines that a public hearing is necessary to the public interest and the proper administration of justice.

- On issuance of an order to disclose test results, the court shall impose appropriate safeguards against unauthorized disclosure, which shall specify the persons who may gain access to the information, the purposes for which the information shall be used, and appropriate prohibitions on future disclosure.

Section 229.25(2) provides that an exception to the general prohibition against disclosing confidential medical records of mentally ill persons is when the information is sought by court order.

KANSAS

Kansas does not have a statute governing subpoena of medical records. However, Kansas Statutes Annotated § 60-234 (1990), entitled Production of Documents, governs subpoena of records generally.

KENTUCKY

Kentucky Revised Statutes Annotated §§ 422.300–422.330 (Baldwin 1991) provide for mailing by certified or registered mail or by personal delivery of certified copies of the medical record to the attorney or the clerk of court, in lieu of originals and of personal appearance by the records custodian.

LOUISIANA

According to Louisiana Revised Statutes § 44:7(c) (1991), whenever the past or present condition, sickness, or disease, physical or mental, of any patient treated in any hospital is at issue or relevant in any judicial proceeding, the charts, records, reports, documents, and other memoranda shall be subject to discovery, subpoena, and introduction into evidence in accordance with the general law of the state relating to discovery, subpoena, and introduction into evidence of records and documents.

Section 13:3174 provides that if a certified copy of the chart or record of any hospital, signed by the hospital administrator or the medical record administrator, is offered into evidence the copy is prima facie proof of its contents. Section 13:3715.1 adds that when a subpoena *duces tecum* is served on the custodian of records, in an action in which the facility is not a party, and such subpoena requires the production of records, the facility is in compliance if the custodian or other officer delivers by registered mail or by hand a true and correct copy of all records described in the subpoena to the clerk of court, together with an affidavit as discussed below. The record shall be separately enclosed in an inner envelope or wrapper and sealed, with the title and number of the action, name of witness, and date of subpoena inscribed thereon. The sealed envelope or wrapper shall be enclosed in an outer envelope or wrapper, sealed, and directed to the clerk or to the court.

The records shall be accompanied by the affidavit of the custodian or other witness stating that

- The affiant is the duly authorized custodian of the records and has authority to certify the records.

- The copy is a true copy of all records described in the subpoena.

- The records were prepared by the personnel of the hospital or facility, staff physicians, or persons acting under the control of either, in the ordinary course of business of the hospital or facility, at or near the time of the act, condition, or event.

Section 37:1278.1 provides that notwithstanding any privilege of confidentiality, no physician or healthcare institution with which such physician is affiliated shall fail or refuse to respond to a lawfully issued subpoena of the board for any medical information.

MAINE

Maine statutes do not discuss any specific requirements for subpoena of medical records in general. However, a party may subpoena medical records subject to confidentiality requirements.[8] Maine Revised Statutes Annotated § 19203-D(5) (1991) provides that medical records containing results of a human immunodeficiency virus (HIV) test may be disclosed, among other reasons, pursuant to a court order on a showing of good cause, provided that the court order limits the use and disclosure of records and provides sanctions for misuse of records or sets forth other methods for assuring confidentiality.

Maine's Regulations Governing the Licensure of General and Specialty Hospitals note that medical records generally are not to be removed from the hospital except on subpoena.[9]

MARYLAND

Maryland Health–General Code § 4-306 (1991) exempts from its rule prohibiting disclosure of medical records the provision of information in accordance with compulsory process, a stipulation by a patient or person in interest, or a discovery request permitted by law to be made to a court, an administrative tribunal, or a party to a civil court, administrative, or health claims arbitration proceeding.

Infectious and contagious disease reports, by physicians (*id.* § 18-201(f)), by institutions (*id.* § 18-202(d)), and by laboratories, (*id.* § 18-205(f)), are only subject to subpoena or discovery in a civil or criminal proceeding pursuant to a court order sealing the court record.

Under § 4-306, professional licensing and disciplinary boards may subpoena medical records for an investigation concerning licensure, certification, or discipline of a health professional or into the improper practice of a health profession.

MASSACHUSETTS

Massachusetts General Laws, ch. 111, § 70 (1992), provides that on proper judicial order, hospitals or clinics may permit inspection and copying of medical records kept by the hospital or clinic on request and payment of a reasonable fee. The exception is the records of a hospital or clinic under the

---

8. LeFay v. Morton Coopersmith, 576 A.2d 192 (Maine 1990).
9. State of Maine, Regulations Governing the Licensing and Functioning of General and Specialty Hospitals, ch. XII, § A (1972).

control of the Department of Mental Health, unless the commissioner determines that disclosure would be in the best interests of the patient, Further, on proper judicial order, except in mental health facility cases when not in the best interest of the patient, such records may be furnished on payment of a reasonable fee. A hospital or clinic served with a subpoena for records of any party named in that proceeding, as shown by the case caption appearing on the subpoena, shall deliver certified copies of the subpoenaed records in its custody to the court or place of hearing. Chapter 233, § 79, adds that copies of records, when duly certified by the person in charge, shall be equally admissible as the originals. The certification must be by affidavit that the record is a true and complete record.

Chapter 231, § 60B, gives medical malpractice tribunals subpoena power.

MICHIGAN

Under Michigan Compiled Laws § 333.5131(1) (1991), disclosure of information pertaining to human immunodeficiency virus (HIV) infection, acquired immune deficiency syndrome (AIDS), or AIDS-related complex (ARC) in response to a court order and subpoena shall be limited to only the following cases and all the following restrictions:

- The court petitioned for an order to disclose the information shall determine both of the following:

  - That other ways of obtaining the information are not available or would not be effective

  - That the public interest and the need for disclosure outweigh the potential for injury to the patient (*id.* § 333.5131(3)(a))

- If a court issues an order for the disclosure of the information, the order shall do all of the following:

  - Limit disclosure to those parts of the patient's record determined by the court to be essential to fulfill the objectives of the order

  - Limit disclosure to those persons whose need for the information is the basis of the order

  - Include such other measures as considered necessary by the court to limit disclosure for the protection of the patient (*id.* § 333.5131 (3)(b))

Under § 333.6113, whether a specific individual is under treatment by a licensed substance abuse treatment and rehabilitation service, a licensed prevention service, an approved service program, or an emergency medical service may be disclosed on order of a court. In all other respects, the confidentiality is the same as the physician–patient relationship. A court may also order disclosure for the purpose of a hearing under § 333.6124 or 6126 (involving review whether substance abuse treatment and rehabilitation is necessary in the case of minors and review of minor's treatment plans).

MINNESOTA

Minnesota does not have a specific statute on subpoena of medical records generally, but medical records can be obtained by subpoena.[10]

Minnesota Statutes § 254A.09 (1991), providing for confidentiality of records of treatment for alcohol or drug abuse, notes that a court may order release of such records if, after review of the records, the court determines that the information is relevant for the purpose requested and weighs the public interest and the injury to the patient, to the treatment relationship in the program and in other similarly situated programs, and the actual or potential harm to the ability of programs to attract and retain patients if disclosure occurs. The court shall order disclosure of only that information that is determined relevant.

Section 144A.12(2), pertaining to confidentiality of convalescent, nursing, and boarding homes residents' records, notes that such records may not be disclosed except, among other reasons, when ordered to do so by a court of competent jurisdiction.

Section 144.054 gives the state commissioner of health subpoena power for his or her investigations into whether a serious health threat exists or to locate persons who may have been exposed to an agent that can seriously affect their health.

MISSISSIPPI

Mississippi permits disclosure without patient consent when pursuant to a valid court order. Mississippi Code Annotated § 41-9-101(a) (1991) notes that hospital records subject to a subpoena do not include x rays, electrocardiograms, and similar graphic matter unless specifically referred to in the subpoena. Sections 41-9-103 through 117 cover the procedure to comply with subpoenas. When a subpoena requires hospital records, the custodian may comply by filing with the court clerk or the officer, body, or tribunal a true and correct copy (which may be a film or a copy created by another reproduction method) of all records described in such subpoena (*id.* § 41-9-103). The records must be separately enclosed in an inner envelope or wrapper, sealed, with the title and number of the action, name of witness, and date of subpoena written thereon and enclosed in an outer envelope (*id.* § 41-9-105). The custodian must enclose an affidavit stating that he or she is the custodian and has the authority to certify the records; that the copy is a true copy of the records described in the subpoena; that the records were prepared by hospital personnel in the ordinary course of business at or near the time of the act, condition, or event reported therein;

---

10. *See,* e.g., Padilla v. State Board of Medical Examiners, 382 N.W.2d 876 (Minn. 1986).

and certifying the amount of the reasonable charges for furnishing the record (*id.* §§ 41-9-109 and 41-9-117).

Section 73-25-27 gives the board of medical licensure the authority to subpoena records.

MISSOURI

Missouri does not have a specific statute relating to subpoena of medical records, but they may be subpoenaed under Rule 57.09 covering subpoenas for documents.[11]

MONTANA

Montana Code Annotated § 50-16-535(1) (1992) discusses the circumstances under which healthcare information is available by compulsory process. It states that a provider may not disclose such information pursuant to compulsory legal process, such as a subpoena or court order, in any judicial, legislative, or administrative proceeding unless

- The patient has consented in writing to the release in response to compulsory process or a discovery request.

- The patient has waived his or her right to claim confidentiality for the information sought.

- The patient is a party to the proceeding and has placed his or her physical or mental condition in issue.

- The patient's physical or mental condition is relevant to the execution or witnessing of a will or other document.

- The physical or mental condition of a deceased patient is placed in issue by any person claiming or defending through or as a beneficiary of the patient.

- A patient's healthcare information is to be used in the patient's commitment proceeding.

- The healthcare information is for use in any law enforcement proceeding or investigation in which a provider is the subject or a party, except that healthcare information so obtained may not be used in any proceeding against the patient unless the matter relates to payment for his health care or is authorized as specified below.

- The healthcare information is relevant to a proceeding brought under §§ 50-16-551 through 50-16-553 (concerning misrepresentation or bribery to examine healthcare information or allowing another to do so).

---

11. Missouri Rules of Civil Procedure 57.09 (1991); Missouri Revised Statute § 491.100(3) (1990); *Baker v. State Farm*, 806 S.W.2d 742 (Mo. 1991).

- A court has determined that particular healthcare information is subject to compulsory legal process or discovery because the party seeking the information has demonstrated that a compelling state interest exists that outweighs the patient's privacy interest.

- The healthcare information is requested pursuant to an investigative subpoena under § 46-4-301.

NEBRASKA

Revised Statutes of Nebraska § 75-511(1) (1990), providing for confidentiality of contagious disease information, specifies that such information shall not be made public on subpoena, discovery proceedings, or otherwise except as permitted by §§ 71-503.01 (requiring reports of communicable diseases) and 71-2017 (concerning Department of Health standards for health services).

Section 44-32,171 notes that data or information pertaining to the diagnosis, treatment, or health of any enrollee or applicant of a health maintenance organization (HMO) is confidential but may be disclosed pursuant to statute or court order for the production of evidence.

NEVADA

Nevada Revised Statutes Annotated § 41A.046(1) (1991) allows the health division to subpoena books, papers, healthcare records, and other materials as may be required by medical malpractice screening panels. Under *id.* § 52.325(1), a custodian of medical records complies with a subpoena if he or she delivers a true and exact photographic, electrostatic, or other acceptable authenticated copy of the original record. If the authenticity of the records is an issue in a discovery proceeding or trial, the court may order production of the original medical record, or personal appearance of the custodian (*id.* § 52.355). The custodian shall not allow anyone to review medical records relevant to a complaint filed with the health division before those records are transferred to the authority issuing the subpoena (*id.* § 41A.053(1)).

NEW HAMPSHIRE

New Hampshire Revised Statute § 329:9-a (1991) provides that medical disciplinary boards have the power to compel, by subpoena *duces tecum,* the production of papers and records. Further, malpractice hearing panels may subpoena evidence including copies of medical records, x rays, and other documents.

NEW JERSEY

New Jersey does not have a specific statute relating to subpoena of medical records, but medical records may be subpoenaed, subject to confidentiality requirements.[12]

New Jersey does, however, have a specific statute for disclosure of acquired immune deficiency syndrome (AIDS) or human immunodeficiency virus (HIV) infection records in New Jersey Revised Statutes § 26:5C-9.

Further, *id.* § 45:9-19.3 provides for release of confidential information concerning the conduct of a physician or surgeon to the State Board of Medical Examiners on court order, and § 45:9-42.39 permits examination of information concerning inspections of clinical laboratories on application to a court.

NEW MEXICO

The *New Mexico Hospital Association Legal Handbook,* ch. V, § C, ¶ 1, art. V-8 (rev. ed. 1991), simply says that hospitals must obey any subpoena to produce medical records or information unless it concerns treatment related to drug or alcohol abuse, child abuse or neglect, certain mental health records, or if the patient is not a party to the action. If the patient is not a party and has not consented to release of the record, the hospital should notify the patient of the request and abide by his or her wishes as to whether to comply with the subpoena. Such records must be released, however, if the hospital receives a court order to do so instead of a subpoena. A court order is necessary to release drug or alcohol abuse information relating to a patient, even if the patient consents.[13] A subpoena is insufficient authority to release drug or alcohol abuse information.

NEW YORK

New York Civil Practice Law and Rules § 2306(a) (McKinney 1992) provides that where a subpoena *duces tecum* is served on a hospital requiring the production of records relating to the condition or treatment of a patient, a transcript or reproduction certified as correct by the superintendent or head of the hospital may be produced, unless otherwise ordered by a court. Such a subpoena shall be served at least 24 hours before the time fixed for the production of the records unless otherwise ordered by a court.

Section 2306(b) further provides that where a court has designated a clerk to receive records described in subdivision (a), delivery may be made to him or her at or before the time fixed for their production. The clerk shall give a receipt for the records and notify the person subpoenaed when they

---

12. *See* Brayshow v. Gelber, 232 N.J. Super. 99, 556 A.2d 788 (1989).
13. New Mexico Statutes Annotated § 43-2-11 (Michie 1992).

are no longer required. The records shall be delivered in a sealed envelope indicating the title of the action, the date fixed for production, and the name and address of the attorney as shown on the subpoena. The records shall be available for inspection pursuant to the rules or order of the court.

The New York Mental Hygiene Law § 33.13(c) (McKinney 1992) provides that confidential clinical records of mental hygiene patients or clients may be released pursuant to a court order on a finding that the interests of justice significantly outweigh the need for confidentiality.

The New York Public Health Law § 2782 (McKinney 1992) permits disclosure of human immunodeficiency virus (HIV)–related information pursuant to court order.

NORTH CAROLINA

North Carolina General Statutes §§ 1A-1 and 8-61 (1991), concerning Rules of Civil Procedure 45, specify that when a subpoena commands any custodian of hospital medical records to appear for the sole purpose of producing certain records in his or her custody, the custodian may, in lieu of a personal appearance, tender to the presiding judge or his or her designee by registered mail or personal delivery certified copies together with the subpoena and an affidavit by the custodian testifying to the identity and authenticity of the records, that they are true and correct copies, and, as appropriate, that the records were made and kept in the regular course of business and that they were made by persons having knowledge of the information set forth. If the custodian doesn't have such records in his or her custody, he or she should submit an affidavit to that effect (*id.*).

Communicable disease information and records may be made available pursuant to a subpoena or court order. On request of the person identified in the record, the judge shall review it *in camera* and may, during the taking of testimony concerning such information, exclude from the courtroom all persons except the officers of the court, the parties, and those engaged in the trial of the case (*id.* § 130A-143).

The Health Maintenance Organization Act (*id.* § 58-67-180) specifies that any data or information pertaining to the diagnosis, treatment, or health of any enrollee or applicant obtained from such person or from any provider by any health maintenance organization (HMO) may be disclosed pursuant to a statute or court order, among other exceptions to the general confidentiality requirement.

NORTH DAKOTA

North Dakota does not have a separate statute governing subpoena of medical records. Its general subpoena for production of documentary evidence is Rule 45(b) of the North Dakota Rules of Civil Procedure.

OHIO

Ohio Revised Code Annotated § 2317.422 (Baldwin 1992) specifies that records of hospitals, nursing or rest homes, or adult care facilities may be qualified as evidence if the custodian, person who made them, or person under whose supervision they were made endorses thereon his or her verified certification identifying such records, giving the mode and time of their preparation, and stating that they were prepared in the usual course of business of the institution and delivers a copy to the attorney of record for each adverse party not less than five days before trial. Ohio's general subpoena statute is contained in Rule 45 of the Ohio Rules of Civil Procedure, and Ohio Revised Code Annotated § 2317.40 (Baldwin 1992) governs records in evidence generally.

OKLAHOMA

Oklahoma does not have any statute pertaining specifically to subpoena of medical records, although they may be subpoenaed under its general discovery statute, Oklahoma Statutes Annotated tit. 12, § 3230 (1991).[14]

OREGON

In a proceeding for commitment the court may order that medical records established by the Mental Health and Developmental Disability Division by rule be made available for review by court-appointed medical examiners (Oregon Revised Statute § 426.075 (1991)).

In a proceeding for imposing a public health measure, the court may order that the medical record of treatment of a person placed in custody as the subject of a petition be made available for review by court-appointed medical examiners. The court shall be fully advised of all drugs and other treatment known to have been administered to the subject of the petition (*id.* § 433.019(9)).

Privileges provided in §§ 40.230 to 40.240 shall not apply to information relevant to the proceeding (*id.* § 433.019(8)).

If the subject of the petition is committed to a facility, medical records and other information deemed necessary by the court shall be delivered to the director of the facility where the person is committed (*id.* § 433.019(22)).

PENNSYLVANIA

When an employee is served a subpoena requiring the production of medical records, he or she may comply by notifying the attorney causing service of the subpoena of the healthcare facility's intention to proceed under 42 Pennsylvania Statutes § 6152(a) (1990), and of the estimated reasonable and actual expenses of reproducing the records (*id.*). Afterward, the healthcare facility

---

14. *See also* Oklahoma v. Lloyd, 787 P.2d 855 (Okla. 1990).

shall hold the originals available and on payment of the costs deliver legible and durable certified copies by certified mail or personal delivery within 10 days (*id.* § 6152(c)). The certification shall be notarized and include a statement as follows:

> The copies of records for which this certification is made are true and complete reproductions of the original or microfilmed medical records which are housed in (name of health care facility). The original records were made in the regular course of business at or near the time of the matter recorded. This certification is given pursuant to [section 61(E)] (relating to medical records) by the custodian of the records in lieu of his personal appearance.

Copies shall be separately enclosed and sealed in an inner envelope or wrapper bearing the legend "Copies of Medical Records" (id. § 6152(d)). When these records are delivered in person, the deliverer should obtain a receipt (id. § 6153).

Under this statute, patients may apply for a protective order limiting access to their records (*id.* § 6155).

If the healthcare facility has none of the charts or records specified in the subpoena, or only a part thereof, § 6154 instructs the custodian of the charts or records to state so in a notarized affidavit and, following notice and payment of expenses, that he or she will hold available the original charts or records that are in the healthcare facility's custody and specified in the subpoena and shall deliver the certified copies together with the affidavit.

Section 6155(A) and (B) gives any patient whose medical charts or records are copied and delivered pursuant to this subchapter, any person acting on such patient's behalf, and the healthcare facility having custody of the charts or records, standing to apply to the court or other body before which the action or proceeding is pending for a protective order denying, restricting, or otherwise limiting access to and use of the copies or original charts or records.

Finally, §§ 6158 and 6159 provide that the original record or personal attendance of the custodian of records shall be required if the subpoena so specifies.

RHODE ISLAND

Rhode Island has a comprehensive statute governing response to legal process concerning confidential healthcare information.[15] Such information is not subject to compulsory legal process, such as a subpoena, in any type of proceeding.[16] A patient or his or her representative may refuse to disclose such information in any such proceeding except:

- When he or she introduces his or her physical or mental condition into evidence

---

15. Rhode Island General Laws § 5.37.3-6 (1991) (Confidentiality of Health Care Information Act).
16. *Id.* § 5.37.3-6(a)(1).

- When, during a commitment proceeding, a physician determines that the individual needs care or treatment in a facility that is appropriate for mental illness

- When a court finds that an individual, after having been informed that the communications would not be privileged, has made communications to a psychiatrist in the course of a psychiatric examination ordered by the court, provided that the communications shall be admissible only on issues involving the individual's mental condition

- When, in a court proceeding, the court determines that an individual's physical or mental condition endangers another

- In actions involving insurance carriers when such information is relevant and material

- When, in a court proceeding, the issue arises whether the individual used intoxicating liquors, toluene, or any controlled substance and such confidential healthcare information is relevant and material. In such cases, the court may issue an order compelling production of information that demonstrates the presence of alcohol in a concentration of one tenth of one percent (0.1%) or more, or the presence of a controlled substance as shown by chemical analysis of blood, breath, or urine, if such test was performed at the direction of a law enforcement official.[17]

However, in Bartlett v. Danti, 503 A.2d 515 (R.I. 1986), the court ruled that this statute was unconstitutional insofar as, in cases in which the patient did not consent to disclosure, the statute precluded litigants from introducing material evidence, thereby preventing them from effectively presenting their claims before the court. Thus, you must check with a Rhode Island attorney as to the current status of any provisions of the Confidentiality of Health Care Information Act.

SOUTH CAROLINA

South Carolina has no specific rules for subpoena of medical records.[18]

SOUTH DAKOTA

South Dakota has no specific rules for subpoena of medical records. Its general statute for subpoenas of records is South Dakota Codified Laws § 15-6-45(b) (1992).

---

17. *Id.* § 5-37.3-6(a)(2).
18. *But see* chapters 9 and 10.

TENNESSEE

Tennessee Code Annotated § 68-11-304(a)(1) (1991), specifying that court records are the property of the various hospitals, notes that they are subject to court order to produce them.

When a custodian receives a subpoena for records in an action in which the hospital is neither a party nor the place where the case arose, the custodian can comply by within five days personally delivering or mailing, by certified or registered mail, to the court clerk or officer, body, or tribunal conducting the hearing, a true and correct copy (which may be reproduced) of all records described in the subpoena. The copy should be enclosed in a sealed inner envelope with the title and number of the action, name of the witness, and date of the subpoena written thereon, enclosed in an outer envelope and accompanied by an affidavit. The affidavit should state that the affiant is the custodian and has authority to certify the records, that they are a true copy of the records described in the subpoena, that hospital personnel prepared them in the ordinary course of business at or near the time of the event, and certifying the charges (*id.* §§ 68-11-401–68-11-408).

TEXAS

Special care facilities may release medical records or information under court order.[19]

Under the Health Maintenance Organization Act, Texas Insurance Code art. 20A.17 (West 1992) requires a showing of good cause to obtain medical, hospital, and health records of enrollees and records of physicians and providers providing service under independent contract with a health maintenance organization (HMO) for examination in accordance with the commissioner's quality of health assurance program (*id.* art. 20A.17(1)).

Texas Health and Safety Code Annotated § 81.062(a) (West 1992) gives the Department of Health the authority to compel the production of documents or request county or district courts to compel the production of a requested document at a hearing involving communicable diseases.

UTAH

Utah Code Annotated § 31A-8-405 (1992) specifies that the Department of Health shall treat medical records of enrollees of an organization and its annual audits as confidential unless a court orders otherwise.

Section 26-25a-101(d) provides an exception to the general rule of confidentiality of communicable disease information, and permits disclosure to the courts. When involving child abuse, the information shall be disclosed *in camera* and sealed by the court at the conclusion of the proceedings (*id.*). Child

---

19. Texas Department of Health Hospital Licensing Standard ch. 12, § 8.7.3.1 (1991).

abuse reports may be made available to a court on a finding that access to the records may be necessary for the determination of an issue before it.

Medical records are the property of the hospital and may not be removed from the hospital's control except by court order or subpoena.[20]

VERMONT

Vermont does not have any specific laws about subpoena of medical records. However, its general subpoena statute for books or writings is Vermont Statutes Annotated tit. 12 § 1691 (1991).

VIRGINIA

While Virginia does not appear to have a specific statutory provision for the subpoena of medical charts and records from healthcare facilities, Virginia Code Annotated §§ 54.1-2922 and 54.1-2923 (Michie 1991) do grant a subpoena power to medical complaint investigation and medical practices audit committees, respectively. This subpoena power extends not only to the person who may be the subject of a complaint and other witnesses but also includes requirements for the production of any documents, records, or other materials that the committee may deem relevant to the inquiry. In addition, § 32.1-320 gives the attorney general's medical services audit and investigation unit the power to issue subpoenas for its audits and investigations.

Supreme Court Rule 4:9 governs subpoenas generally, and Virginia Code Annotated § 8.01-506.1 and § 16.1-89 (Michie 1991) concerns subpoena *duces tecum.*

Results of tests for human immunodeficiency virus (HIV) are confidential and may only be released to any person allowed access to such information by a court order (*id.* § 32.1-38).

WASHINGTON

Revised Code of Washington § 71.05.630(2)(d) (1991) notes that confidential treatment records of mental illness patients may be released pursuant to a lawful order of a court.

With respect to disclosure of human immunodeficiency virus (HIV) antibody tests or treatment of sexually transmitted diseases, *id.* § 70.24.105(2)(e) and (f) provides that a person may be allowed access to the record by a court order granted after a showing of good cause.[21]

Records of alcoholics and intoxicated persons treated for such conditions may be disclosed if authorized by an appropriate order of a court of competent jurisdiction after application showing good cause (*id.* § 70.96A.150).

---

20. Utah Administrative Rules 432-100-7.404(D) (1990).
21. *See also* Chapter 10.

WEST VIRGINIA

West Virginia Code §§ 57-5-4b through 57-5-4i (1992) cover providing copies of hospital records in compliance with subpoenas. They provide that when a record custodian receives a subpoena *duces tecum* in an action in which the hospital is neither a party nor the place where the action arose, he or she can comply by filing with the court a true copy of the records described in the subpoena (*id.* § 57-5-4b). The copy of the records shall be enclosed separately in an inner envelope or wrapper, sealed and labeled clearly, with the style (case name) and number of the action, the name of the witness, and the date of the subpoena. The sealed envelope or wrapper shall then be enclosed in an outer envelope or wrapper, sealed, and directed as follows:

- If the subpoena directs attendance in court, to the clerk of such court or to the judge

- If the subpoena directs attendance at a deposition, to the officer before whom the deposition is to be taken, at the place designated in the subpoena for the taking of the deposition, or at his or her place of business

- In other cases, to the officer, body, or tribunal conducting the hearing, at a like address (*id.* § 57-5-4c).

The custodian is required to prepare an affidavit stating that the records are true copies of the records described in the subpoena, that the affiant is a duly authorized custodian of the records and has authority to certify the records, and that the records were prepared by the personnel of the hospital, staff physicians, or persons acting under their control, in the ordinary course of hospital business at or near the time of the act, condition, or event recorded. Finally, the affidavit must certify the amount of the reasonable charges the hospital incurred in furnishing the copies of the subpoenaed records. If the hospital does not have all or any part of the records, the custodian must so state (*id.* § 57-5-4e).

Confidential communications and information obtained in the course of treatment or evaluation of a mentally ill patient may be disclosed in court proceedings to disclose the results of involuntary examinations, and pursuant to court orders based on a finding that the information is sufficiently relevant to a proceeding before the court to outweigh the importance of maintaining confidentiality (*id.* § 27-3-1).

When a court grants an order to disclose human immunodeficiency virus (HIV) test results or the identity of the subject it must properly maintain the records' confidentiality.[22]

---

22. *See* Chapters 7 and 10.

Section 33-25A-26(4) provides an exception to the general rule of confidentiality of data or information pertaining to the diagnosis, treatment, or health of any enrollee or applicant in the possession of a health maintenance organization (HMO) for court orders for the production of evidence.

WISCONSIN

Patient healthcare records may be released under a lawful order of a court (Wisconsin Statutes §§ 146.82(2)(4) and 146.025(5)(a)(8\9) (1991)).

Results of human immunodeficiency virus (HIV) tests may be released under a lawful order of a court except as provided under § 901.05 (making such test results inadmissible during a civil, criminal, or administrative proceeding as evidence of a person's character for the purpose of proving he or she acted in conformity with that character (*id.* § 146.025(5)(a)(9)).

Alcohol, drug abuse, developmental disabilities, and mental health treatment records may be released pursuant to a lawful order of a court (*id.* § 51.30(4)(b)(4)).

The Department of Health and Social Services has subpoena power under § 49.45(3)(h)(1) for the purposes of any audit, investigation, analysis, review, or other authorized function with respect to the medical assistance program.

WYOMING

Wyoming's only references to subpoenas do not specify special requirements for subpoena of medical records. Wyoming Statutes § 1-36-109(a) (1991) allows subpoena of records in civil actions.

CHAPTER 12

Disclosure for Medical Research

Introduction

Most states allow medical staff access to patients' records for medical research. In such cases, you should be careful to delete from any research reports all information that would identify the patient unless the patient has consented to being identified.

You should have written procedures documenting your policy on use of records for research covering, for example, access for staff, for nonphysician healthcare providers, and for investigators; approval authority; and security controls.

Federal Laws

Alcohol and drug abuse programs must maintain confidentiality certificates to protect the privacy of research subjects. Retention is not specified.[1]

The Social Security Administration (SSA) and Health and Human Services Department (HHS) release information held by them for research and statistical studies. The Privacy Act, 5 U.S.C. § 522a (1988), allows disclosure of records held by these departments, but the records may not contain personal identifiers unless the identifiers are necessary for the research project and the Department receives assurance from the requesting party that assures the privacy of the individuals subject to the records. The departments will also release personal identifiers if the recipient guarantees the records' safety and submits to on-site inspection of those safeguards.[2]

HHS also has procedures to protect the privacy of research subjects in federally funded research studies.[3]

---

1. 29 C.F.R. § 2a (1991).
2. 20 C.F.R. § 401.325 (1991).
3. *Id.* (found at 45 C.F.R. § 46.102 *et seq.* (1991)).

State Laws

ALABAMA

Alabama has no specific requirements for medical records used for medical research other than those discussed in Chapter 7.

ALASKA

Alaska Administrative Code tit. 7, § 13.130(b)(3) (April 1984), states that patient records and information may be released without consent for research projects authorized by the governing board, if provision is made to preserve anonymity in the reported results.

ARIZONA

Arizona Revised Statutes § 36-509(A) (1991), concerning the confidentiality of records, states that all information and records obtained in the course of evaluation, examination, or treatment shall be kept confidential and not as public records, except as the requirements of a hearing may necessitate a different procedure. Information and records may only be disclosed pursuant to rules established by the Department of Health Services, among others, to persons doing research or maintaining health statistics, provided that the Department establishes rules for the conduct of such research as will ensure the anonymity of the patient (*id.* § 36-509(A)(5)).

Section 36-664 also provides that otherwise confidential communicable disease information may be disclosed for the purpose of research.

ARKANSAS

Arkansas Code Annotated § 20-9-304 (Michie 1992) covers the use of records for medical research. All information, interviews, reports, statements, memoranda, or other data of the State Board of Health, Arkansas Medical Society, allied medical societies, or in-hospital staff committees of licensed hospitals, but not the original medical records of patients used in the course of medical studies for the purpose of reducing morbidity or mortality, shall be strictly confidential and shall be used only for medical research. Any authorized person, hospital, sanatorium, nursing home, rest home, or other organization may provide such information relating to the condition and treatment of any person to the entities listed above for use in the course of studies for the purpose of reducing morbidity or mortality without incurring liability for damages or other relief. However, in any event, the patient's identity is confidential and will not be released under any circumstances.

CALIFORNIA

You may release medical information to researchers if the director of mental health or developmental disabilities designates, by regulation, rules for the conduct of research, and requires such research to be first reviewed by the appropriate institutional review board. The rules shall include the requirement that all researchers sign an oath of confidentiality (California Welfare and Institutions Code § 5328 (e) (Deering 1992)).

California Civil Code § 56.10(c)(7) allows healthcare providers to disclose information to public agencies, clinical investigators, healthcare research organizations, and accredited public or private nonprofit educational or healthcare institutions for bona fide research purposes. However, the recipient may not further disclose the information in any way that would permit identification of the patient.

COLORADO

Colorado Revised Statutes § 27-10-120 (1991) notes that records for care and treatment of the mentally ill may be released if the Department of Institutions has promulgated rules for the conduct of research. Such rules shall include the requirement that all researchers sign an oath of confidentiality. All identifying information concerning individual patients, including names, addresses, telephone numbers, and social security numbers, shall not be disclosed for research purposes.

CONNECTICUT

Connecticut General Statutes § 19a-25 (1990) provides for confidentiality of records concerning morbidity and mortality. No disclosure is authorized except as may be necessary for the purpose of furthering the research project to which it relates.

Section 52-146g provides that a person engaged in research may have access to psychiatric communications and records that identify patients where needed for such research, if such person's research plan is first submitted to and approved by the director of the mental health facility or his or her designee. The communications and records shall not be removed from the mental health facility that prepared them. Coded data or data that does not identify the patient may be removed from a mental health facility, provided the key to the code remains on the premises. The facility and the researcher are responsible for the preservation of the anonymity of the patients.

DELAWARE

Delaware Code tit. 16, § 1203 (1991), authorizes disclosure of human immunodeficiency virus (HIV) tests to health facility staff committees or accreditation or oversight review organizations conducting program monitoring, program evaluation, or service reviews.

DISTRICT OF COLUMBIA

District of Columbia Code Annotated § 32-255 (1991) provides that medical records without names for patients at D.C. General Hospital may be made available to federal, state, and local agencies authorized to conduct utilization review or research with prior consent from the D.C. General Hospital Commission.

FLORIDA

Florida Statutes ch. 381.004(8) (1991) allows disclosure of human immunodeficiency virus (HIV) test results to authorized medical or epidemiological researchers, who may not further disclose any identifying characteristics or information.

GEORGIA

Georgia has no specific requirements concerning disclosure of medical record information for research.

HAWAII

Hawaii's only reference to confidentiality of research data is in Hawaii Revised Statute § 321-43 (1991), which provides that mortality and morbidity data of the Department of Health regarding cancer is confidential, except that researchers may use the names of patients when requesting additional information for research studies when such studies have been approved by the Cancer Commission of the Hawaii Medical Association.

IDAHO

Idaho Code § 39-1392b (1992) provides that all records relating to research, discipline, or medical study of any in-hospital medical staff committees or medical society are confidential. Section 39-1392d adds that all records used in a research, discipline, or medical study project are the property of the hospital or medical society that obtains or compiles them. In addition, *id.* § 39-308 provides for an exception to the general rule of confidentiality of records of alcoholics or intoxicated or addicted persons receiving treatment. The director may make available information from such records for the purposes of research into the causes and treatment of alcoholism or drug addiction (*id.* § 39-308 (1)). However, information from such research shall not be published in a way that discloses patients' names or other identifying information (*Id.* § 39-308(2)).

ILLINOIS

Illinois has no specific requirements regarding disclosure of medical information for research purposes, except that under Illinois Revised Statutes ch. 111½, ¶ 7408(a)(2) (1991), sexually transmissible disease information, including acquired immune deficiency syndrome (AIDS), may be disclosed for statistical purposes and medical or epidemiologic information if summarized so that no one can be identified and no names are revealed.

INDIANA

Indiana Code §§ 16-4-9-5–16-4-9-8 (Michie 1991) provides for the confidentiality of information for cancer research purposes. Generally, any disclosure cannot identify individual patients.

Section 16-1-9.5-2 prohibits the inclusion of the name or other identifying characteristics of the individual tested for human immunodeficiency virus (HIV) or acquired immune deficiency syndrome (AIDS). The board may adopt rules under § 4-22-2 concerning the compilation for statistical purposes of other information collected under this section.

A case report concerning the HIV infection that does not involve a confirmed case of AIDS, which is submitted to the State Medical Board, may not include the name or other identifying characteristics of the person tested if it involves

- An individual enrolled in a formal research project for which a written study protocol has been filed with the state board

- An individual tested anonymously at a designated counseling or testing site

- An individual tested by a healthcare provider permitted by rule by the State Medical Board to use a number identifier code

Section 16-1-9.5-7(a) provides that a person may not disclose or be compelled to disclose medical or epidemiological information involving a communicable disease or other disease that is a danger to general health. This information may not be released or made public on subpoena or otherwise, except under the following circumstances:

- Release may be made of medical or epidemiological information for statistical purposes if done in a manner that does not identify any individual.

- Release may be made of medical or epidemiological information with the written consent of all individuals identified in the information released.

- Release may be made of medical or epidemiological information to the extent necessary to enforce public health laws, laws described in § 35-38-1-7,[4] or to protect the health or life of a named party.

Further, release of such information is prohibited unless:

- Release shall be made of the medical records concerning an individual to that individual, or to a person authorized in writing by that individual to receive the medical records (*id.* § 16-1-9-7(d)).

- An individual may voluntarily disclose information about his or her communicable disease (*id.* § 16-1-9.5-9).

Any person responsible for recording, reporting, or maintaining information required to be reported under this section who recklessly, knowingly, or intentionally discloses or fails to protect medical or epidemiological information classified as confidential under this section commits a Class A misdemeanor. In addition, any public employee who violates this section is subject to discharge or other disciplinary action under the personnel rules of that governmental agency (*id.* § 16-9.5-7(c) and (e)).

IOWA

Iowa's general statute regarding disclosure for medical research is Iowa Code § 135.40 (1991), which provides that any person, hospital, sanatorium, nursing or rest home, or other organization may provide information, interviews, reports, statements, memoranda, or other data relating to the condition and treatment of any person to the Department of Public Health, the Iowa Medical Society, any of its allied medical societies, the Iowa Osteopathic Medical Society, or any in-hospital staff committee, to be used in the course of any study for the purpose of reducing morbidity or mortality.

While § 125.37 makes records of chemical substance abuse confidential, it does, however, permit disclosure for purposes of research into the causes and treatment of substance abuse. Such information shall not be published in a way that discloses patients' names or other identifying information.

Section 229.25 specifies that one of the exceptions to the requirement that medical records of mentally ill persons be confidential is that they may be released by the chief medical officer when requested for the purpose of research into the causes, incidence, nature, and treatment of mental illness. However, information shall not be provided in a way that discloses patients' names or identity.

KANSAS

Kansas Statutes Annotated § 65-5525(a)(2)(C) (1990) provides a specific authorization for disclosure of patients' records for purposes of research into

---

4. Section 35-38-1-7 has been repealed.

the causes and treatment of drug abuse. Researchers may not publish such information in any way that may disclose a patient's identity.

Similarly, § 65-177 provides for the secretary of health and environment to receive otherwise confidential data in connection with medical research studies conducted for the purpose of reducing morbidity or mortality from maternal, perinatal, and anesthetic causes.

KENTUCKY

Kentucky has no specific requirements governing access to medical records for research purposes.

LOUISIANA

Louisiana has no specific requirements regarding disclosure of medical information for research.

MAINE

Maine Revised Statutes Annotated tit. 5, § 19203-D(3) (West 1991) permits access to medical records concerning human immunodeficiency virus (HIV) infection for utilization review and scientific research, provided the individual patient is not identified.

MARYLAND

Maryland Health–General Code Annotated § 4-102 (1991) specifies that state confidential research records may only be used for the research and study for which they were assembled or obtained and may not be disclosed to any person not engaged in the research. However, statistics, information, or other material that summarizes or refers to confidential records in the aggregate, without disclosing the identity of any individual, may be published.

MASSACHUSETTS

Massachusetts General Laws ch. 111, § 24A (1992), specifies that all information procured in connection with scientific studies authorized by the commissioner of the Department of Public Health is confidential and shall be used solely for the purposes of medical or scientific research.

MICHIGAN

Michigan Compiled Laws § 333.6113 (1991) provides for disclosure of a patient record without the patient's consent to, among others, qualified personnel for the purpose of conducting scientific statistical research, financial audits, or program evaluation, but the personnel shall not directly or indirectly identify an individual.

Section 333.2361 mandates that information of an organization that has been designated as a medical research project by the department is confidential. Further, § 333.2632 provides that medical research project data is inadmissible in evidence and may not be disclosed except as is necessary for the purpose of furthering the medical research project.

Section 333.5111 requires the Department of Health to promulgate rules to provide for the confidentiality of reports, records, and data pertaining to research, among others, associated with communicable diseases or infections. Reports, records, and data pertaining to testing, care, treatment, reporting, and research associated with serious communicable diseases or human immunodeficiency virus (HIV) infection, acquired immune deficiency syndrome (AIDS), and AIDS-related complex (ARC) are confidential and may be released only as provided in the statute (*see* Chapter 7; *id.* § 333.5131).

MINNESOTA

Minnesota Statutes § 144.053(1) (1991) provides that data of the state commissioner of health or of the commissioner and other persons, agencies, and organizations, held jointly, for the purpose of reducing morbidity or mortality is confidential and shall be used solely for the purposes of medical or scientific research. No person participating in the research shall disclose the information except in strict conformity with the research project. Violation of the nondisclosure requirements is a misdemeanor.

Section 254A.09 provides for confidentiality for individuals who are the subject of alcohol or drug abuse research by the state authority.

Tests and personal information involving genetics and metabolic disease programs is confidential (*id.* §§ 144.053(2) and 144.91).

MISSISSIPPI

Mississippi has no specific requirements for disclosure of medical information for research.

MISSOURI

Missouri has a few references to medical information used for research. Revised Statutes of Missouri § 191.656(4) (1990) requires that the identity of any subject of human immunodeficiency virus (HIV) testing participating in a research project approved by an institutional review board shall not be reported to the Department of Health by the physician conducting the research project. Under § 192.067, the Department of Health may receive information from patients' medical records for the purpose of conducting epidemiological studies to be used in promoting and safeguarding health, but shall maintain the confidentiality of such information.

MONTANA

Montana Code Annotated § 50-16-529(6) (1992) notes that a healthcare provider may disclose healthcare information without the patient's authorization to the extent that the recipient needs to know the information if the disclosure is, among others, for use in a research project that an institutional review board has determined

- Is of sufficient importance to outweigh the intrusion into the privacy of the patient that would result from disclosure

- Is impracticable without the use or disclosure of the healthcare information in individually identifiable form

- Contains reasonable safeguards to protect the information from improper disclosure

- Contains reasonable safeguards to protect against directly or indirectly identifying any patient in any report of the research project

- Contains procedures to remove or destroy at the earliest opportunity, consistent with the purposes of the project, information that would enable the patient to be identified, unless an institutional review board authorizes retention of identifying information for purposes of another research project

Section 50-16-204 adds that in-hospital medical staff committees shall use or publish information from records only for, among other reasons, research and statistical purposes. The name or identity of patients whose records have been studied will not be disclosed.

Section 53-21-166 provides that an exception to the general rule of confidentiality of medical records of the mentally ill is for research, if the Department of Corrections and Human Services has promulgated rules for the conduct of research, including the requirement that all researchers sign an oath of confidentiality.

Section 50-16-102(1) permits use of information on infant morbidity and mortality for advancing medical research or medical education in the interest of reducing infant morbidity or mortality. Such data is privileged but may be given to the Department of Health and Environmental Sciences, the Montana Medical Association, an allied society of the Association, a committee of a nationally organized medical society or research group, or an in-hospital staff committee.

NEBRASKA

Revised Statutes of Nebraska § 71-3402 (1990) provides that the Department of Health, the Nebraska State Medical Association or any of its allied medical societies, or any in-hospital staff committee shall use or publish patient ma-

terial for the purpose of medical research or education for reducing morbidity and mortality only for those purposes, except that a summary may be
released for general publication. In all events, the identity of any person
whose condition or treatment has been studied shall be confidential and shall
not be revealed under any circumstances.

NEVADA

Nevada Revised Statutes Annotated § 457.260(1) (1991) allows the health
division to make appropriate use of material related to cancer reporting to
advance research and education concerning cancer and to improve treatment
of the disease.

NEW HAMPSHIRE

New Hampshire Revised Statutes Annotated §§ 318-B:12-a and 172:8-a (1991)
provide that if the patient gives written consent, records of alcohol and drug
abuse treatment may be used for research.

Section 141C:10 specifies conditions under which communicable disease
information may be disclosed to researchers. It requires that the researchers
demonstrate a need that is essential to health-related research, and any release of information shall be conditioned on personal identities of patients
remaining confidential. Section 141-B:9 contains virtually identical language
concerning disclosure of cancer information for research.

NEW JERSEY

New Jersey has no specific requirements concerning disclosure of medical
records information for research except for such disclosure by the State Department of Health.[5]

NEW MEXICO

New Mexico Statutes Annotated § 14-6-1(c) (Michie 1992) notes that statistical
studies and research reports based on confidential information may be published or released to the public as long as they do not identify individual
patients either directly or indirectly or in any way violate the privileged and
confidential nature of the relationship and communications between practitioner and patient.

The *New Mexico Hospital Association Legal Handbook* adds that in determining what restrictions should be placed on staff access to medical records
for reasons not required by medical care, the hospital must balance the
patients' privacy interests against medical staff interest in medical research or
the learning value of a particular case. It further adds that without written

---

5. *See* New Jersey Revised Statutes § 26:1A-37.2 (1991).

patient consent, records related to drug and alcohol treatment may be disclosed only to qualified personnel for the purpose of conducting scientific research, management audits, financial audits, or program evaluation, but such personnel may not identify, directly or indirectly, any individual patient in any report of such research or report.[6]

New Mexico Statutes Annotated §§ 24-2B-1 through 24-2B-8 (Michie 1992), the Human Immunodeficiency Virus Test Act, permit disclosure of otherwise confidential test results and the identity of any person tested to authorized medical or epidemiological researchers, who may not further disclose any identifying characteristics or information (*id.* § 24-2B-6(G)).

NEW YORK

New York Mental Hygiene Law § 33.13(b) and (c) (McKinney 1992) permit disclosure of confidential mental hygiene client records to qualified researchers on the approval of an institutional review board or other committee specially constituted for the approval of research projects at the facility, provided that the researcher shall in no event disclose information tending to identify a patient or client.

Human immunodeficiency virus (HIV)–related information may be disclosed to health facility staff committees or accreditation or oversight review organizations authorized to access medical records, provided that such committees or organizations may only disclose confidential HIV-related information

- Back to the facility or provider of a health or social service

- To carry out the monitoring, evaluation, or service review for which the information was obtained

- To a federal, state, or local government agency for the purpose of monitoring health or social services (*id.* § 2782).

NORTH CAROLINA

Confidential communicable disease information, whether publicly or privately maintained, which identifies a person who has acquired immune deficiency syndrome (AIDS) virus infection or who has or may have a reportable disease or condition, may be disclosed for bona fide research purposes. Or a provider may release specific medical or epidemiological information for statistical purposes in such a way that no person can be identified (General Statutes of North Carolina § 130A-143 (1991)).

---

6. Healthcare Financial Management Association, *New Mexico Hospital Association Legal Handbook*, ch. V, § C, ¶ 1-3, at V-6–V-8 (rev. ed. 1991).

Section 130A-212 provides that while the clinical records or reports of cancer patients are confidential, the Commission shall provide by rule for their use for medical research.

NORTH DAKOTA

North Dakota Century Code § 23-07.5-05 (1991) specifies that a provider of blood may disclose human immunodeficiency virus (HIV) test results to a person who conducts research if the researcher

- Is affiliated with the test subject's healthcare provider

- Has obtained permission to perform the research from an institutional review board

- Provides written assurance to the person disclosing the test results that the information requested is only for the purpose for which it is provided to the study, the information will not be released to a person not connected with the study, and the final research product will not reveal information that may identify the test subject unless the researcher has first received informed consent for disclosure from the test subject

OHIO

Ohio has only a few references to disclosure of medical record information for research. Ohio Revised Code § 3701.261 (Baldwin 1992) permits disclosure of information with respect to a case of malignant disease furnished to a cancer registry for statistical, scientific, and medical research for the purpose of reducing the morbidity or mortality of malignant disease. Under § 3793.13, patients' records of drug treatment programs may be disclosed without their consent to qualified personnel for the purpose of conducting scientific research, management, financial audits, or program evaluation, but these personnel may not identify, directly or indirectly, any individual patient in any report of the research, audit, or evaluation or otherwise disclose a patient's identity in any manner.

OKLAHOMA

Oklahoma Statutes Annotated tit. 63, § 1-1709 (1991), specifies that any authorized person, hospital, sanatorium, nursing home or rest home, or other organization may provide information relating to the condition and treatment of any person to the State Board of Health; the Oklahoma State Medical Association, or any committee or allied society thereof; the American Medical Association, or other national organization approved by the State Board of Health, or any committee or allied medical society thereof; or any in-hospital staff committee for use in studies for the purpose of reducing morbidity or mortality. Recipients shall use or publish such information or material only for the purpose of advancing medical research or education in the interest of reducing morbidity or mortality, except that a summary of such studies may be released for general publication. In all events, the identity of any person whose condition or treatment has been studied shall be confidential and not revealed under any circumstances. Any information furnished shall not contain the name of the person whose records are furnished, and shall not violate the confidential relationship of patient and physician. All such information and the findings and conclusions of such studies are privileged and not admissible in evidence (*id.*).

OREGON

Under Oregon Revised Statutes § 179.505(4)(b) (1991), a public healthcare provider may release, without patient consent, written medical records such as case histories, clinical records, x rays, progress reports, treatment charts, and other similar patient records maintained by the provider, to persons engaged in scientific research at the discretion of the responsible officer.

The provider shall not disclose patient identities except when essential to the research. When a patient's identity is disclosed, the provider shall include in the patient's permanent record a written statement detailing the reasons for the disclosure, what was disclosed, and recipients of the information (*id.* § 179.505(5)).

PENNSYLVANIA

Pennsylvania has no specific requirements concerning disclosure of medical record information for research.

RHODE ISLAND

Rhode Island General Laws § 5-37.3-4(b)(3) (1991) exempts from the general prohibition against disclosure of confidential healthcare information release to qualified personnel to conduct scientific research, provided they do not disclose patient identities.

SOUTH CAROLINA

South Carolina Code Annotated § 44-1-110 (Law. Co-op. 1990) permits the Department of Health and Environmental Control to investigate the causes, character, and means of preventing the epidemic and endemic diseases the state may suffer from. Thus, it has, on request, full access to the medical records, tumor registries, and other special disease record systems maintained by physicians, hospitals, and other health facilities as necessary to carry out its investigation of these diseases. The Department must keep patient-identifying information confidential.

Section 44-52-190(3), which establishes confidentiality of records that identify drug and alcohol abuse patients, permits disclosure for research conducted or authorized by the State Department of Mental Health or the South Carolina Commission on Alcohol and Drug Abuse. Section 44-52-170(f) permits disclosure in the same circumstances of records of such patients' commitment.

Section 44-29-135, which mandates confidentiality of sexually transmitted disease records, permits disclosure of medical or epidemiological information for statistical purposes in such a manner that no person can be identified.

Concerning the statewide Alzheimer's disease and related disorders registry, the School of Public Health and all persons to whom data is released shall keep all patient information confidential. No publication of information, biomedical research, or medical data may identify the patients (*id.* § 44-36-30).

SOUTH DAKOTA

South Dakota Codified Laws § 34-14-1 (1992) makes information obtained in medical studies for the purpose of reducing morbidity or mortality confidential. Disclosure of information from a medical study constitutes a misdemeanor (*id.* § 34-14-3).

TENNESSEE

Under Tennessee Code Annotated § 68-10-113(1) (1991), records or information concerning sexually transmitted disease held by health departments are confidential, but may be released for statistical purposes in such a form that no individual person can be identified.

Section 68-3-504 specifies that reports of fetal deaths are to be used only for medical, health, and research purposes.

TEXAS

Texas Revised Civil Statute art. 4495b, § 5.08(n)(3) (West 1992), lists disclosure of medical information to qualified personnel for research as one of the exceptions to the physician-patient privilege. However, personnel may not identify, directly or indirectly, a patient in any report of the research or otherwise disclose identity in any manner.

Under Texas Health and Safety Code Annotated § 161.021(a) (West 1992), a person, including a hospital, nursing home, medical society, or other organizations, may provide information relating to the condition and treatment of any person for studies to reduce morbidity or mortality or to identify to various organizations and practitioners persons who may need immunization. The recipients may only use such data to advance medical research or medical education in the interest of reducing morbidity or mortality, except that they may release a summary of the studies for general publication. However, the identity of a person whose condition or treatment has been studied is confidential and may not be revealed except to identify persons who need immunization. The information and any findings or conclusions resulting from that study are privileged (*id.* § 161.022(b)–(c)).

Medical personnel may disclose an acquired immune deficiency syndrome (AIDS), human immunodeficiency virus (HIV), or other related disorders test result for statistical summary purposes without the written consent of the person tested only if the researcher removes information that could identify the subject (*id.* § 81.103(e)).

UTAH

Utah Code Annotated § 26-25-1 (1992) states that any person or health facility may, without incurring liability, provide information, interviews, reports, statements, memoranda, or other data relating to the condition and treatment of any person to the Department of Health, to the Division of Mental Health within the Department of Social Services, to research organizations, to peer review committees, to professional review organizations, to professional societies and associations, or to any health facility's in-house staff committee for use in any study with the purpose of reducing morbidity or mortality or for the evaluation and improvement of hospital and health care. Such data is confidential and privileged. Section 26-25-2 provides that the Department of Health, the Division of Mental Health of the Department of Human Services, scientific and healthcare research organizations affiliated with institutions of higher education, the Utah State Medical Association or any of its allied medical societies, peer review committees, professional review organizations, professional societies and associations, or any health facility's in-house staff committee may only use or publish data received or gathered under § 26-25-1 for the purpose of advancing medical research or medical education in the interest of reducing morbidity or mortality, except that a summary of studies may be released for general publication.

Section 26-25a-101(2)(b), (c), and (e) through (i) provide that specific medical or epidemiological information regarding communicable or reportable diseases may be released to authorized personnel within the Department of Health, local health departments, official health agencies in other states, the U.S. Public Health Service, or the Centers for Disease Control, when necessary to continue patient services or to undertake public health efforts to interrupt the transmission of disease, presumably including research.

Section 62A-4-513(1)(g) provides that otherwise confidential child abuse reports and information may be disclosed to a person engaged in bona fide research when approved by the director of the division, if the information does not contain names and addresses.

VERMONT

Vermont's Bill of Rights for Hospital Patients, contained in Vermont Statutes Annotated tit. 18, § 1852(7) (1991), in delineating a patient's right to privacy, notes that medical personnel or individuals under the supervision of medical personnel researching the effectiveness of a given medical treatment shall have access to the patient's medical records without the patient's consent.

VIRGINIA

Virginia Code Annotated § 32.1-36.1(A)(6) (Michie 1991), which provides for confidentiality of tests for human immunodeficiency virus (HIV), specifies that such test results may be released to medical or epidemiological researchers for use as statistical data only.

Section 32.1-40 permits the commissioner of health or his or her designee to examine and review any medical records in the course of investigation, research, or studies of diseases or deaths of public health importance. Section 32.1-41 requires the commissioner or designee to preserve the anonymity of each patient and practitioner of the healing arts whose records are examined pursuant to § 32.1-41, except that the commissioner, at his or her sole discretion, may divulge the identity of such patients and practitioners if pertinent to an investigation, research, or study. Any person to whom such identities are divulged shall preserve their anonymity.

WASHINGTON

Revised Code of Washington § 42.48.020(1) (1991) provides that a state agency may authorize or provide access to or provide copies of an individually identifiable personal record for research purposes, if informed written consent for the disclosure has been given to the appropriate department secretary, the president of the institution, or his or her designee, by the person to whom the record pertains, or, in the case of minors and legally incompetent adults, the person's legally authorized representative. This statute also provides detailed guidelines for such disclosure without patient consent (*id.* § 42.48.020(2)). In addition, § 42.48.040 provides for confidentiality of research records and specifies the conditions under which individually identifiable records may be disclosed. Unauthorized disclosure is a misdemeanor (*id.* § 42.48.050).

Section 70.96A.150(2) and (3) permit the secretary of the Department of Social and Health Services to receive information from alcoholic and intoxicated patients' records for purposes of research into the causes and treatment of alcoholism and other drug addiction, verification of eligibility and appropriateness of reimbursement, and the evaluation of alcoholism and other drug treatment programs. Such information shall not be published in a way that discloses patients' names or identities. Section 71.05.630 permits disclosure of mental illness patient records for research.

WEST VIRGINIA

West Virginia Code § 16-3C-2(e)(2) (1992) permits disclosure of the performance of a human immunodeficiency virus (HIV)–related test for the purpose of research if the testing is performed in a manner by which the identity of the test subject is not known and may not be retrieved by the researcher.

WISCONSIN

Wisconsin Statutes § 146.82(2)(b) (1990), governing confidentiality of healthcare records, permits access without informed consent for purposes of research if the researcher is affiliated with the healthcare provider and provides written assurances to the custodian of the patient healthcare records that the information will be used only for the purposes for which it is provided to the researcher, the information will not be released to a person not connected with the study, and the final product of the research will not reveal information that may serve to identify the patient whose records are being released without the informed consent of the patient. The private pay patient may deny such access by annually submitting to the healthcare provider a signed, written request on a form provided by the Department of Health and Social Services.

Wisconsin Administrative Code § HSS 92.04(3) (June 1986), relating to confidentiality of treatment records of persons treated for mental illness, developmental disabilities, or alcohol or drug abuse, permits access to medical records without patient consent for authorized research.

Section 146.025(4), relating to confidentiality of acquired immune deficiency syndrome (AIDS) testing information, permits use of confidential data for research if the researcher is affiliated with a healthcare provider, has obtained permission to perform the research from an institutional review board, and provides written assurance to the person disclosing the test results that use of the information is only for the purpose for which it is provided to the researcher, the information will not be released to a person not connected with the study, and the final research product will not reveal information that may identify the subject unless the researcher has first received informed consent for disclosure from the subject.

WYOMING

Under Wyoming Statutes § 35-2-609(a)(vii) (1991), a hospital may disclose healthcare information about a patient without the patient's authorization to the extent that the recipient needs to know the information for use in a research project that an institutional review board has determined

- Is of sufficient importance to outweigh the intrusion into the privacy of the patient that would result from the disclosure

- Is impracticable without the use or disclosure of healthcare information in individual identifiable form

- Contains reasonable safeguards to protect against identifying, directly or indirectly, any patient in any report of the research project

- Contains procedures to remove or destroy at the earliest possible opportunity, consistent with the purposes of the project, information that would enable the patient to be identified, unless an institutional review board authorizes retention of identifying information for purposes of another research project

In addition, subject to bylaws and control by the hospital governing body, the medical staff committees of any hospital shall have access to the records, data, and other information relating to the condition and treatment of patients in that hospital for the purpose of evaluating, studying, and reporting on matters relating to the care and treatment of patients and for research, mortality reduction, and prevention and treatment of diseases, illnesses. and injuries (*id.* § 35-2-609(c)).

PART IV

How Do You Dispose of Your Medical Records?

You may have to dispose of your medical records in one (or both) of two situations. The more common way is pursuant to a proper record retention schedule as discussed in Chapter 3. Chapter 13 tells you how to accomplish the actual destruction of medical records to avoid any legal pitfalls. Chapter 14 discusses the rarer, although recently more prevalent, situation of disposing of records during mergers, acquisitions, and closings.

How Do You Destroy Your Medical Records?

Introduction

You may destroy medical records in one of two situations: pursuant to your record retention plan or on a one-time basis. The latter is often necessary to eliminate old, worthless medical records that your retention program does not cover. Because courts look on any records destruction that is not part of a records retention plan with suspicion, you must be certain that you conduct such a one-time destruction properly.

When it is time to destroy records, you can't just take them out and throw them away. A lot more is involved. If you are conducting a one-time destruction of a group of records, rather than destroying records pursuant to your records retention program destruction schedule, you must first review the records to make certain that you really want to destroy them. An excellent technique is to send out notices to interested parties, such as your hospital directors, staff attorney, and the like, that you are going to destroy the named records, telling them that if they do not respond within a certain time, you will destroy the records without further discussion. If your records are on computer media, such as floppy disks, you should print out a hard copy to review. Then you should destroy both the printout and the electronic media—the tape, disk, and so forth. On your review, take out any records that you should retain, like minors' records, records involved with litigation or government investigation or audit, and records that someone has requested. Also, you should not destroy any records during a one-time destruction that should be retained under your retention schedule.

State or federal statutes or regulations will normally prescribe how you must destroy records, usually by burning or shredding. Often, the controlling law will require you to create an abstract of any pertinent data in medical records prior to destroying the record.

If you use a commercial document destruction company, you should do so under a contract that sets forth how to destroy the records, how to avoid breaching confidentiality, including indemnification from loss due to unauthorized disclosure, and requires documentary proof of the destruction.

Regardless of whether you destroy records yourself or hire someone to do it, you must be certain that the records are completely destroyed and keep dated certificates of destruction of the records permanently. These certificates may be used as evidence in court or before a government agency to show that you destroyed the records in the regular course of business instead of in an attempt to hide something or gain an advantage in a litigation. Make certain that you destroy all records pursuant to your usual procedure. In a malpractice case, for example, the judge might allow the jury to infer that your destroying medical records in some way other than your usual procedure would show malpractice.

Federal Laws

44 U.S.C. §§ 3301-3303 and 3308-3314 (1988) (§§ 3304–3307 have been repealed) contain the provisions for destruction of government records. Nothing is specific as to types of records or the act's application outside the federal government.

State Laws

ALABAMA

Alabama has no specific provisions governing destruction of medical records.

ALASKA

Alaska has repealed Alaska Administrative Code tit. 7, § 12.010(f)(2)(H), which had specified that a hospital may not dispose of any records without the approval of the Department of Health and Social Services.

ARIZONA

Arizona's Department of Health Services suggests that when you destroy records, you keep a careful report including the date of destruction, the name of the person or organization doing the destruction, and a list of the names of patients whose records were destroyed.

ARKANSAS

After the 10-year retention period, you may destroy medical records, provided you retain the following for 99 years:

- Basic information including dates of admission and discharge
- Name of physician(s)
- Record of diagnosis and/or operations performed
- Operative reports; tissue (pathology) reports
- Discharge summaries for all admissions[1]

---

1. Arkansas Register Part 6, § III (E).

CALIFORNIA

The California Department of Health Services approves destruction by shredding, recycling, incineration, and even disposal in landfills on acceptance of an approved plan. The Department retains the right to approve unusual methods of destruction.

Skilled nursing facilities must inform the health department within three business days, in writing, whenever patient health records are defaced or destroyed before termination of the required retention period.[2]

In addition, the following other types of facilities must inform the department of any premature destruction of patient records[3]:

- Intermediate care facilities[4]

- Home health agencies[5]

- Primary care clinics[6]

- Psychology clinics[7]

- Psychiatric health facilities[8]

COLORADO

Colorado Administrative Regulations, 6 Code of Colorado Regulations § 1011-1, ¶ 4.2.2 (1977), requires healthcare facilities to establish procedures to notify patients whose records are to be destroyed prior to actually destroying such records.

CONNECTICUT

The draft Record Retention and Disposition Schedule of the Connecticut State Library's Medical Records/Case Files User Committee states that agencies may destroy records only after receiving approval in the form of a signed "Records Disposal Authorization" from the Department of Health Services. If the institution is not subject to inspection by the Department, it may destroy records after notification of compliance from the Joint Commission on Accreditation of Healthcare Organizations.

DELAWARE

Delaware has no specific rules governing destruction of medical records.

---

2. California Code of Regulations tit. 22, § 72543(d) (1991).
3. *Id.*
4. *Id.* § 73543(d).
5. *Id.* § 74731(e).
6. *Id.* § 75055(d).
7. *Id.* § 75343(d).
8. *Id.* § 77143(b).

DISTRICT OF COLUMBIA

The District has no specific rules governing destruction of medical records.

FLORIDA

Florida General Records Schedule for Hospital Records details provisions for disposal of any records possessed by a state agency that appear on a General Records Schedule.[9] The agency must initiate a Records Destruction Request, with Form LS5E107, submit multiple copies to the appropriate governmental office, and await authorization before proceeding with destruction.

GEORGIA

Georgia has no specific rules governing destruction of medical records.

HAWAII

Hawaii Revised Statute § 622-58(d) (1990) specifies that medical records may be destroyed after the seven-year retention period or after being reproduced in miniature form (minification), in a manner that will preserve the confidentiality of the information in the record, provided that the healthcare provider retains basic information from the record (as defined in Chapter 1). The provider or its successor must retain this basic information for 25 years after the last entry, or for the period of minority of a minor patient plus 25 years.

IDAHO

Hospitals may destroy records relating to patient care after the retention period by burning, shredding, or other effective method in keeping with the confidential nature of their contents. Destruction must be in the ordinary course of business, and no record may be destroyed on an individual basis.[10]

ILLINOIS

Illinois has no specific requirements for the destruction of medical records.

INDIANA

Prior to microfilming and destruction of original records, the facility shall prepare and keep on file a written program for microfilming and destruction of original records that ensures that the confidential nature of the records is maintained, that the responsibility for destruction is retained by the hospital, and that given records can be obtained on short notice when out of files for

---

9. Department of State Division of Library and Information Services Records Management Program, General Records Schedule for Hospital Records E-1, § III (March 1988).
10. Idaho Code § 39-1394(d) (1991).

microfilming, that the microfilmed records are readily available for reference and can be furnished when needed (Indiana Administrative Code tit. 410, 15-1-9(2)(a) and (c) (1988)).

IOWA

Iowa does not specify any particular requirements for destruction of records.

KANSAS

Kansas regulations require hospitals to maintain a summary of medical records that have been destroyed on file for at least 25 years. Such a summary must contain

- Name, age, and date of birth of patient

- Name of nearest relative

- Names of attending and consulting physicians

- Surgical procedure and date, if applicable

- Final diagnosis[11]

KENTUCKY

Kentucky has no specific requirements governing destruction of medical records.

LOUISIANA

Louisiana has no specific statutory provisions regarding destruction of medical records. However, Opinion of the Attorney General, January 8, 1964, noted that after the six-year retention a public hospital could destroy the record and may, but need not, microfilm it for permanent preservation prior to destruction.

MAINE

Maine has no specific regulations governing destruction of medical records.

MARYLAND

Maryland Health–General Code § 4-403 (1990) covers destruction of medical records. Except for minor patients' records, § 4-403 prohibits destruction, unless the patient is notified, of medical records, laboratory reports, or x-ray reports for five years after the record is made. Minor patient records may not be destroyed until the patient reaches the age of majority plus three years or for five years, whichever is later, unless the parent or guardian is notified or

---

11. Kansas Administrative Regulations § 28-34-9a(d)(3) (1990).

unless the minor is notified when his or her care was provided (*id.* §§ 20-102(c) or 20-103(c)). Notice must be by first-class mail sent to the patient's last known address and must include a statement that the record or a synopsis thereof may be retrieved at a designated location within 30 days of the proposed date of destruction.

If a sole practitioner dies, his administrator must forward the required notice to the patient's last known address and publish a notice in a daily newspaper with local circulation for two consecutive weeks, before destroying or transferring medical records.

MASSACHUSETTS

Massachusetts General Law ch. 111, § 70 (1992), provides that whenever preexisting records have been photographed or microphotographed and indexed and filed, a hospital or clinic may destroy the original on notifying the supervisor of public records.

MICHIGAN

Michigan Compiled Laws § 750.492a (1990), discussed in Chapter 6, which makes it a felony to destroy medical records for the purpose of concealing responsibility for a patient's injury, sickness, or death, notes that destruction is permissible if all of the information contained in or on the record or chart is otherwise retained by means of photography, mechanical or electronic recording, chemical reproduction, or other equivalent techniques that accurately reproduce all of the information contained in or on the original. This statute would not, however, appear to prohibit the destruction of medical records after the expiration of the retention period and in the regular course of business.

MINNESOTA

Minnesota Statute § 145.32 (1990) specifies that the superintendent or other chief administrative officer of a public or private hospital, with the consent of the board of directors or other governing body, may divest the files and records of that hospital of any individual case records bearing dates more than three years prior to the date of the divestiture and destroy them, provided they have first been recorded on photographic film of convenient size for preservation as evidence.

However, in Minnesota the commissioner of health defines what comprises an individual permanent medical record, which must be maintained permanently (*id.*). In 1988, the commissioner issued a revised rule specifying that an individual's permanent medical record must consist of all the following elements of the hospital record applicable to that patient:

- Identification data, which includes the patient's name, address, date of birth, sex, and if available, the patient's social security number

- Medical history, which includes details of the present illness, the chief complaint, relevant social and family history, and provisional diagnosis. For obstetrical patients, the medical history shall include prenatal information when available. For newborns, a birth history consisting of a physical examination report and delivery record as it pertains to the newborn must be included.

- A physical examination report

- A report of operations that includes the preoperative diagnosis, the names of all surgeons and assistants, the anesthetic agent, a description of the specimens removed and the resultant pathology findings, a description of the surgical findings, the technical procedures used, and the postoperative diagnosis

- A discharge summary, which includes the reason for hospitalization, summary of clinical observations, procedures performed, treatment rendered, significant findings (for example, pertinent laboratory, x-ray, and test results), and condition at discharge. For newborns or others for whom no discharge summary is available, a final progress note must be included.

- Autopsy findings[12]

This rule sets out the minimum information that the hospital must retain if it chooses to destroy a portion of the patient's medical record.

MISSISSIPPI

The Mississippi Code has comprehensive provisions for early retirement and destruction of hospital records.

Any hospital may, in its discretion, retire a record prior to the expiration of the retention period if the patient and the physician consent in writing. If the physician is no longer alive, the patient's consent is sufficient. In no event is such consent valid, however, if given within one year from the date of discharge (Mississippi Code Annotated § 41-9-71 (1990)). Section 41-9-61 defines "retirement" as "the withdrawal from current files of hospital records, business records or parts thereof on or after the expiration of the applicable minimum period of retention." However, no such record is subject to retirement where otherwise required by law to be kept as a permanent record.

Upon retiring any record, or part thereof, the hospital shall make an abstract of any pertinent data where so required by the rules of the licensing agency or as the hospital finds proper. The record so retired will be destroyed or otherwise disposed of by burning, shredding, or other effective method in keeping with its confidential nature (id. § 41-9-75).

A hospital may also, in its discretion, reproduce any hospital record on

---

12. Minnesota Rules 4642.1000 (1991).

film or other material and, after three years from the patient's discharge, retire the originals (*id.* § 41-9-77).

MISSOURI

Missouri's County/District Hospitals *Records Manual* states that selling of nonconfidential or valueless records as waste is permissible. But you should destroy confidential data under the supervision of competent persons designated or appointed to see that no records fall into unauthorized hands. A record of the disposition of records should be preserved in some permanent document, which includes the description and quantity of the record series disposed of, manner of destruction, inclusive dates covered, and the date of destruction.

Missouri Revised Statute § 109.156 (Supp. 1992) authorizes a business to destroy the original after it has microfilmed or otherwise reproduced a record.

MONTANA

The Montana Hospital Association notes that when you destroy records, you should keep a careful report of the date, the name of the organization or person performing the destruction, a list of the names of the patients' records destroyed, and prepare a patient summary card. The fully completed face sheet of the patient's record may be substituted for the summary card.[13]

NEBRASKA

Department of Health Regulations and Standards for Hospitals, Nebraska Administrative Rules and Regulations 175-9-003.04A6 (1979), provides that records may be destroyed only when they are more than 10 years old. In order to ensure the patient's right of confidentiality, licensed hospitals must destroy medical records by shredding, mutilation, burning, or other equally effective protective measures.

The regulation governing intermediate care facilities adds that the facility must permanently retain records or documentation of the actual fact of medical record destruction (*id.* 175-8-003.04A3).

NEVADA

No specific Nevada provisions govern destruction of medical records.

NEW HAMPSHIRE

New Hampshire Licensure Rules of the Department of Health and Human Services simply require that each hospital have a written policy in regard to the disposition of records.[14]

---

13. Montana Hospital Association, *Montana Hospital Association Manual,* ch. 23-7, § 7.1 (1981).
14. New Hampshire Code of Administrative Rules and Regulations, Department of Health and Human Services He-P 802.11(c) (1986).

NEW JERSEY

No specific New Jersey provisions govern destruction of medical records.

NEW MEXICO

New Mexico law provides that anytime after the retention period specified in the statute, a hospital may, without thereby incurring liability, destroy medical records by burning, shredding, or other effective method in keeping with the confidential nature of their contents, provided that the destruction is in the ordinary course of business and that no record is destroyed on an individual basis.[15]

NEW YORK

No specific New York provisions govern destruction of medical records.

NORTH CAROLINA

Nursing homes must have plans for destruction of medical records, identifying information to be retained and the manner of destruction to ensure confidentiality.[16]

NORTH DAKOTA

North Dakota has no specific rules governing destruction of medical records.

OHIO

Ohio's only reference to procedures for destroying medical records is that the Department of Mental Retardation and Developmental Disabilities shall adopt and promulgate rules with respect to the systematic and periodic destruction of residents' records.[17]

OKLAHOMA

Oklahoma has no specific requirements governing destruction of medical records.

OREGON

Records of nursing homes for the mentally retarded may not be destroyed without the written approval of the Health Division.[18]

---

15. New Mexico Statutes Annotated § 14-6-2 (D) (Michie 1991).
16. North Carolina Administrative Code tit. 10, r. 3H.0607(c) (March 1983).
17. Ohio Revised Code § 5123.89 (Baldwin 1991).
18. Oregon Administrative Rules § 333-92-095(5) (1986).

PENNSYLVANIA

Prior to destruction, public notice must be provided to permit former patients or their representatives to claim their records. The notice must be both legal notice and display advertisement in a newspaper of general circulation.[19] If the facility wants to destroy the original records after microfilming, it may not do so until the medical records department has had an opportunity to review the processed film for content.[20]

RHODE ISLAND

Rhode Island has no specific requirements for destruction of medical records.

SOUTH CAROLINA

Hospitals may destroy medical records after 10 years, except those of minors, which must be retained until after the expiration of the period of election following achievement of majority as prescribed by statute, which is one year,[21] so long as the hospital retains an index, register, or summary cards providing such basic information as dates of admission and discharge, name of responsible physician, and record of diagnoses and operations for all records so destroyed.[22]

The Department of Health and Environmental Control, Records Series Retention/Disposition Schedule DHEC-CHD-75(R) (Sept. 6, 1990) provides that county health departments should screen files for records of patients who have not been treated or serviced in the preceding four years. In tuberculosis (TB) and acquired immune deficiency syndrome (AIDS) cases, the TB nurse and district medical director, respectively, must screen the records prior to transfer to the State Records Center. After removal of all material no longer needed for immediate medical or reference purposes, the clinical health records may be transferred to the State Records Center, if space is available, held there for 20 years, and then destroyed.

SOUTH DAKOTA

South Dakota has no specific requirements concerning destruction of medical records.

TENNESSEE

On retirement of the record after the retention period, the facility may destroy records by burning, shredding, or other effective method in keeping with the confidential nature of their contents. The facility must destroy records

---

19. 28 Pennsylvania Code § 115.23 (1989).
20. *Id.* § 563.7.
21. South Carolina Code Annotated § 15-3-40 (Law. Co-op. Supp. 1991).
22. South Carolina Code of Regulations 61-16, § 601.7(A) (1982).

in the ordinary course of business and may not destroy any record on an individual basis.[23] Tennessee Code Annotated § 68-11-302 defines "retirement" as "the withdrawal from current files of hospital records, business records, or parts thereof on or after the expiration of the applicable period of retention." Tennessee's Department of Health and Environment, Board for Licensing Health Care Facilities Rules, Tennessee Compilation of Rules and Regulations tit. 1200, ch. 8-4-.03(f)(1), adds that records shall not be destroyed except by shredding or incineration. When you destroy records, you must record the date and time of such destruction and make an entry on the patient index card (*id*. ch. 8-4-.03(f)(1) and 8-6-.07(c)).

TEXAS

Texas Health and Safety Code Annotated § 577.012 (West 1992) specifies that private mental hospitals may not destroy medical records that relate to any matter involved in litigation if the hospital knows the litigation has not been finally resolved. Section 241.103 of the Health and Safety Code has identical provision for hospitals, as does § 262.030 for municipal hospitals and § 281.073 for hospital districts.

Texas's Hospital Licensure Rules do not specify how to destroy records, but provide that the facility may not destroy medical records that relate to any matter involved in litigation if the hospital knows the litigation has not been finally resolved.[24]

UTAH

For hospitals and general healthcare facilities, prior to destroying a medical record, you must make a summary to be retained. The summary must include patient's name; medical record number; date of birth, admission, and discharge; nearest relative, if available; attending physician; final diagnosis; surgical procedure or procedures; and pathology findings. Destroy the medical record completely to maintain confidentiality.[25]

Mental retardation facilities, small healthcare facilities, abortion clinics, and end-stage renal disease facilities shall notify the Department of Health in writing within 10 business days whenever client records are inadvertently defaced or destroyed.[26] Freestanding ambulatory surgical centers shall immediately document in the medical record when patient records are inadvertently destroyed.[27]

---

23. Tennessee Code Annotated § 68-11-305(c) (1990) (general statute); Tennessee Compilation of Rules and Regulations tit. 1200, ch. 8-6-.07(c) (1990).
24. Texas Department of Health, Hospitals Licensing Standards ch. 1, § 221.3 (1991).
25. Utah Administrative Rules 432-100-7.406 (1990).
26. *Id*. at 432-152-4.203(E), 432-200-6.102(E), and 432-600-6.104(E).
27. *Id*. at 432-500-6.104(E).

VERMONT

Vermont has no specific requirements governing destruction of medical records.

VIRGINIA

Virginia has no specific requirements governing destruction of medical records.

WASHINGTON

During final disposal of records, each hospital shall prevent retrieval and subsequent use of any data permitting identification of individuals in relation to personal or medical information.[28]

WEST VIRGINIA

West Virginia has no specific requirements for destruction of medical records.

WISCONSIN

Wisconsin has no specific requirements for destruction of medical records except that providers may not destroy fetal monitor tracings unless they provide notice to the patient 35 days prior to the destruction.

WYOMING

Wyoming has no specific requirements for destruction of medical records.

---

28. Washington Administrative Code 248-18-440(11)(h) (1986).

CHAPTER 14

Disposing of Records During Acquisitions, Mergers, and Closings

Introduction

What do you do with your records when your healthcare facility ceases operation, either because another facility acquires your facility, you merge with another facility, or you close your facility?

Some states have statutory or regulatory guidelines that tell you what to do if your facility closes or is merged with another facility. If not, you may want to review the guidance, listed below, that other states provide. Most states specify that if a healthcare facility is taken over by another, the new operator will maintain the old facility's records as if there had been no change of ownership. In the case of a merger, the new entity should merge the old entity's active records with its own records and prepare a retention schedule for inactive records so as to maintain them as required by law, regulations, or necessity[1] and destroy them as indicated by the retention schedule. You should include a provision in your merger or other agreement detailing which party is responsible for records.

State laws vary more concerning disposition of records during closings. Some states, such as Arizona, require the closing provider to store the records for the required period. Other states, such as Indiana, require the hospital to turn over records to other hospitals or to a health authority in the vicinity. Still others, such as Mississippi, require the facility to turn over its records to the licensing authority. Regardless of the appropriate recipient of such records, many states require you to either inform the licensing agency or get its permission to dispose of your records in a particular way on an acquisition, a merger, or a closing. If your state does not have any rules concerning disposition of records in such circumstances, you should arrange for the safe retention of those that should not be destroyed and the proper destruction of those that may be destroyed,[2] and query your licensing authority as to whether your arrangements are satisfactory.

Federal Laws

Federal laws do not specify any requirements for disposition of medical records on acquisition, merger, or closing of a facility.

---

1. *See* Chapter 3.
2. *See* Chapter 16.

State Laws

ALABAMA

Rule 420-5-7.07 of the Alabama State Board of Health Division of Licensure and Certification states that when a hospital ceases to operate as a hospital, the medical records shall be disposed of as directed by the State Board of Health. When a hospital ceases to operate, either voluntarily or by revocation of its license, the governing body (licensee) at or prior to such action shall develop a proposed plan for the disposition of its medical records. Such plan shall be submitted for review and approval to the division of Licensure and Certification and shall contain provisions for the proper storage, safeguarding, confidentiality, and transfer or disposal of patient medical records and x-ray files. The following options are provided for use in the development of such plans:

- Option A. The governing body may, through mutual agreement with other hospitals in the service area, transfer patients' medical records and x-ray files to other licensed hospitals. Such an arrangement may be preferable in the case of a replacement facility where the medical staff assumes staff responsibilities at the new facility.

- Option B. The governing body may develop a formal plan for the retention of medical records through microfilm or microfiche reproduction, provided the plan includes provision for a safe storage area, the designation of responsibility for the withdrawal of records, and for screening of records at regular intervals to allow for timely destruction in accordance with the following schedule:

  - Retain as original medical records any files under litigation.

  - Retain medical records of patients under majority as original or as microfilm for the period of minority plus one year, or as a minimum for six years, as complete medical records, after which they may be destroyed.

  - Retain records of patients having reached majority (19 years of age at time of discharge) as originals or as microfilm for a period of three years to a minimum period of 20 years after any injury arose.

  - X-ray film may be destroyed after five years from date of exposure, provided the written and signed findings of a physician who has read such film are retained as part of the medical record.

  - At the discretion of the governing authority, nurses' notes may be deleted from the reproduction of medical records.

ALASKA

Alaska Statutes § 18.20.085(c) (1990) provides that if a hospital ceases operation, it shall make immediate arrangements, as approved by the Department of Health and Social Services, for the preservation of its records. Likewise, 7 Alaska Administrative Code tit. 7, § 43.030 (April 1984), requires that healthcare providers to Medicaid recipients notify the Department so as to receive instructions as to the disposition of Medicaid records. Section 12.040(i)(2) requires nursing homes that close or transfer ownership to apply to the Department for instructions as to the disposition of admission and death records.

ARIZONA

Arizona Compilation Administrative Rules and Regulations 9-10-221(R) provides that if a facility ceases operation, the facility shall arrange for preservation of records to ensure compliance with these regulations. The Department shall be notified, in writing, concerning the arrangements.

ARKANSAS

Arkansas has no specific requirements for disposition of medical records on acquisition, merger, or closing of a facility.

CALIFORNIA

Licensed providers of health services have an obligation, if the licensee ceases operation, to preserve records for a minimum of seven years following discharge of the patient, except that the records of unemancipated minors shall be kept at least one year after the minor has reached the age of 18 years, and in any case, not less than seven years. The department or any person injured as a result of the licensee's abandonment of health records may bring an action in a proper court for any damages suffered as a result. In the event that the licensee is a corporation or partnership that is dissolved, the person injured may take action against that corporation's or partnership's principal officers of record at the time of dissolution. The term "abandoned" means leaving patients treated by the licensee without access to medical information to which they are entitled pursuant to California Health and Safety Code § 1795.12.[3]

California Code of Regulations tit. 22, § 70751(d) (1991) states that if a hospital ceases operation, it shall notify the Department of Health within 48 hours of the arrangements made for safe preservation of patient records. If the hospital changes ownership, both the previous and the new licensee shall, prior to the change of ownership, provide the Department with written documentation that the new licensee will have custody of

---

3. California Health and Safety Code § 1795.26 (Deering 1992).

patient records, provide for safe preservation of the records, and that they are available to both the new and former licensees and other authorized persons (*id.* § 70751(e)).

In addition to general acute care hospitals, Title 22 provides substantially similar requirements for record preservation during closings of the following various other types of facilities:

- Acute psychiatric hospitals (*id.* § 71551(d) and (e))

- Skilled nursing facilities (*id.* § 72543(c) and (e))

- Intermediate care facilities (*id.* § 73543(c) and (e))

- Home health agencies (*id.* § 74731(d) and (f))

- Primary care clinics (*id.* § 75055(c) and (e))

- Psychology clinics (*id.* § 75343(c) and (e))

- Psychiatric health facilities (*id.* § 77143(d) and (e))

- Chemical dependency recovery hospitals (*id.* § 79351(d) and (e))

COLORADO

Colorado has no specific requirements for disposal of records during acquisitions, mergers, or closings.

CONNECTICUT

Connecticut has no specific requirements for disposal of records during acquisitions, mergers, or closings.

DELAWARE

Delaware has no specific requirements for disposal of records during acquisitions, mergers, or closings.

DISTRICT OF COLUMBIA

District of Columbia has no specific requirements for disposal of records during acquisitions, mergers, or closings.

FLORIDA

Florida Administrative Code r. 10D-28.153(8) (1991) requires the licensee to notify the department of impending closure of a licensed hospital 90 days prior to such closure. The hospital must advise the licensing agency as to the placement of patients and disposition of medical records.

GEORGIA

Georgia has no specific requirements for disposal of records during acquisitions, mergers, or closings.

HAWAII

Hawaii law notes that healthcare provider successor providers are liable for the preservation of basic information (defined in Chapter 1) from the medical record for 25 years after the last entry, except that in the case of minors, they are responsible for retention for the period of minority plus 25 years. If a healthcare provider is succeeded by another entity, the burden of compliance with this law rests with the successor. Before a provider ceases operations, it shall make immediate arrangements, subject to the approval of the Department of Health, for the retention and preservation of its medical records.[4]

IDAHO

Idaho has no specific regulations governing disposal of medical records during acquisitions, mergers, and closings.

ILLINOIS

Illinois Administrative Code tit. 77, § 250.1510(d) (1991), mandates that the hospital shall have a policy for the preservation of patient medical records in the event of the closure of a hospital.

INDIANA

The Hospital Licensure Rules of the Indiana State Board of Health Indiana Administrative Code tit. 410, r. 15-1-9(2) (1988), requires that, on closure of a hospital, the facility will transfer the microfilmed medical records, when possible, to a local public health department or public hospital in the same geographic area. When the facility cannot do so, it should send the microfilmed records to the Board of Health.

IOWA

Iowa regulations provide that records shall be retained in the facility on change of ownership and when the facility ceases to operate, the facility shall release residents' records to facilities to which they are transferred. If no transfer occurs, the facility shall release the record to the individual's physician.[5]

---

4. Hawaii Revised Statute § 622-58(e) (1990).
5. Iowa Administrative Code r. 481-59.19(135C) (1990) (skilled nursing facilities); *id.* r. 481-63.17(135C) (residential care facilities for the mentally retarded); *id.* r. 481-57.16(3) (residential care facilities); *id.* r. 481-58.15(5) (intermediate care facilities); *id.* r. 481-62.18(4) (residential care facilities for persons with mental illness).

Rule 441-81.9(249A) of the Iowa Administrative Code specifies that records will be maintained in nursing facilities upon change of ownership.

KANSAS

Under Kansas regulations, if a hospital discontinues operation, it shall inform the licensing agency as to the location of its records.[6]

KENTUCKY

902 Kentucky Administrative Regulation 20:016, § 3(11)(3) (1991), states that hospitals shall provide for written designation of special locations for the storage of medical records in the event the hospital ceases to operate because of disaster, or for any other reason.

LOUISIANA

Louisiana Revised Statutes § 40:2109(E)(1) (1990), concerning healthcare rules, regulations, and minimum standards, provides that

- The secretary shall adopt rules, regulations, and minimum standards providing for the disposition of patients' medical records on closure of a hospital.

- When a hospital is closing, it may need to submit a plan for the disposition of patients' medical records to the secretary for approval.

- Notwithstanding the provisions of Louisiana Revised Statute 40:2144, the secretary may approve any plan that he or she deems to be in the best interest of the patients.

MAINE

Maine has no specific requirements governing disposal of medical records during acquisitions, mergers, or closings.

MARYLAND

Maryland has no specific requirements governing disposal of medical records during acquisitions, mergers, or closings except in the case of home health agencies. However, healthcare providers must make provisions for retention of clinical records when they cease operation.[7]

MASSACHUSETTS

Massachusetts General Laws ch. 111, § 70 (1992), provides that in the event of a transfer of ownership of a hospital, an institution for unwed mothers, or a

---

6. Kansas Administrative Regulations § 28-34-9a(d)(2) (1990).
7. Code of Maryland Regulations tit. 10, § .07.10.11(6) (1991).

clinic, the new owner shall maintain all medical records as if there were no change in ownership. In the event of a permanent closing, the institution will arrange for preservation of such medical records for the thirty-year retention period.

MICHIGAN

Michigan does not specify what to do with medical records in the event of an acquisition, merger, or closing.

MINNESOTA

Minnesota does not specify what to do with medical records in the event of an acquisition, merger, or closing.

MISSISSIPPI

As part of its comprehensive statutory scheme for regulating hospital records, Mississippi Code Annotated § 41-9-79 (1990) provides that when a hospital is closed, it must turn over its hospital records to any other hospital or hospitals in the vicinity willing to accept and retain them. If no such hospital exists, the closing hospital shall deliver properly indexed records to the licensing agency.

MISSOURI

Missouri's only reference to mergers, acquisitions, or closings is in Missouri Revised Statutes § 198.052 (Supp. 1992), relating to convalescent, nursing, and boarding homes. It requires new operators of such a facility to retain the original medical records of residents.

MONTANA

Montana Code Annotated § 50-16-529 (1991) specifies that a healthcare provider may disclose healthcare information about a patient without the patient's consent to a healthcare provider who is the successor in interest to the healthcare provider maintaining the information.

NEBRASKA

Nebraska law provides that in cases in which a hospital ceases operation, all medical records shall be transferred to the licensed hospital or other licensed healthcare facility to which the patient is transferred. All other records shall be disposed of.[8] The regulations have identical language for intermediate care facilities.[9]

---

8. Nebraska Administrative Rules and Regulations 175-9-003.04A6 (1979) (Department of Health Regulations and Standards for Hospitals).
9. *Id.* 175-8-003.04A3.

NEVADA

Nevada has no specific guidance for disposing of records during acquisitions, mergers, and closings.

NEW HAMPSHIRE

New Hampshire Code Administrative Rules, Department of Health and Human Services He-P 806.10 (1986), state that, in the event an outpatient clinic ceases operation, it must provide for the safe preservation of clinical records, as does He-P 807.07 for residential treatment and rehabilitation facilities, and He-P 809.07 for home health service providers.

NEW JERSEY

If a hospital discontinues operations for any reason, the governing authority must, before closing, notify the Department of Health, in writing, where it will store and service its medical records.[10]

In addition, the Administrative Codes of the State Board of Medical Examiners[11] provide that when a licensee ceases to engage in practice or anticipates remaining out of practice for three months or more, he or she shall

- Establish a procedure by which patients can obtain treatment records or acquiesce in the transfer of those records to another licensee or healthcare professional who is assuming the responsibilities of that practice

- Publish a notice of the cessation and the established procedure for the retrieval of records in a newspaper of general circulation in the geographic location of the licensee's practice, at least once each month for the first three months after the cessation

- Make reasonable efforts to directly notify any patient treated during the six months preceding the cessation, providing information concerning the established procedure for retrieval of records

NEW MEXICO

New Mexico has no specific requirements for disposing of records during acquisitions, mergers, or closings.

NEW YORK

New York has no specific requirements for disposing of records during acquisitions, mergers, or closings.

---

10. New Jersey Administrative Code tit. 8, § 34B-7.4(b) (1985).
11. *Id.* tit. 13, § 35-6.5.

NORTH CAROLINA

Nursing homes' policies with regard to retention of medical records shall ensure that either the original or a copy of each patient's or resident's medical record is kept in the facility regardless of a change of ownership or administrator, in accordance with state statutes of limitations for both adults and minors.[12]

NORTH DAKOTA

North Dakota has no specific requirements for disposing of records during acquisitions, mergers, or closings.

OHIO

Ohio has no specific requirements for disposing of records during acquisitions, mergers, or closings.

OKLAHOMA

Oklahoma has no specific requirements for disposing of records during acquisitions, mergers, or closings.

OREGON

Oregon Administrative Rule 333-505-050(14) (1991) provides that if a hospital or related institution changes ownership, its medical records must remain therein and become the responsibility of the new owner. Rule 333-505-050(15) states that if a hospital is closed, its medical records may be turned over to any other hospital or hospitals in the vicinity willing to accept and keep them.

   If a long-term care facility (LTCF) changes ownership, the medical records shall remain at the LTCF. The new owner shall be responsible to protect and maintain the records (*id.* § 333-86-055(7)). If the LTCF is closed, the administrator shall notify the Health Division of the location of the medical records (*id.* § 333-86-055(8)).

PENNSYLVANIA

If a hospital discontinues operation, it shall inform the Department of Health where its records are stored. The storage facility must offer retrieval services for at least five years after the closure date. Prior to destruction, public notice must be provided to permit former patients or their representatives to claim their records. The notice must be both legal notice and display advertisement in a newspaper of general circulation (28 Pennsylvania Administrative Code § 115.23 (1989)). Section 563.6 requires the same procedures for ambulatory surgical facilities.

---

12. North Carolina Administrative Code tit. 10, r. 3H.0607(b) (March 1983).

Section 601.36(a) requires long-term care nursing facilities that close to transfer patient medical records with the patient if the patient is transferred to another healthcare facility. If not, the owners of the facility shall make provision for the safekeeping and confidentiality of the records and shall notify the Department of how the records may be maintained.

Home health agencies shall have policies that provide for retention even if the agency discontinues operation. If the patient is transferred to another home healthcare agency, a copy of the record or abstract shall accompany the patient (*id.* § 606.36(b)).

RHODE ISLAND

Rhode Island has no specific requirements for disposition of medical records on acquisition, merger, or closing.

SOUTH CAROLINA

The South Carolina Department of Health and Environmental Control's regulations specify that, if hospitals or institutional general infirmaries change ownership, they must transfer all medical records to the new owners.[13] If the hospital or institutional general infirmary closes, it must arrange for preservation of the records and notify the Department, in writing, of its arrangements therefor.[14]

South Carolina Code Regulation 61-14, § 504.3, is similar, except that it states that upon the closing of an intermediate care facility, the medical records "will be kept intact or legally disposed of." Regulations governing nursing care facilities have identical language (*id.* 61-17).

The regulations covering mental retardation facilities state that on closure of a facility, the licensee must maintain the health record and all other required records (id. 61-13, § 503).

SOUTH DAKOTA

South Dakota has no specific requirements for disposal of records during acquisitions, mergers, or closings.

TENNESSEE

Tennessee Code Annotated § 68-11-308 (1990) states that if any hospital closes, it shall deliver and turn over its hospital records, in good order and properly indexed, to the Department of Health and Environment.

---

13. South Carolina Code Regulations 61-16 § 601.7(D) (1982).
14. *Id.*

TEXAS

Texas Department of Health Hospital Licensing Standards do not discuss changes of ownership of hospitals, but ch. 1, § 22.1.6, notes that if a hospital closes, it shall notify the licensing agency of the disposition of medical records, including the location of the record storage and the identity of the custodian of the records. Chapter 12, § 8.7.6, states that in the event of change of ownership of special care facilities, the new management will maintain proof of the medical information required for the continuity of services to residents.

UTAH

Hospitals and general healthcare facilities that cease operations must provide for appropriate safe storage and prompt retrieval of all medical records, patient indexes, and discharges for the 10-year retention period of Utah Administrative Rule 432-100-7.406(A) (1990). The hospital may arrange for storage with another hospital or may return patient medical records to the attending physician if he or she is still in the community. In any event, the facility will notify the Department of Health in writing within three business days of closure, detailing the provisions for the safe storage of the records and their location and publish the location of all hospital medical records in the local newspaper (*id.* at 432-100-7.406(D)). Other facilities, such as mental retardation facilities (Rule 432-152-4.203), small healthcare facilities (Rule 432-200-6.102), freestanding ambulatory surgical centers (Rule 432-500-6.104), abortion clinics (Rule 432-600-6.104), end-stage renal disease facilities (Rule 432-650-3.206), and home health agencies (without the publication requirement, Rule 432-700-3.705), have the same requirements.

VERMONT

Vermont has no specific requirements for disposition of medical records on acquisition, merger, or closing.

VIRGINIA

Virginia's regulations do not specify what a hospital must do with its medical records upon closing, but its Rules and Regulations for the Licensure of Nursing Homes § 24.7 (1980) states that nursing home records should be transferred with the patient if the patient is transferred to another licensed healthcare facility. Otherwise, the owners shall make provisions for the safeguarding and confidentiality of all medical records. When a nursing home changes ownership, it must make adequate provision for the orderly transfer of all medical records.

WASHINGTON

If any hospital ceases operations, it shall make immediate arrangements as approved by the Department of Social and Health Services for preservation of its records.[15]

Washington's administrative code amplifies the statutory guidance by providing that in the event of transfer of ownership of a hospital, the hospital shall keep patients' medical records, registers, indexes, and analyses of hospital services in the hospital to be retained and preserved by the new owner in accordance with state statutes and regulations. If the hospital ceases operation, the hospital shall make immediate arrangements for preservation of its medical records and other records of or reports on patient care data in accordance with applicable state statutes and regulations and obtain approval of the department for the planned arrangements prior to the cessation of operation.[16]

WEST VIRGINIA

West Virginia has no specific rules governing disposal of records during acquisitions, mergers, and closings.

WISCONSIN

Wisconsin has no specific rules governing disposal of records during acquisitions, mergers, and closings.

WYOMING

Wyoming has no specific rules governing disposal of records during acquisitions, mergers, and closings.

---

15. Revised Code of Washington § 70.41.90 (Supp. 1992).
16. Washington Administrative Code § 248-18-440 (1986).

PART V

Healthcare Business Records

Because healthcare providers are businesses as well as services, they must maintain not only medical records but business records as well. The proper maintenance of business records is important for many of the same reasons as is the maintenance of medical records: to comply with the law, to provide better health care, and to minimize litigation losses.

The need to comply with the many statutes, executive orders, and agency regulations is obvious. Governmental power to require record keeping carries with it the power to inspect to ensure compliance and to enforce sanctions, such as fines, for failure to keep required records. Keeping medical records properly is a more obvious need for providing quality health care, but maintaining good business records helps ensure quality health care as well, by assisting the facility administration to operate efficiently and on a sound fiscal basis. Good business records also facilitate successful lawsuits against others, such as collection actions for overdue accounts, and minimize harm from lawsuits against the institution, as for failure to comply with statutory or regulatory requirements.

However, the first principle of keeping business records is that you should keep them primarily to meet your needs rather than merely to meet legal requirements. Setting up your records management system to support your needs will meet many of the legal requirements as well. To help do so, Chapter 15 defines healthcare business records, Chapter 16 tells you the federal and state requirements for what business records to maintain and for how long, and Chapter 17 tells you what media you may preserve your business records on.

What Are Healthcare Business Records?

Business Records Generally

Section 1 (c) of the Uniform Preservation of Business Records Act defines business records as

> books of account, vouchers, documents, canceled checks, payrolls, correspondence, records of sales, personnel, equipment and production reports relating to any or all of such records and other business papers.

HEALTHCARE BUSINESS RECORDS

Many states have definitions of business records, but only a few define healthcare business records. Perhaps Mississippi provides the best definition of healthcare business records. Code § 41-9-61, which regulates hospitals, defines "business records" as those books, ledgers, records, papers, and other documents prepared, kept, made, or received in hospitals that pertain to the organization, administration, or management of the business and affairs of hospitals, but do not constitute hospital records. Hospital records are basically medical records.

Federal Laws

Federal law does not define healthcare business records. The Business Records Act, 28 U.S.C. 1732, defines records as ". . . any memorandum, writing, entry, print, representation or combination thereof, of any act, transaction, occurrence or event. . . in the regular course of business. . . ."

State Laws

ALABAMA

Code of Alabama § 13A-9-45 (1991), which makes it a crime to falsify business records, defines them as any writing or article kept or maintained by an enterprise for the purpose of evidencing or reflecting its condition or activity. Chapter 420-5-7.07 (1990) of the Rules of Alabama State Board of Health

Division of Licensure and Certification lists hospital documents and records other than medical records that hospitals must maintain.[1]

ALASKA

Alaska defines "business record" as a writing or article kept or maintained by an activity for the purpose of evidencing or reflecting its condition or activity in its statute making falsifying business records a crime.[2]

ARIZONA

Arizona's statute governing admissibility of business records defines "business" as every kind of business, profession, occupation, calling, or operation of institutions whether or not carried on for profit (Arizona Revised Statutes Annotated § 12-2262(A) (1991)). Arizona does not define healthcare business records, but § 36-447.09 lists a number of records other than patient records that nursing care institutions must maintain. Arizona Compilations Rules and Regulations R9-10-213 (1982) lists records and reports hospitals must maintain.[3]

ARKANSAS

Arkansas does not define healthcare business records but defines "business" expansively in Arkansas Statutes §§ 16-46-101 and 25-18-101 (1991) to include business, industry, profession, occupation, and calling of every kind.

CALIFORNIA

California Civil Code § 1799 (Deering 1992) defines "record" as any item, collection, or grouping of information about an individual or business entity. "Business entity" means a sole proprietorship, partnership, corporation, association, or other group, however organized and whether or not organized to operate at a profit, but does not mean a financial institution.

California Evidence Code § 1270 defines "a business" to include every kind of business, governmental activity, profession, occupation, calling, or operation of institutions, whether carried on for profit or not.

California Revenue and Tax Code § 997 defines "records" to include all written documents and photographic reproductions thereof, recorded data, research notes, calculations, and indices maintained or utilized by persons engaged in a business or profession.

California Code Regulations tit. 8, § 3204(c)(10) (1992) (governing industrial relations), defines a "record" as any item, collection, or grouping of information regardless of the form or process by which it is maintained.

---

1. *See* Chapter 16.
2. Alaska Statutes § 11.46.630 (1991).
3. *See* Chapter 16.

COLORADO

Colorado's Uniform Photographic Records Act, Colorado Revised Statutes § 13-26-102 (1991), covers any business, institution, or member of a profession or calling. Colorado does not define healthcare business records.

CONNECTICUT

Connecticut's statute governing business record admissibility into evidence defines "business" to include business, profession, occupation, and calling of every kind.[4]

DELAWARE

Delaware does not define healthcare business records or business records generally, but Delaware Code Ann. tit. 6 § 1502 (1991), which defines terms used in Delaware's partnership laws, defines business as including every trade, occupation, or profession.

DISTRICT OF COLUMBIA

See federal laws, above.

FLORIDA

The Florida Evidence Code, Florida Statutes § 90.803(7) (1990), defines a record of regularly conducted business activity as a memorandum, report, record, or data compilation (in any form) of acts, events, conditions, opinion, or diagnosis, made at or near the time by, or from information transmitted by, a person with knowledge, if it was the regular practice of that business activity to make such memorandum, report, record, or data compilation, all as shown by the testimony of the custodian or other qualified witness, unless the sources of information or other circumstances show lack of trustworthiness. The term "business" as used here includes a business, institution, association, profession, occupation, and calling of every kind, whether or not conducted for profit.

GEORGIA

In its statute making business records admissible, Georgia defines "business" as every kind of business, profession, occupation, calling, or operation of institutions, whether carried on for profit or not. Business records are any writing or record, whether in the form of an entry in a book or otherwise, made as a memorandum or record of any act, transaction, occurrence, or event.[5]

---

4. Connecticut General Statutes § 52-180(d) (1990).
5. Official Code of Georgia 23-4-14(a) and (b) (Michie 1991).

HAWAII

Hawaii's statute prohibiting falsifying business records defines them as any writings or articles kept or maintained by an enterprise for the purpose of evidencing or reflecting its condition or activity.[6]

IDAHO

Idaho does not define healthcare business records, but its statute providing for admissibility of business records defines "business" as including every kind of business, profession, occupation, calling, or operation of institution, whether carried on for profit or not.[7]

ILLINOIS

Illinois does not define healthcare business records but defines "business" broadly to include business, occupation, and calling of every kind in its statute making business records admissible.[8] Illinois has also adopted the Uniform Preservation of Private Business Records Act, which defines business to include every kind of private business, profession, occupation, calling, or operation of private institutions, whether carried on for profit or not. Business records include books of account, vouchers, documents, canceled checks, payrolls, correspondence, records of sales, personnel, equipment and production, reports relating to any or all of such records, and other business papers.[9]

INDIANA

Indiana does not specifically define healthcare business records, but Indiana Administrative Code tit. 410, r. 15-1-8 (1988), requires hospitals to keep documents and records that show ownership and compliance with local, state, and federal laws and regulations and adherence to bylaws and regulation of the facility including the records listed in Chapter 16.

IOWA

Iowa does not define healthcare business records, but its administrative code rules setting minimum standards for various healthcare facilities list records, other than medical records, various types of facilities must maintain.[10]

---

6. Hawaii Revised Statutes § 708-872 (1990).
7. Idaho Code § 9-413 (1991).
8. Illinois Revised Statutes, Chapter 110A, ¶ 236 (Supp. 1991).
9. *Id*. Chapter 116, ¶ 59.
10. *See* Chapter 16.

KANSAS

Kansas Statutes § 60-460 (1990), discussing subpoena of business records of a business not a party to the lawsuit as evidence, defines business to include every kind of business, profession, occupation, calling, or operation of institutions, whether carried on for profit or not. Business records are defined as writings made by personnel or staff of a business or persons acting under their control, including memoranda or records of acts, conditions, or events made in the regular course of business at or about the time of the act, condition, or event recorded. Section 60-459, relating to the business record exception to the hearsay rule, has a similar definition of business.

KENTUCKY

Kentucky does not define healthcare business records. However, Kentucky Revised Statutes Annotated § 422.105 (Baldwin 1992) provides that if any business, institution, or member of a profession or calling in the regular course of business keeps any memorandum, writing, entry, print, or representation of any act, transaction, occurrence, or event, and in the regular course of business records, copies, or reproduces the original by any process that accurately reproduces the original, the entity may destroy the original unless its preservation is required by law. Such reproduction is admissible in evidence.

LOUISIANA

Louisiana does not define business records specifically, but Louisiana Statutes Revised § 13.3733 (West 1990), discussing reproduction of documents, states that "Any business may cause any or all records kept by such business in the regular course of its operation" to be reproduced and disposed of as specified.[11]

MAINE

Maine does not define healthcare business records but 16 Maine Revised Statutes, governing admissibility of reproductions specifies that if any business or governmental activity keeps or records any memorandum, writing, entry, print, representation, or combination thereof in the regular course of business, such will be admissible in evidence.[12]

MARYLAND

Maryland does not define healthcare business records, but Maryland Courts and Judicial Process Code Annotated § 10-101 (1990), discussing proof of

---

11. *See* Chapter 16 for full text of § 3733.
12. Maine Revised Statutes Annotated tit. 16, § 356 (West 1991).

accounts or records, defines "business" as including a business, profession, and occupation of every kind. While the statute is limited to business records, business is defined broadly to include the records of institutions and associations like hospitals. Maryland Code Article 15B, § 1, the Uniform Preservation of Private Business Records Act, defines "business records" to include books of account, vouchers, documents, canceled checks, payrolls, correspondence, records of sales, personnel, equipment, and production reports relating to any or all of such records, and other business papers.

MASSACHUSETTS

Massachusetts does not specifically define healthcare business records, but Massachusetts Regulations Code tit. 105, § 150.013 (1990), lists clinical and related records long-term care facilities must maintain. *Id.* tit. 105, § 140.301, lists administrative records clinics must maintain. And *id.* § 142.503 lists administrative records birth centers must maintain.[13]

MICHIGAN

Michigan's evidence rules define business as including any business, profession, occupation, and calling of every kind. Michigan Compiled Laws § 600.2146 (1991) notes that business records, for purposes of admissibility, include all existing records including, but not limited to, checks, bills, notes, acceptances and all other types of commercial instruments, passbooks, deposit slips, and statements furnished to depositors (*id.* §§ 600.2146 and 600.2147). Although Michigan does not define healthcare business records, the Department of Public Health lists administrative records of hospitals in Michigan Administrative Code r. 325.1028 (1989), required records for nursing homes and nursing care facilities in *id.* r. 325.2110, and general records for homes for the aged in *id.* r. 325.1851.[14]

MINNESOTA

Minnesota does not define healthcare business records, but Minnesota Administrative Code R. 4640.1100 (1991) requires hospitals to maintain the "hospital records" listed in Chapter 16. *Id.* R. 4615.3000 requires maternal and infant health grantees to maintain "full and complete records concerning operation."

MISSISSIPPI

Mississippi Code § 41-9-61 (1990), which regulates hospitals, defines "business records" as those books, ledgers, records, papers, and other documents prepared, kept, made, or received in hospitals that pertain to the organization, administration, or management of the business and affairs of hospi-

---

13. *See* Chapter 16.
14. *See* Chapter 16.

tals, but do not constitute hospital records. Hospital records are basically medical records.

MISSOURI

Missouri does not define healthcare business records, but Revised Statute of Missouri, governing admissibility of business records, defines "business" as including every kind of business, profession, occupation, calling, or operation of institutions, whether carried on for profit or not.[15] Melton v. St. L.P.S. Co., 363 Mo. 474 (1952), held that a hospital was a business within this statute.

MONTANA

In its statute making records of regularly conducted activities admissible, Montana defines "business" as including a business, institution, association, profession, occupation, and calling of every kind, whether or not conducted for profit.[16]

NEBRASKA

Nebraska does not define healthcare business records, but its regulations and standards for various types of facilities specify records, other than medical records, they must maintain.[17]

NEVADA

Nevada has no specific provisions.

NEW HAMPSHIRE

New Hampshire does not define healthcare business records, but business records in general include books of account, vouchers, documents, canceled checks, payrolls, correspondence, records of sales, personnel, equipment, and production, reports relating to any or all of such records, and other business papers. A business includes every kind of private business, profession, occupation, calling, or operation of private institutions, whether carried on for profit or not.[18]

NEW JERSEY

New Jersey does not define healthcare business records, but its Standards for Hospital Facilities requires hospitals to maintain such additional records, other

---

15. Missouri Code Annotated § 13-1-151 (1990).
16. Montana Code Annotated § 10.803 (1990).
17. *See* Chapter 16.
18. New Hampshire Revised Statutes Annotated §§ 337-A:1 and 337-A:2 (1990), Preservation of Private Business Records.

than medical records, as shall be required to fully document the overall operation and to provide statistical data that may be required by the Department of Health.[19]

NEW MEXICO

The closest New Mexico comes to defining healthcare business records is the definition of "records" in New Mexico Statute Annotated § 30-44-2 (Michie 1991), the Medicaid Fraud Act, as "any medical or business documentation, however recorded relating to the treatment or care of any recipient, to services or goods provided to any recipient or to reimbursement for treatment, services, or goods, including any documentation required to be retained by regulations of the program." Obviously, this definition does not cover all business records a provider should maintain.

NEW YORK

In connection with its statutes criminalizing false written statements, New York defines a business record as any writing or article, including computer data or a computer program, kept or maintained by an enterprise for the purpose of evidencing or reflecting its condition or activity. An enterprise is an entity of one or more persons, corporate or otherwise, public or private, engaged in business, commercial, professional, industrial, eleemosynary, social, political, or governmental activity.[20]

New York's statute governing admissibility of business records speaks of any writing or record, whether in the form of an entry in a book or otherwise, made as a memorandum or record of any act, transaction, occurrence, or event (New York Civil Practice Law and Rules § 4518 (McKinney 1992)). Subsection (b) of this statute notes that a hospital bill is admissible in evidence under this rule.

NORTH CAROLINA

North Carolina does not define healthcare business records. It does, however, in its statute making photographic reproductions of business records admissible in evidence, include any business, institution, or member of a profession or calling that has kept or recorded any memorandum, writing, entry, print, representation, x ray, or combination thereof, of any act, transaction, occurrence, or event.[21]

NORTH DAKOTA

North Dakota does not define healthcare business records, but its Century Code § 31.08-01.1 (1991), governing admissibility of business records, speaks

---

19. New Jersey Administrative Code tit. 8, § 43B-7.3 (1985). *See* Chapter 16.
20. New York Penal Law § 175.00 (McKinney 1992).
21. North Carolina General Statute § 8-45.1 (1991).

of any business, institution, or member of a profession or calling who kept a memorandum, writing, entry, print, representation, or combination thereof, of any act, transaction, occurrence, or event.

OHIO

Ohio defines "business" as including every kind of business, profession, occupation, calling, or operation of institutions, whether carried on for profit or not, in its records as evidence statute.[22]

OKLAHOMA

Oklahoma defines "business records" as including books of account; vouchers; documents; canceled checks; payrolls; correspondence; records of sales, personnel, equipment, and production; reports relating to any or all of such records; and other business papers. "Business" includes every kind of private business, profession, occupation, calling, or operation of private institutions, whether carried on for profit or not.[23] Several Oklahoma statutes specify records healthcare providers must make available for public inspection.[24]

OREGON

Oregon does not define healthcare business records, but business records in general include any writing or article kept or maintained by an enterprise for the purpose of evidencing or reflecting its condition or activities.[25]

PENNSYLVANIA

Pennsylvania does not define healthcare business records. It does, however, in its statute making photographic reproductions of business records admissible in evidence, include any business, institution, member of a profession or calling that has kept or recorded any memorandum, writing, entry, print, representation, or combination thereof, of any act, transaction, occurrence, or event.[26]

RHODE ISLAND

Rhode Island does not define either healthcare business records or business records. Its Rules of Evidence provide that records of regularly conducted activity, kept in the regular course of business, are admissible in court.[27]

---

22. Ohio Revised Code Annotated § 2317.40 (Baldwin 1992).
23. Uniform Preservation of Private Business Records Act, Oklahoma Statutes Annotated tit. 67, § 251 (1992).
24. *See* Chapter 16.
25. Oregon Revised Statutes § 165.075 (1989).
26. 42 Pennsylvania Consolidated Statutes § 6109 (1991).
27. Uniform Rules of Evidence 803(6) and 1003 (1990).

SOUTH CAROLINA

South Carolina does not define healthcare business records. It does, however, in its statute making photographic reproductions of business records admissible in evidence, include any business, institution, or member of a profession or calling that has kept or recorded any memorandum, writing, entry, print, representation, or combination thereof, of any act, transaction, occurrence, or event.[28]

SOUTH DAKOTA

In its Photographic Copies of Business and Public Records as Evidence Act, South Dakota speaks of any business, institution, member of a profession or calling, or any department or agency of government, recording any memorandum, writing, entry, print, representation, or combination thereof, of any act, transaction, occurrence, or event.[29]

TENNESSEE

According to Tennessee Code Annotated § 68-11-302(2) (1990), health facility business records comprise all those books, ledgers, records, papers, and other documents prepared, kept, made, or received at hospitals that pertain to the organization, administration, or management of the business and affairs of hospitals, but that do not constitute hospital records (i.e., medical records).

TEXAS

The Texas statute governing retention of business records defines them as letters, words, sounds, or numbers, or their equivalent recorded in the operation of a business by handwriting, typewriting, printing, photostat, photograph, magnetic impulse, mechanical or electronic recording, or other form of data compilation.[30]

UTAH

Utah does not define healthcare business records, but its Health Facility Licensure Rules specify other records various facilities must maintain.[31]

VERMONT

Vermont does not define healthcare business records, but Vermont Statutes tit. 12, § 1701 (1991), the Uniform Photographic Copies of Business and Public Records as Evidence Act, talks of any business, institution, member of

---

28. South Carolina Code § 19-5-610 (Law. Co-op. 1992).
29. South Dakota Codified Laws § 19-7-12 (1991).
30. Texas Business and Commerce Code § 35.48 (West 1991).
31. *See* Chapter 16.

a profession or calling, or any department or agency of government, which in the regular course of business or activity has kept or recorded any memorandum, writing, entry, print, representation or combination thereof, of any act, transaction, occurrence, or event, and in the regular course of business has caused any or all of the same to be recorded, and so forth (*see* Chapter 17). Such records are admissible in evidence.

VIRGINIA

Virginia does not define healthcare business records. Virginia Code Annotated § 8.01-391 (Michie 1991), governing admissibility of copies, specifies that if any business or member of a profession or calling in the regular course of business or activity copies a record, it is admissible in evidence.

WASHINGTON

Washington does not define healthcare business records, but Revised Code of Washington § 5.46.010 (1990), which permits photographic copies of business records to be used as evidence if made in the regular course of business, talks about any business, institution, or member of a profession or calling.

WEST VIRGINIA

West Virginia does not define healthcare business records, but West Virginia Legislature, Title 64 West Virginia Legislative Rule 16-5C, Department of Health: Hospital Licensure, series 13, §§ 8.8, 7.9, and 7.10, respectively, list general healthcare recordkeeping requirements, administrative records, and personnel records. West Virginia Code § 16-29B-3 (Supp. 1991), governing the West Virginia Health Care Cost Review Authority, defines "records" as accounts, books, and other data related to healthcare costs at healthcare facilities subject to the provisions of the statute, which does not include privileged medical information, individual personal data, confidential information, the disclosure of which is prohibited, and any information that if disclosed would be an invasion of privacy.

WISCONSIN

Wisconsin does not define healthcare business records specifically, but Wisconsin Administrative Code § HSS 134.47(5)(c) (July 1, 1988), Facilities for the Developmentally Disabled Rules, requires such facilities to retain all records "not directly related to health care for at least two years."

WYOMING

Wyoming does not define healthcare business records or business records.

CHAPTER 16

Which Business Records Must You Keep and for How Long?

Introduction

Determining which business records you must keep and for how long is very similar to determining which medical records you must keep and for how long, as discussed in Chapter 3. Again, you look at statutes of limitation, federal laws and regulations, and state laws and regulations. However, as with medical records, which business records you keep and for how long should be determined primarily by your need for them, unless a law or regulation mandates a specific retention period. And you are always free to keep a record longer than required if you need to. Just make certain that you develop a records retention schedule, have it reviewed by your officers and your attorney, and only retain and destroy records pursuant to that schedule during the regular course of business. Never destroy business records selectively, especially if they are involved with anticipated or pending litigation.

Some states have comprehensive statutory or regulatory guidance, or both, on what business records a healthcare facility must keep. Others have little or no guidance on healthcare business records, but detail requirements for general business records. Others have little or no guidance on either healthcare business records or general business records. You may also use the guidance in chapters 5 and 6 to help you store and correct business records because few states specify requirements for those aspects of business record retention.

Federal Law Summary

The federal government has many requirements for keeping business records, either by express guidance or by implication, in order to prove compliance with a law or regulation.

DEPARTMENT OF LABOR

Employers subject to the Fair Labor Standards Act must keep for three years employment records relating to wages, hours, sex, occupation, conditions of employment, and so forth, as well as records containing employment information, payrolls, and certificates. Records that should be kept for two years include basic employment and earnings records, wage rate tables, work time schedules, order shipping and billing records, job evaluations, merit or seniority systems, or other matters that describe or explain the basis for any wage differentials to employees of the opposite sex in the same establishment, and records of deductions from or additions to pay.[1]

Employers with an employee benefit or pension plan must file a summary of the plan with the Department of Labor under the Employee Retirement Security Act of 1974 (ERISA), 29 U.S.C. §§ 1001 through 1461 (1988), and keep sufficient records to provide in sufficient detail the basic information and data for not less than six years after filing the required reports.[2]

The regulations concerning the Welfare and Pension Plans Disclosure Act, 29 U.S.C. § 1024(a) (1988), require the retention for five years of annual reports, plan descriptions, summary plan descriptions, and modifications and changes.[3]

Physicians and hospitals treating federal employees covered by the Federal Employees' Compensation Act must keep records of all injury cases they treated sufficient to supply the Office of Federal Employees' Compensation with a history of the employee's accident; the exact description, nature, location, and extent of injury; the degree of disability arising therefrom; the x-ray findings if x-ray examination has been made; and the nature of the treatment rendered and the degree of disability arising from the injury. The department has not specified a retention period.[4]

Hospitals and institutions employing patient workers must maintain records of disability, productivity, prevailing wage, production standards, evaluation and training records, work activities and group minimum wage records, and patient worker exceptions.[5] The facility must keep payroll records; certificates, agreements, plans, notices, and so forth, of collective bargaining agreements, plans, trusts, and employee contracts; and sales and purchase records concerning such employees for at least three years.[6] Supplementary basic records including basic employment and earnings records and wage rate tables must be preserved for at least two years.[7]

Hospitals and institutions employing patient workers must maintain records of disability, productivity, wage, production standards, evaluation and training records, work activities and group minimum wage records, patient worker exceptions, and other records as provided in 29 C.F.R. § 525.16 (1991).

Applicable retention periods are specified in 20 C.F.R. § 516.

Facilities using nonimmigrant aliens as registered nurses (RNs) must maintain complete supporting documentation on substantial disruptions (lay-

---

1. 29 C.F.R. §§ 516.2, 516.3, 516.5, 516.6, 516.11-516.29 (1991).
2. 29 U.S.C. § 1027 (1988).
3. 29 C.F.R. Part 486 (1991).
4. 20 C.F.R. § 10.410 (1991).
5. 20 C.F.R Part 519 (1991).
6. 20 C.F.R. § 516.2(a) (1991).
7. 20 C.F.R. § 516.6.

offs and nursing shortages); facilities nursing position, wages, and state employment security agency determination; collectively bargained wage rates; determination of pay and total compensation; facility/employer wages; and other information concerning the employees.

The documentation must be available for public inspection within a reasonable time after an oral or written request. No retention period is specified.[8]

Employers subject to the Employee Polygraph Protection Act of 1988 must retain a copy of the statement that sets forth the specific incident or activity under investigation and the basis for testing a particular employee, if an employee is requested to submit to a polygraph in connection with an ongoing investigation involving economic loss or injury. Maintain records specifically identifying the loss or injury in question and the nature of the employee's access to the person or property in question. Keep all opinions, lists, and other records relating to polygraph tests of persons, and maintain records of the number of exams conducted each day and other records as required by the section. Such records must be retained for three years.[9]

EQUAL EMPLOYMENT OPPORTUNITY COMMISSION

Employers subject to the Civil Rights Act must maintain personnel, employment, and other records having to do with hiring, promotion, demotion, transfer, layoff, termination, pay, and selection for training or apprenticeship. Such records must be maintained for six months after making the record or the personnel action that necessitates the record, whichever is longer.[10]

Employers subject to the Equal Pay Act are required by the Fair Labor Standards Board to keep all records as required in 29 C.F.R. § 516.[11]

Employers subject to the Age Discrimination Act must keep (1) records for each employee containing name, address, date of birth, occupation, rate of pay, and compensation earned each week; (2) personnel or employment records relating to applications, promotion, discharge, recruitment, aptitude tests, other employer-administered tests, results of physical exams considered in connection with personnel actions and advertisements; (3) records relating to employee benefit plans; and (4) copies of applications for temporary positions. These records must be retained for the following periods: (1) three years; (2) one year; (3) one year after termination of the plan; and (4) 90 days.[12]

INTERNAL REVENUE SERVICE

The statute of limitations for the commencement of collection actions for income tax is three years from the due date of the return (i.e., April 15, 19yy),

---

8. 20 C.F.R. § 655.310 (1991).
9. 29 C.F.R. § 801.30 (1991).
10. 29 C.F.R. § 1602.14 (1991).
11. 29 C.F.R. § 1620.32 (1991).
12. 29 C.F.R. § 1627.3 (1991).

or the date the return is filed (if filed late or pursuant to an extension), whichever is longer.[13] In cases where more than 25 percent of the gross income has not been reported, an assessment or a collection proceeding may be commenced at any time within six years after the return was filed.[14] The term "gross income" means the total amounts received or accrued from the sale of goods or services prior to diminution by the cost of such sales or services.[15] In cases where a return has not been filed, or a filed return contains insufficient information to constitute a return, or the return was falsely or fraudulently filed with the intent to evade tax, or if any willful attempt in any manner to defeat or evade tax, the statute of limitations does not commence and the Commissioner of Internal Revenue could assess or collect the tax at any time.[16]

In the case of the exchange of or distribution of corporate property pursuant to sales of assets or corporate reorganization, the Commissioner of Internal Revenue must assess a tax before three years from the date the Commissioner is notified of the exchange or distribution pursuant to the applicable notification provisions of the Internal Revenue Code.[17]

In the case of a deficiency arising because of a net capital loss, a net operating loss, or an unused business credit, the Commissioner can assess a deficiency at any time before the expiration of the period within which the deficiency for the tax year of the net capital loss, net operating loss, or unused business credit carryback may be assessed.[18]

In the event an organization believes in good faith that it is a tax-exempt organization and files a return to that effect, and is later determined to be a taxable organization for the year in which the return was filed, that return will be held to be the return of the organization for purposes of the statute of limitations, necessitating retention of records concerning tax-exempt status for at least three years.[19]

Lastly, the organization will need to maintain all records necessary to support the basis and current depreciation amounts of all depreciated property for time limits identified above. The IRS has the ability to review the depreciation schedules for all assets depreciated during a timely filed assessment or collection proceeding. In other words, if the IRS audits the 1992 tax return, and in that year depreciation was deducted for a building (or other like kind asset) that was properly placed in service 18 years ago, the taxpayer would be required to provide all documentation necessary to support the original basis of the property, capital improvements, and current depreciation deduction amounts.

---

13. 26 U.S.C. § 6501 (1992).
14. *Id.* § 6501(e)(1)(A).
15. *Id.* § 6501(e)(1)(A)(i).
16. *Id.* § 6501(c)(1-3).
17. *Id.* § 6501(c)(8) (1986).
18. *Id.* § 6501(h); § 301.6501(a)-1(b).
19. *Id.* § 6501(g)(2).

OCCUPATIONAL SAFETY AND HEALTH ADMINISTRATION

Employers must make available to all employees, their designated representatives and the Occupational Safety and Health Administration (OSHA) all exposure records, medical records for examination and copying, and any analyses using employee exposure or medical records. This informantion must be retained for 30 years.[20]

Each employer must maintain a separate log at each business establishment of all recordable occupational injuries or illnesses. The employer must record any injury or illness within six days of the incident. An employer may maintain a central log or a log using data processing (computer) if, at the location of the log, enough information exists to be able to update and record any injuries or illnesses within six days of the incident and if the employer keeps a copy of the log, current to within 45 calendar days, at each business establishment. This information must be retained for five years.[21]

OSHA mandates that all records be maintained on a calendar year basis.[22]

In addition to the log required by 29 C.F.R. § 1604.2, each employer must maintain, and have available for inspection within six days of any injury or illness, a separate record of all occupational injuries or illnesses at each establishment. Worker's compensation insurance forms or other records may suffice. This information must be retained for five years.[23]

If a state plan concerning occupational safety and health is an approved plan, then state record-keeping requirements satisfy the federal requirements of OSHA.[24]

FOOD AND DRUG ADMINISTRATION

Hospitals and other authorized dispensers of methadone must keep clinical records on each patient including the dates, quantities, and batch or code mark of methadone dispensed for three years.[25]

Sponsors of methadone maintenance programs must maintain for each patient an admission evaluation and records consisting of personal and medical history, physical examinations, and other information as necessary.[26]

Collectors and processors of blood must maintain a manual of procedures and methods to be followed by employees to determine the suitability of donors. These organizations also must maintain a list of the names and qualifications of people who supervise an employee's determination of suitability when a physician is not present, without specifying a retention period.[27]

---

20. 29 C.F.R. § 1910.20 (1991).
21. 29 C.F.R. §§ 1904.2 and 1904.6 (1991).
22. *Id.* § 1904.3.
23. 29 C.F.R. § 1904.4 (1991).
24. 29 C.F.R. § 1904.10 (1991).
25. 21 C.F.R. § 291.505 (1991).
26. *Id.* § 291.505.
27. *Id.* § 600.12.

Collectors and processors of blood must maintain on the premises, and file with the Center for Biologics Evaluation and Research, a manual of standard procedures and methods approved by the Director of the Center for Biologics Evaluation and Research that shall be followed by all employees who collect blood. Additionally, all centers must maintain records indicating the name and qualifications of the people immediately in charge of employees when a physician is not present.[28]

HEALTH AND HUMAN SERVICES DEPARTMENT

Medicare contract and reimbursement requirements include 42 C.F.R. § 417.236 (1991), which requires that contracts with health maintenance organizations (HMOs) contain provisions that the HMO maintain books and records as required by 42 C.F.R. § 417.244.

42 C.F.R. § 417.244 (1991) states that HMOs must maintain sufficient financial records and statistical data for proper determination of costs payable by Medicare. Standard definitions, accounting procedures, and statistical and reporting practices followed by the healthcare industry are followed, so no special records must be made or kept.

42 C.F.R. § 417.236 (1991) requires that HMOs meet the requirements of the Privacy Act and keep confidential the information obtained on enrollees.

All contracts for medical assistance, including contracts with private, nonmedical institutions and with insurers, must contain provisions requiring the contractor to maintain appropriate record systems for services provided to enrolled recipients, and to provide that the contractor safeguard the information in the records (*id.* § 434.6).

42 C.F.R. § 417.107 (1991) outlines organization and operation requirements for HMOs participating in Medicare. Each HMO must disclose to its members descriptions of benefits provided, coverage information, rate information, procedures to follow to obtain benefits, grievance procedures, participating provider information, and service area information.

Additionally, while maintaining confidentiality, each HMO must provide a procedure to develop, compile, evaluate, and report to its members, the public, and the secretary of the Health Care Finance Administration (HCFA) statistics relating to the HMO's cost of operations, financial position, utilization and availability of services, and developments in the health status of its members. A copy of this report must be filed with HCFA within 180 days after the end of an HMO's fiscal year.

Also, within 180 days after the end of its fiscal year, each HMO must file with HCFA a report describing significant business transactions (sales, leases of equipment, and so forth) (*id.*).

Providers of services under Medicare must retain copies of all physician certification and recertification statements.[29]

---

28. *Id.* § 240.2.
29. 42 C.F.R. § 424.11 (1991).

Each long-term care facility participating in Medicare is subject to the resident rights requirements of 42 C.F.R. § 483.10 (1991). The section requires each facility to establish and maintain a system that ensures separate accounting for residents' personal funds entrusted to the facility. The system must preclude commingling of resident funds with facility funds or the funds of other residents.

The residents' rights section also requires that the facility protect the privacy and confidentiality of resident personal and clinical records and that the resident has the right to refuse disclosure of clinical or personal information unless the resident is transferred to another facility or the disclosure is required by either law or third-party payment contract.[30]

42 C.F.R. § 413.20 (1991) requires that providers of services must maintain sufficient financial records and statistical data to determine costs payable under the Medicare program. Costs reports are required from providers on an annual basis. The methods used to determine cost involve making use of a provider's basis accounts. Standard definitions, accounting, and statistical and reporting practices followed by the healthcare industry are followed; therefore, changes in these practices are not necessary to determine costs payable.

The records required include, but are not limited to, provider ownership data; organization and operating data; fiscal records; medical records; tax records; asset sale, acquisition, or lease records; patient service charge schedules; records pertaining to operating costs; amounts of income received; and funds flow information. No retention period is specified.

Basically, access to a provider's books is necessary to determine reimbursement, and no changes or special records need be kept.

42 C.F.R. § 413.24 (1991) outlines various methods of determination and reporting of costs, all based on the records outlined in 42 C.F.R. § 413.20.

Ambulatory surgical centers must also maintain adequate financial data to determine payment rates for surgical services provided.[31]

Outpatient dialysis centers are required to keep records and submit cost reports as outlined in 42 C.F.R. § 413.20 and 42 C.F.R. § 413.24. 42 C.F.R. § 413.174 deals specifically with these providers.

As to reimbursement requirements, rural health clinics must maintain adequate financial and statistical data to determine payment for services provided. Additionally, clinics must submit annual reports that include actual and estimated costs incurred to help determine payments.[32]

Recipients of Health and Human Services (HHS) grants must maintain financial records, supporting documents, statistical records, accords for equipment purchased under the grant, and any other records pertinent to the grant. this information must be retained for three years from date of submission of an annual or final expenditures report or three years after any audit by the Department. Records may be kept on microfilm or other media.[33]

---

30. 42 C.F.R. § 483.10(e) (1991).
31. 42 C.F.R. § 416.40 (1991).
32. 42 C.F.R. § 405.2429.
33. 45 C.F.R. § 74.20 (1991).

Recipients of HHS grants subject to the age discrimination act must maintain records to ascertain compliance with the act.[34]

Institutions participating in health profession or nursing student loan programs must retain the records found at 42 C.F.R. § 57.125 for five years.[35]

Applicants for project grants for public medical facility construction and modernization must keep accounting and bookkeeping records concerning the use of federal funds.[36]

42 C.F.R. contains many specific records retention requirements for various healthcare programs administered by the Public Health Service, including

- § 52.8. Individuals or institutions receiving grants for research projects

- § 52.8. Public or nonprofit private hospitals or schools of medicine or other agencies receiving National Heart, Lung, and Blood Institute grants for National Research and Demonstration Centers

- § 52b.6. Agencies receiving National Cancer Institute grants

- § 52d.8. Schools of medicine, osteopathy, dentistry, or public health affiliated teaching hospitals, or specialized cancer institutes receiving grants under the National Cancer Institute Clinical Cancer Education Program

- § 57.215. Institutions participating in the health professions and the nursing student loan programs

- § 57.2913. Institutions receiving grants for training U.S. citizen foreign medical students

- § 60.42: Health Education Assistance Loan (HEAL) Program lenders

- § 64.4. Institutions receiving federal grants for National Institutes of Health and National Library of Medicine training

- §§ 74.2, 74.50, 74.52, 74.53. Clinical laboratories

- § 124.8. Applicants for project grants for public medical facility construction and modernization

These regulations also have detailed requirements for various categories of health professions schools and for institutions receiving federal health insurance other than those mentioned above.

MEDICAL WASTE TRACKING ACT

The Demonstration Medical Waste Tracking Program[37] gives the Environmental Protection Agency authority to promulgate various regulations and

---

34. 45 C.F.R. § 91.34.
35. 42 C.F.R. § 57.315 (1991).
36. 42 C.F.R. § 124.8.
37. 42 U.S.C § 6992 (1988).

record-keeping requirements on generators, transporters, treatment, disposal, and destruction facilities that handle medical wastes. The effective dates of the program were June 22, 1989, to June 22, 1991, but the program may be extended or reinstated. The various record-keeping and retention requirements imposed upon generators of medical wastes are summarized here. Healthcare providers should, however, check to see whether states in which they do business have their own such requirements.

The record-keeping requirements imposed upon generators of medical waste are found at 40 C.F.R. § 259.54 (1991) and are best analyzed according to how much waste is produced and what is done with it.

Definitions of regulated medical waste are found at 40 C.F.R. § 249.30. The covered states (participants under the original act) include Louisiana, Connecticut, New Jersey, New York, Rhode Island, the District of Columbia, and Puerto Rico.[38]

Pre-Transport Requirements

Generators must place medical waste in strong, sealed, leakproof containers and indicate whether the waste is treated or untreated medical waste.[39]

40 C.F.R. § 259.55 requires that the containers must be labeled with the generator's name; state permit, if applicable; the transporter's name and state permit, if applicable, the date of the shipment; and an indication that the contents are medical waste. If the container has any smaller containers within it, the inner containers must also be labeled with the generator's name and state permit.

All generators of more than 50 pounds of medical waste per month are subject to the tracking form requirements of 29 C.F.R. § 259.52. If a generator uses a transporter to ship medical waste, the transporter is required to provide the tracking forms; if not, the forms can be obtained from the state where the waste was generated, or the generator can use the tracking form found at 40 C.F.R. § 259 Appendix I. The generator must prepare enough copies of the tracking form to provide the generator, each transporter, and intermediate handler with one copy, and the final destination facility with two copies. The generator and the initial transporter must sign the tracking form, and the generator must keep copies of all tracking forms for at least three years after the shipment date.

Post-transport Record-keeping Requirements

All generators of more than 50 pounds of regulated medical waste were subject to the tracking form requirements of the program,[40] and must keep copies of all tracking forms for at least three years after the date the waste was accepted by a transporter. Additionally, if the generator submitted any

---

38. 40 C.F.R. § 259.20.
39. 40 C.F.R. § 259.44.
40. 40 C.F.R. § 259.52.

exception reports as outlined in 40 C.F.R. § 259.55 (reports filed for failure to receive return tracking forms from a treatment or disposal facility within 45 days after shipment) these reports should be kept for at least three years after the date the waste was accepted by a transporter.

Generators of less than 50 pounds of regulated medical waste were exempt from using the tracking forms, but must keep, for three years after the date of shipment, any tracking forms used voluntarily.

Generators who used transporters to ship wastes must also keep the log mandated by 40 C.F.R. § 259.54 for at least three years from the date of the shipment of waste. The log, as an alternate to the tracking forms, must contain the following information: transporter's name and state permit/ID number (if required by the state), quantity of waste shipped, date of the shipment, and the signature of the person who accepted the waste for the transporter.

Generators who transported regulated medical wastes between their own facilities must keep copies of the logs mandated by 40 C.F.R. § 259.54. The logs were required at both the point of shipment of waste (generation point) and point of destination. The generation point log was to contain the date of the shipment, the weight of the shipment, the signature of the employee who shipped the waste, and the address of the destination point. The destination point was to contain the date of receipt of the waste, the quantity received, the address of the generation point, and the signature of the employee who received the waste.

Generators of less than 50 pounds per month who shipped waste directly to a healthcare facility or to a treatment, destruction, or disposal site, must keep the log, which contains the name and address of the destination of the waste, quantity of waste shipped, date of shipment, and signature of the generator.

Generators of less than 50 pounds of waste per month who shipped via U.S. mail must keep copies of the original USPS receipt, the return mail receipt, and the shipment log required by 40 C.F.R. § 259.54 for three years after the date of the shipment. The log was to contain the name of the recipient of the waste, the date, and quantity shipped.

Requirements for On-site Destruction or Incineration

Generators who treat or destroy wastes on site, other than by incineration, must keep logs of the quantity of waste treated or destroyed, an estimate of the percent of the waste that was regulated medical waste, and the dates of acceptance, treatment, and destruction. The log must be kept for three years after the date of the destruction.[41]

Generators who incinerate waste on site are subject to the record-keeping requirements of 40 C.F.R. § 259.61 and must keep an operation log at least of the dates of each incineration cycle, the quantity of waste incinerated per cycle,

---

41. 40 C.F.R. § 259.60.

and an estimate of the percent of the waste incinerated that was regulated medical waste until June 22, 1992, and all other records for at least three years.

Generators with on-site incinerators who also accepted waste from other generators must keep logs of the date the waste was accepted; the name of the generator the waste was accepted from; that generator's state permit, if applicable; the quantity of waste accepted; and the signature of the person who accepted the waste. Generators must also keep any tracking forms relating to accepted wastes. The retention period for the log and forms is three years after the date the waste was incinerated.[42]

On-site incinerators must also file incineration reports (during the life of the program) that summarized the information in the operating logs mandated by part 259.61.[43]

NUCLEAR REGULATORY COMMISSION

The Nuclear Regulatory Commission (NRC) places record-keeping requirements on establishments that use nuclear materials, such as radiopharmaceuticals, for medical uses. The requirements center around the procedure or use of a radioactive byproduct, equipment, radioactivity levels, and safety regulations. Each record required by NRC must be legible, but can be a copy, reproduction, microform, or electronic record, so long as all information required by NRC is contained. All records must be safeguarded from loss or unauthorized use.[44]

Licensees must maintain records of all misadministration of radiopharmaceuticals for 10 years. The record must contain the names of all parties involved (patient, physicians, technicians, and so forth), the patient's social security number or ID number, if assigned, a description of what happened, and any steps taken to prevent recurrence of a similar misadministration.[45]

10 C.F.R. § 35.50 outlines various tests licensees must perform on dose calibrators to ensure that they are working properly, and the records required to be kept concerning these tests.

Tests to ensure that survey and detection instruments are working properly and the records required to document the tests are described in 10 C.F.R. § 35.51.

Licensees must measure the activity of certain radiopharmaceutical dosages and maintain records that include the name of the radiopharmaceutical, the patient's name and ID number, the patient's dosage and activity of the dosage, date and time of the measurement, and the initials of the person who measured the dosage. No retention period is specified.[46]

---

42. 40 C.F.R. §§ 259.61–259.62 (1991).
43. 229 C.F.R. § 259.62.
44. 10 C.F.R. § 35.5 (1991).
45. 10 C.F.R. § 35.33.
46. 10 C.F.R. § 35.33.

The Code of Federal Regulations requires facilities to keep records of the following for at least three years:

- Leak testing procedures and applicable record-keeping requirements concerning sealed sources of radioactive materials are contained in 10 C.F.R. § 35.59.

- 10 C.F.R. § 35.70 contains various requirements outlining where and how often a licensee must survey locations with a detection device to measure radioactivity levels. This part also outlines the record-keeping requirements concerning these surveys.

- Licensees providing mobile nuclear medicine services must carry detection devices and survey client locations to ensure that all radiopharmaceuticals and wastes have been removed. The mobile provider must retain a record of the survey for three years. The record must contain the date of the survey, measurements, plans of the location surveyed, the detection device, and the initials of the person who performed the survey (10 C.F.R. § 35.80).

- Measurement and administration requirements pertaining to radiopharmaceuticals containing molybdenum-99 are found at 10 C.F.R. § 35.204. Licensees must measure and record levels of molybdenum-99 and keep the records for three years.

- Safety precautions regarding providers of radiopharmaceutical therapy, including testing of individuals who help prepare and administer radiopharmaceuticals, are contained in 10 C.F.R. § 35.315. People who assist the administration of radiopharmaceuticals must be examined, and records of the examinations must be made. No retention period is specified for these records.

- Implanted sources of radioactive materials. After removing the last implant from a patient, the area in which the procedure was performed must be surveyed with a detection device. A record must be made that contains the date of the survey, plans of the area, the detection device, measurements, and the initials of the person who performed the survey. These records must be retained for three years (10 C.F.R. § 35.415).

- 10 C.F.R. § 35.610 outlines various safety instructions that must be given to operators of teletherapy units and the record-keeping requirements applicable to these instructions.

- 10 C.F.R. § 35.615 outlines safety precautions that relate to teletherapy and various records that must be kept concerning these precautions.

- Teletherapy units must perform periodic spot checks to ensure compliance with safety regulations. Records relating to these spot checks must be kept three years (10 C.F.R. § 35.634).

- 10 C.F.R. § 35.641 outlines radiation survey and measurement requirements concerning teletherapy services and the record-keeping requirements imposed by the surveys.

- Teletherapy units must be fully inspected by NRC or the state every five years and must keep a record of the inspection for the life of their license (10 C.F.R. § 35.647).

VETERANS ADMINISTRATION

Contractors providing medical resources or services to the Veterans Administration (VA) must keep all records required by the contract for the life of the contract plus three years.[47]

State Law Summary

ALABAMA

Rules of the Alabama State Board of Health Division of Licensure and Certification, Chapter 420-5-7.07 (1990), require each hospital to maintain:

- Administrative Records and Documents

  - Articles of incorporation or certified copies thereof

  - Current copy of the approved constitution, bylaws, or both, of the governing authority, with a current roster of the membership of the governing authority

  - A copy of the minutes of the governing authority

  - Current copy of the approved constitution, bylaws, or both, and rules and regulations of the medical staff, with a current roster of the membership of the medical staff

  - Minutes of the meetings of the medical staff and/or services, departments, or committees or other basis of the clinical experience of the staff

  - Narcotic permit

  - Narcotic records[48]

  - Current personnel records

  - License or registration number of each employee, such as nurses, therapists, technicians, and so forth, who has such credentials

---

47. 41 C.F.R. §§ 8-16.9503 and 8-16.95043 (1991).
48. Chapter 420-5-7.11(i) states that records shall be kept of all stock supplies of all controlled substances, giving an accounting of all items received and dispensed.

- A current record on each member of the medical staff, which includes his or her application for membership on the staff, privileges granted by the governing authority, and so forth

- Reports. The following reports shall be made by each hospital:

  - Vital statistics report

  - Destitute children

  - Annual report

As to hospital personnel records, Chapter 420-5-7.06(a) and (b), *Personnel,* Rules of Alabama State Board of Health Division of Licensure and Certification (1990), requires hospitals to keep the following records:

- Physician examinations. Personnel absent from duty because of any communicable disease shall not return to duty until examined by a physician for freedom from any condition that might endanger the health of patients or employees. Documentation of freedom from communicable disease shall be available in facility records.

- Personnel records. As a minimum, the record shall include

  - Application for employment, which contains information regarding education, training, experience, and if applicable, registration or licensure information, or both, of the applicant

  - Record of physical examinations

A current roster of medical staff members shall be maintained in the hospital. At its discretion, the State Board of Health may request that a copy of this roster be placed on file with the Board.[49]

Under Chapter 420-5-7.05(1)(e) when the medical staff is organized, a copy of the approved medical staff bylaws, rules, and regulations, with any amendments, shall be maintained in the hospital. At its discretion, the State Board of Health may request that a copy of this medical staff organization be placed on file with the Board.

Under Chapter 420-5-7.05(2)(a), *Medical Staff Organizations,* the bylaws, rules, and regulations of the medical staff shall, at a minimum, specifically provide that medical staff meetings be held at regular intervals and that minutes of each meeting shall be kept as a permanent record.

Chapter 420-5-7.16, *Food Service,* Rules of Alabama State Board of Health Division of Licensure and Certification (1990), requires that the current week's menu shall be displayed in the food service area of each hospital and shall be kept on file for the following two weeks.

---

49. Chapter 420-5-7.05(1)(d), *The Medical Staff,* Rules of Alabama State Board of Health Division of Licensure and Certification.

As to nursing homes, Chapter 420-5-10-.16 (1990) requires them to maintain copies in the business office of vital statistics reports, employees' health certificates, and reports of physical examination.

Nursing homes must keep personnel records as detailed in Chapter 420-5-10-.04, *Personnel,* Rules of Alabama State Board of Health Division of Licensure and Certification (1990):

- Personnel records. Each nursing home shall maintain a personnel record for each employee. As a minimum, the record shall include

  - Application for employment, which contains information regarding education, training, experience, and if applicable, registration or licensure information, or both, of the applicant

  - A job description

  - General administrative and job-related orientation

  - Record of physical examinations

In Alabama, nonprofit corporations must keep correct and complete books and records of account and shall keep minutes of the proceedings of its members, board of directors, and committees having any of the authority of the board of directors. Each nonprofit corporation also shall keep at its registered office or principal office in Alabama a record of the names and addresses of its members entitled to vote, directors, and officers. All books and records of a corporation may be inspected by any member, director, or officer, or his or her agent or attorney, for any proper purpose at a reasonable time.[50]

ALASKA

Alaska Administrative Code tit. 7, § 43.030 (Apr. 1984), requires providers receiving payment for medical services under the Medicaid program to retain all fiscal, patient care, and related records for three years following the year in which the services were provided, except when specifically requested by the department to be retained for a longer period. This requirement applies to facilities that are sold by the original provider, even if the facility does not continue to participate in the Medicaid program.

Alaska Statutes § 10.06.430 (1991) requires corporations to keep correct and complete books and records of account; minutes of proceedings of its shareholders, board, and committees of the board; and a record of its shareholders.

Section 10.20.131 requires nonprofit corporations to keep correct and complete books and records of account and minutes of the proceedings of its members, board of directors, and committees having any of the authority of the board of directors. Nonprofit corporations must also keep a record of the

---

50. Code of Alabama § 10-3A-43 (1991).

names and addresses of members entitled to vote in the corporation's registered office or principal office in the state.

Under § 18.20.220, employers must maintain records on age, sex, and race under the antidiscrimination unlawful employment practices laws.

ARIZONA

Arizona Compilation Administrative Rules and Regulations R9-10-213 (1982) discusses what records a hospital must maintain.

- Records and reports. The following documents or copies shall be available in the hospital:

  - Bylaws of the governing body

  - Bylaws and rules and regulations of the medical staff

  - Policies and procedures for all established hospital services

  - Reports of all inspections and reviews related to licensure for the preceding five years, together with corrective actions taken

  - Contracts and agreements related to licensure to which the hospital is bound

  - Appropriate documents evidencing control and ownership

  - A current copy of Title 9 Health Care Regulations available from the Office of the Secretary of State

    - Chapter 1, Article 4, Codes and Standards referenced

    - Chapter 8, Article 1, Food and Drink

    - Chapter 9, Articles 1, 2, 3, Health Care Institutions: Establishment and Modification

    - Chapter 10, Article 1, Health Care Institutions: Licensure

    - Chapter 11, Articles 1, 2, Health Care Institutions: Rates and Charges

- Personnel records. A record of each employee shall be maintained, which includes the following:

  - Employee's identification, including name, address, and next of kin

  - Resume of education and work experience

  - Verification of valid license if required, education and training

  - Payroll and attendance records for the preceding 12-month period shall be available for review by Arizona Department of Health Services personnel.

- Every position shall have a written description that describes the duties of the position.

Rule 9-10-219, concerning disaster preparedness, requires hospitals to write a disaster plan that includes the establishment of an emergency treatment record for external disasters such as mine explosions, bus accidents, floods, earthquakes, and so forth. The section also has specifications for internal disasters.

Rule 9-10-220 requires hospitals to maintain records to ensure that appropriate inspections and maintenance of equipment of the hospital physical plant are periodically accomplished by qualified personnel.

Arizona Revised Statutes § 36-447.09 (1991) requires nursing care institutions to maintain the following records for inspection by the Department:

- All current required operating licenses, permits, and certificates

- Patient medical records (*see* Chapter 3)

- A listing of current rates and charges

- Reports of all inspections and reviews, and copies of reports showing corrective actions taken, shall be retained for a period of two years.

- Reports of fire and disaster drills held during the previous two years

- Records of pharmaceuticals destroyed during the previous two years

- A copy of Department nursing care institution regulations and interpretive guidelines

- Documents evidencing control and ownership of the facility

- Monthly calendars of activities scheduled during the previous two years

- Copies of all current contracts for services that relate to patient care, if applicable

- Up-to-date medically approved confirmation for each nursing care institution patient and employee showing freedom from current pulmonary tuberculosis disease

- Records showing that each person providing nursing care services has received in-service training averaging two hours per month for the most recent reporting period

- A record of each patient care plan

- Current nursing staffing records

- Records of meals served and schedules of meal times

- Records of food purchased

- A copy of the current nursing care institution emergency services plan

- Patient accident reports

Rule 9-14-111 covers personnel records. They must be maintained on a current basis and include a complete resume of each employee's training, experience, duties, and date or dates of employment. Attendance records shall be maintained for each employee for a period of one year.

ARKANSAS

Rules and Regulations for Hospitals and Related Institutions in Arkansas note that such facilities must maintain an individual file on each physician containing his or her age; year and school of graduation; date of licensure; statement of postgraduate or special training, and experience; statement of the type of medicine the applicant desires to practice; a pledge that if appointed he or she will comply with the rules and regulations of the hospital; and a statement of special qualifications. The file shall also include all actions taken by the medical staff and governing board indicating the type of privileges granted and other applicable data. Medical staff bylaws shall include provision for maintenance of written minutes of the meetings of the staff, including committee reports.

An accurate daily patient census count as of midnight shall be available to the Department of Health at all times. Hospitals shall also maintain written reports of disaster drills.

Personnel records shall contain current and background information covering qualifications for employment and records of all required health examinations and evidence of current registration, certification, or licensure.[51]

Arkansas Department of Health, Adopted Rules for Licensure of Long Term Care Nursing Homes 016.06.84.024(303) (1984), also requires an accurate daily census sheet as of midnight to be available, as well as a personnel file for each employee. Results of skin tests for tuberculosis must be on file in the facility.

Arkansas Department of Health, Human Services–Social Services Regulation of Long-Term Care Residential Care Facilities 016.06.85—003(700) (1985), requires operators of such facilities to provide for the maintenance and submission of such statistical, financial, or other information, records, or reports as the Office of Long Term Care may require.

CALIFORNIA

A provider shall make available, during regular business hours, all pertinent financial books and all records concerning the provision of healthcare services to a Medi-Cal beneficiary, and all records required to be made and retained by this section, to any duly authorized representative of the depart-

---

51. Arkansas Department of Health, Rules and Regulations for Hospitals and Related Institutions, 007.05.79001, ch. II, part 1.

ment acting in the scope and course of employment including, but not limited to, employees of the Attorney General, Medi-Cal Fraud Unit, duly authorized and acting within the scope and course of their employment. Failure to produce records may result in sanctions, audit adjustments, or recovery of overpayments.

Under California Code Regulations tit. 32, § 51476.1 (1991), providers must keep readily retrievable pharmacy records, including written prescription orders and records of oral orders reduced to writing. Such records describing the provision of a pharmaceutical service to a Medi-Cal beneficiary must include

- Full beneficiary name

- Name, category of professional licensure, and license number of the prescriber

- Name, strength, and quantity of the drug or medical supply dispensed, as applicable

- Direction for use of the drug or medical supply

- Name of the principal labeler of any multisource drug or medical supply dispensed when not specifically identified by the brand name of the drug dispensed

- Date of service

- Name or initials of the pharmacist who provided the service

- A unique number to identify each pharmaceutical service billed to the program. This number shall be the "prescription number" required on the form

Pharmacy records shall include documentation of compliance with Code I restrictions for medical supplies and drugs.

Clinical laboratories must maintain for at least two years

- Records of specimens received and tested, including identification of the patient, name of the submitter, dates of receipt and report, type of test performed, and test results

- Records of inspection, validation, calibration, repair, and replacement to ensure proper maintenance and operation of equipment and proper reactivity of test materials

- Manuals, card files, or flow charts for each procedure performed in the laboratory, which include

  - Name of procedure

  - Source or reference for the test method

- Date the procedure was last reviewed or modified by the director or supervisor

- Current specific instructions for test performance

- The standards and controls required

- Instructions for collecting and handling specimens to ensure test reliability

- Records of quality control procedures in use in the various technical areas of the laboratory, including results on standards and reference materials and action limits when appropriate (*id.* tit. 17 § 1050(f)(1))

- Additional requirements for cytology. The laboratory shall retain all cytology slides and cell blocks for a minimum of five years and all cytology reports for a minimum of 10 years (*id.* tit. 17 § 78.1(f)(1)).

Under Title 17 § 1050(f)(2), the laboratory shall maintain records indicating the daily accession of specimens, each of which is numbered, and an appropriate cross-filing system according to patient's name.

As to other than medical records, Title 22 § 70733 requires each hospital to maintain, subject to inspection by the department

- Articles of incorporation or partnership agreement

- Bylaws or rules and regulations of the governing body

- Bylaws and rules and regulations of the medical staff

- Minutes of the meetings of the governing body and the medical staff

- Reports of inspections by local, state, and federal agents

- All contracts, leases, and other agreements required by these regulations

- Patient admission roster

- Reports of unusual occurrences for the preceding two years

- Personnel records

- Policy manuals

- Procedure manuals

- Minutes and reports of the hospital infection control committee

- Any other records deemed necessary for the direct enforcement of these regulations by the department

Title 22 § 70725 requires hospitals to maintain personnel records for all employees for at least three years following termination of employment. The record shall include the employee's full name; social security number; the license or registration number, if any; brief resume of experience; employment classification; date of beginning employment; and date of termination of employment. The facility shall also keep records of hours and dates worked by all employees during at least the most recent six-month period. In addition, Title 22 § 70723(c) requires hospitals to keep employee health records, including records of all required health examinations, for a minimum of three years following termination of employment.

COLORADO

Colorado Code Regulations 1011-1, ¶ 33 (1977), requires hospitals to maintain written records of medical staff meetings. Section 4.9 requires hospitals to maintain the following records:

- Daily census

- Hospital services statistics

- Admissions and discharges analysis record

- Register of all deliveries including live and stillbirths

- Register of all surgeries performed, entered daily

- Diagnostic index

- Operative index

- Physician index

- Number index

- Death register

- Patient master card file

- Register of outpatient and emergency room admissions and visits

Section 5.3 requires hospitals to keep personnel records on each person on the hospital staff, including employment application and verification of credentials.

CONNECTICUT

State Department of Health Regulation, Connecticut Agencies Regulations § 19-13-D1 (1972), governs hospitals, child day-care centers, other institutions, and children's general hospitals. Hospices must keep records of medical staff and departmental meetings (*id.* §§ 19-13-D1 and 19-13-D5). A condition of licensure for hospices is maintenance of all records, memos, and reports, medical or otherwise, including personnel and payroll records (*id.* § 19-13-D4b). Long-term hospitals must also keep records of staff meetings (*id.* § 19-13-D5).

Connecticut Agencies Regulation § 19-13-D8t (1972) requires chronic and convalescent nursing homes and rest homes with nursing supervision to maintain a patient roster and census of all patients admitted or discharged. Such facilities must also keep records of the medical director's visits and statements, including the date of visit, the names of patients audited, and a summary of problems discussed with the staff. Facilities will maintain minutes of the meetings of the medical staff, records of nurse's aide training and competence for three years from the completion of the training, written and signed summaries of nursing staff actions, documentation of emergency preparedness training, and orientation.

Connecticut General Statutes § 31-128a (1990) defines a personnel file as papers, documents, and reports pertaining to a particular employee, which are used or have been used by an employer to determine the employee's eligibility for employment, promotion, additional compensation, transfer, termination, and disciplinary or other adverse personnel action, including employee evaluations or reports relating to such employee's character, credit, and work habits.

DELAWARE

Delaware defines personnel records for purposes of determining compliance with employment practices laws as any application for employment; wage or salary information; notices of commendations, warning, or discipline; authorization for a deduction or withholding of pay; fringe benefit information; leave records; and employment history with the employer, including salary information, job title, dates of changes, retirement record, attendance records, performance evaluations, and medical records (Delaware Code Annotated tit. 19, § 731 (1991)).

Section 1108 requires every employer of more than three employees to make, keep, and preserve for a period of not less than three years the records specified in the chapter, including wage and hour records, in or about the premises or place of business or employment or at one or more central record-keeping offices. *Id.* § 907 requires every employer to preserve for not less than three years a record of the name, address, and occupation of employees; the rate of pay and the amount paid each pay period to each employee; and the hours worked each day and each work week.

Delaware Code Annotated tit. 29, § 7202 (1991), requires hospitals that furnish medical or surgical care and attention to any indigent person to keep a record showing the number of such indigent sick receiving medical or surgical care and attention, the name and residence of such person, the dates the person was admitted and discharged, and an itemized list showing all expenses incurred by the hospital for medical or surgical care and attention.

Delaware State Board of Health, Nursing Home Regulations for Skilled Care, § 57.705 (1986), requires such facilities to keep current, available personnel records for each employee supporting placement in the position to which assigned. *Id.* § 57.706 requires a report of screening tests for tuberculosis for employees, including volunteers, to be kept on file at the facility. *Id.* § 57.502 requires written records of attendance and content of fire drills. *Id.* § 57.810 requires filing of accident reports at the facility.

DISTRICT OF COLUMBIA

Concerning personnel records, District of Columbia Code Annotated § 1-632.1 (1991), which is part of the statute governing the administration of the District, provides that all official personnel records of the District government shall be kept and disposed of so as to ensure the greatest degree of privacy for applicants and employees while allowing the District to conduct its operations.

Section 1-632.5 provides that the official personnel record of an employee of the District shall be disclosed to that employee or a chosen representative. However, the following information shall not be disclosed to any employee: (1) information received on a confidential basis; (2) medical information that would, in the opinion of the employee's physician, be injurious to the employee's health if disclosed; (3) criminal investigative reports; (4) suitability reports, confidential questionnaires, and tests and examination materials that may continue to be used for selection and promotion purposes.

Section 1-2523, which covers prohibited acts of discrimination within the government of the District, requires preservation of regularly kept business records for six months from the date of making the record. If a record is relevant to a charge of discrimination, it must be retained until final disposition of the charge.

All employers are required by District of Columbia Code § 36-1213 (1991) to keep records and report information that will enable the mayor to develop information regarding the causes and prevention of occupational accidents and illnesses. Employers must maintain accurate records of work-related deaths, injuries, and illnesses, other than minor injuries requiring minimal treatment. In addition, employers must maintain accurate records of employee exposure to potentially toxic materials or harmful physical agents. Information contained in these records may be made public without the disclosure of any individual's identity.

FLORIDA

The State of Florida publishes a comprehensive General Records Schedule for Hospital Records E-1, which is available from the secretary of state. Schedule E-1 details the retention requirements for all types of hospital records. Following is a list of some common business records and the E-1 retention requirements for same:

- Accounts payable/receivable: three fiscal years

- Annual financial reports: permanent; microfilm optional

- Annual audit reports: permanent; microfilm optional

- Budgets: permanent

- Communicable disease reports: five calendar years

- Contracts, leases, and agreements: five fiscal years

- Drug inventory records: five calendar years

- Drug requisitioning and dispensing records: two years from date of disbursement

- Equipment maintenance records: one year after disposition

- Employee health examinations: five calendar years

- Incident reports: seven calendar years

- Insurance claims: five fiscal years

- Internal risk management records: five calendar years

- Journals, general accounting: five fiscal years

- Personnel records: 50 years after termination; microfilm optional

Florida Administrative Code Annotated r. 10D-66.060(1) (1990) requires licensed emergency medical services to retain records for five years.

Rule 12A-1.093(2) specifies that persons subject to Florida Sales and Use Taxes shall keep and preserve tax records for three years. Rule 12C-1.021(2) requires corporations subject to Florida corporate income tax to retain copies of tax records as long as the contents are material.

Rule 38B-2.005(1) requires employing units to maintain employment records for five years, subject to reasonable inspection and examination by the Department of Unemployment Compensation Tax and Claims.

Rule 10E-14.002 requires contractors providing mental health or drug or alcohol abuse rehabilitative services to retain all financial and program records, supporting documents, statistical records, and other records necessary to document the expenditures, income, and assets of the contractor. Contractors must retain such records for five years.

Florida Statutes § 400.191(2) (1990) requires each nursing home facility licensee to retain cost reports required by any regulatory agency for not less than five years from the date the reports are filed or issued.

Florida Statutes § 893.04(1)(d) (1990) requires pharmacists to retain written prescriptions for controlled substances for two years.

Florida Administrative Code r. 7G-1.017 (1991) requires healthcare service pools to maintain the following business records, which shall be available for inspection by the department on request:

- Copies of corporate articles and bylaws, if applicable

- Records documenting the work performed by personnel referred by the pool

- Copies of written employment contracts and any other agreements between the pool and each healthcare worker

- Copies of contracts between the pool and any client healthcare facility

- Copies of all records required by the U.S. Internal Revenue Service to be prepared by the pool for their employees or independent contractors

Rule 7G-1.018 requires healthcare service pools to maintain a personnel file for each worker, which shall be available for inspection by the department on request, containing the following information:

- Evidence of the worker's skills, qualifications, and previous training

- Employment, health, and medical history records of the worker

- Documentation to verify the worker's employment eligibility in compliance with U.S. immigration laws

- Documentation of any known complaints to the pool involving the worker and the follow-up action taken

Rule 10A-6.006(5)(b) requires adult day care facilities to establish and maintain a personnel file for each employee, including

- Name, home address, and phone number

- Name, address, and phone number of physician(s) or other persons to be contacted in case of emergency

- Education and experience

- Job assignment and salary

- Evaluation of performance at least yearly

- Dates of employment and termination

- Character references

- Evidence that the employee is free from communicable tuberculosis

Florida Statutes § 443.171(7) (1990) requires each employing unit to keep true and accurate work records, containing such information as the Unemployment Compensation Division may prescribe. Such records shall be open to inspection and may be copied by the division at any reasonable time and as often as may be necessary. Information thus obtained or obtained from any individual shall be confidential and shall not be published or be open to public inspection.

Florida Administrative Code r. 38B-2.005(3) (1990) requires employing units to maintain personnel records best suited to the business transacted, clearly showing the following information with reference to each worker:

- Name and social security number

- Place of employment

- Number of hours worked for each pay period

- Beginning and end dates of each pay period

- Wages payable and paid for each pay period

- Time lost each week due to incapacity

- Date hired, rehired, or returned to work after temporary separation

- Special payments of any kind, such as annual bonuses, gifts, and so forth

- Wages earned each day on an hourly or piece rate basis

- Each day on which any services were performed in employment

Rule 38B-2.005(5) also requires that employing units keep records showing the total amount of any wages paid for employment during each pay period, and the address of each place of business where payroll records are maintained.

Florida Statutes § 400.191(2) (1990) requires each nursing home facility licensee to maintain as public information, available on request, records of all cost and inspection reports pertaining to that facility that have been filed with, or issued by, any governmental agency. Copies of such reports shall be retained in such records for not less than five years from the date the reports are filed or issued. Section 400.191(3) requires any records of a nursing home facility determined by the department to be necessary and essential to establish lawful compliance with any rules or standards to be available to the department on the premises of the facility.

Florida Administrative Code r. 10D-38.025(1) (1990) requires intermediate care facilities to maintain fiscal records in accordance with the requirements of Chapters 393 and 400, Florida Statutes.

Rules 12C-1.021(1) and 12C-1.021(2) require every corporation subject to Florida corporate income tax to keep such permanent books of account and records as will be sufficient to establish the tax base. Such records must be available for inspection by the Department of Revenue as long as the contents are material, but for at least three years.

Florida Statutes § 407.02(5) (1990) allows the Florida Health Care Cost Containment Board to inspect and audit hospital books and records, and records of individual or corporate ownership, including books and records of related organizations with which a hospital had transactions, for compliance with cost containment laws and regulations. Such records include leases, contracts, debt instruments, itemized patient bills, medical record abstracts, and related diagnostic information necessary to evaluate the case mix of a hospital and to identify actual charges and lengths of stay associated with specific diagnostic groups; necessary operating expenses; appropriate expenses incurred for rendering services to patients who cannot or do not pay; all properly incurred interest charges; and reasonable depreciation expenses based on the expected useful life of the property and equipment involved.

Florida Statutes § 407.31 requires nursing homes to file with the cost containment board, on forms adopted by the board and based on the uniform system of financial reporting, their actual audited experience for that fiscal year, including revenues, expenditures, and statistical measures, within 120 days after the end of their fiscal year.

Florida Statutes § 607.1601 details the requirements for corporate record keeping in Florida. A corporation must keep the following records:

- Permanent records of minutes of all meetings of its shareholders and board of directors, a record of all actions taken by the shareholders or board of directors without a meeting, and a record of all actions taken by a committee of the board of directors in place of the board of directors on behalf of the corporation

- Accurate accounting records

- A record of its shareholders in a form that permits preparation of a list of the names and addresses of all shareholders in alphabetical order by class of shares showing the number and series of shares held by each

A corporation must also keep a copy of the following records:

- Articles or restated articles of incorporation and all amendments to them currently in effect

- Bylaws or restated bylaws and all amendments to them currently in effect

- Resolutions adopted by its board of directors creating one or more classes or series of shares and fixing their relative rights, preferences, and limitations, if shares issued pursuant to those resolutions are outstanding

- The minutes of all shareholders' meetings and records of all action taken by shareholders without a meeting for the past three years

- Written communications to all shareholders generally or all shareholders of a class or series within the past three years, including the financial statements furnished for the past three years

- A list of the names and business street addresses of its current directors and officers

- Most recent annual report delivered to the Department of State

- Excerpts from minutes of any meeting of the board of directors

- Records of any action of a committee of the board of directors while acting in place of the board of directors on behalf of the corporation

- Minutes of any meeting of the shareholders, and records of actions taken by the shareholders or board of directors without a meeting

- Accounting records of the corporation

- The record of shareholders

- Any other books and records

Florida Statutes § 617.1601(1) requires nonprofit corporations to keep as permanent records correct and complete books and records of account and to keep minutes of the proceedings of its members, board of directors, and committees having any of the authority of the board of directors. If a corporation has members entitled to vote, it must keep at its registered office in this state a copy of its articles of incorporation, its bylaws and any amendments thereto, and a record of the names and addresses of such members in alphabetical order. All books and records may be inspected by any member, or his or her agent or attorney, for any proper purpose at any reasonable time.

Florida Statutes § 620.106 requires limited partnerships to keep the following records:

- A current list of the full names and last known business addresses of all partners, identifying in alphabetical order the general partners and the limited partners

- A copy of the certificate of limited partnership and all certificates of amendment thereto, together with executed copies of any powers of attorney pursuant to which any certificate was executed

- Copies of the limited partnership's federal, state, and local income tax returns and reports, if any, for the three most recent years

- Copies of any then-effective written partnership agreements and of any financial statements of the limited partnership for the three most recent years

- Unless contained in a written partnership agreement, a writing setting out

  - The amount of cash and a description and statement of the agreed value of the other property or services contributed by each partner and that each partner has agreed to contribute

  - The times or events on which any additional contributions agreed to be made by each partner are to be made

- Any right of a partner to receive distributions, or of a general partner to make distributions to a partner, that include a return of all or any part of the partner's contribution

- Any events on which the limited partnership is to be dissolved and its affairs wound up

Florida Statutes § 465.0156(1)(d) requires a nonresident pharmacy to demonstrate that it maintains its records of medicinal drugs dispensed to patients in this state so that the records are readily retrievable from the other business records of the pharmacy and from the records of other medicinal drugs dispensed.

Florida Statutes § 893.04 details extensive requirements for pharmacist and practitioner prescriptions of controlled substances. Section 893.04(1)(d) requires pharmacists to retain written prescriptions for controlled substances for two years.

Florida Statutes § 893.07 requires every person who engages in the manufacture, compounding, mixing, cultivating, growing, or by any other process producing or preparing, or in the dispensing, importation, or, as a wholesaler, distribution, of controlled substances to make a complete and accurate record of all stocks of controlled substances on hand. Such persons must also maintain, on a current basis, a complete and accurate record of each substance manufactured, received, sold, delivered, or otherwise disposed of. The record of controlled substances received shall show

- The date of receipt

- The name and address of the person from whom received

- The kind and quantity of controlled substances received

- The record of all controlled substances sold, administered, dispensed, or otherwise disposed of shall show

  - The date of selling, administering, or dispensing

  - The correct name and address of the person to whom or for whose use, or the owner and species of animal for which, sold, administered, or dispensed

  - The kind and quantity of controlled substances sold, administered, or dispensed

Every such required inventory or record, including prescription records, shall be maintained separately from all other records of the registrant, or alternatively, in the case of Schedule III, IV, or V controlled substances, in such form that required information is readily retrievable from the ordinary business records of the registrant. In either case, records shall be kept and made available for a period of at least two years for inspection and copying by law enforcement officers whose duty it is to enforce the laws of this state relating to controlled substances.

Each person must maintain a record that shall contain a detailed list of controlled substances lost, destroyed, or stolen, if any; the kind and quantity of such controlled substances; and the date of the discovering of such loss, destruction, or theft.

Florida Administrative Code r. 10D-28.161(3)(a) (1991) requires laboratories to keep records on file indicating the receipt and distribution of all blood provided to patients in the facility.

Rule 10D-28.162(4) requires each hospital to maintain a hospital formulary or drug list, which shall be regularly updated. Rule 10D-28.162(6) requires each hospital to have written policies and procedures governing the receipt, distribution, administration, and record keeping of all drugs, including provisions for maintaining patient confidentiality.

Rule 10D-28.170(8) requires each hospital to maintain a list of licensed personnel, including private duty and per diem nurses, with each individual's current license number, documentation of hours of employment, and the unit of employment within the hospital.

Rule 10D-29.104(6)(e)(1) requires nursing homes to maintain the following written records:

- Admission and discharge register

- Census record

- Composite record for each resident

- Record of all accidents or unusual incidents

- Personnel record for each employee

- Fiscal records as required by applicable Florida statutes

Rule 10D-38.023(1) requires intermediate care facilities to maintain the following written records:

- Admission and discharge register

- Census record

- Personal admission record for each client

- General fiscal record for each client

- Accident and incident record

- Financial records indicating all income by source and expenditures by category

Rule 10D-45.069(2) requires drug manufacturers to keep written records of major equipment cleaning and maintenance. Rule 10D-45.069(7) requires laboratory records to include complete data from all tests necessary to ensure compliance with established specifications and standards.

Rule 10D-66.060(1) requires licensed emergency medical services to file and maintain records and submit reports to the department as requested. The licensee shall maintain the following administrative records:

- Current service license

- Vehicle registration

- Personnel records for each employee

- Accurate records of each call in which patient care is rendered

GEORGIA

Official Code of Georgia § 10-11-2 (Michie 1991) provides that unless a specific period is designated by law for their preservation, business records that the law requires persons to keep may be destroyed after the expiration of three years from the making of such records without violating such laws. This section does not apply to minute books of corporations or to records of sales or other transactions involving weapons or poisons capable of use in the commission of crimes.

Rules of the Department of Human Resources, Public Health, require hospitals to keep patient statistics and hospital operational records current and in such a way as to ensure rapid location with easy access to the following information:

- Daily admission and disposition record

- Monthly and yearly totals of admissions and discharges, excluding newborn

- Number of patient days per month and year

- Monthly and annual occupancy rate

- Number of beds and bassinets

- Number of births and fetal deaths

- Number of deaths

- Average census, daily, monthly, and annual

- Number of autopsies (Rules of the Department of Human Resources, Public Health, Georgia Compilation Rules and Regulations r. 290-5-6-11(h) (Nov. 21, 1973))

Rule 290-5-6-.10(2) requires hospitals to maintain a separate personnel folder for each employee, containing all personal information concerning the employee, including the application and qualifications for employment, physical examination (including laboratory and x-ray reports), and job description.

Georgia hospitals must also maintain accurate records of their costs of care for providing health services for nonresident indigent patients and report the total cost to the commissioner.

Health maintenance organizations (HMOs) must maintain records of written complaints about their healthcare services for five years after they were filed and submit summary reports concerning the complaints to the insurance commissioner (Georgia Code § 33-21-9 (Michie 1991). They must also provide annual reports under § 33-21-15 to the insurance commissioner. Their accounts and financial and other records are subject to inspection by the insurance commissioner and the commissioner of human resources (§ 33-21-17).

HAWAII

Hawaii does not specify required business records for hospitals. Its Business Corporation Act requires corporations to keep accurate and complete books and records of account, which include accounts of the corporation's assets, liabilities, receipts, disbursements, gains, and losses. It must also maintain minutes of the proceedings of its shareholders and board of directors and a book registering the name of all shareholders and the number of shares they hold.[52]

Hawaii's Nonprofit Corporation Act[53] requires nonprofit corporations to keep correct and complete books and records of account and minutes of the proceedings of its members, board of directors, and a record of the names and addresses of its members entitled to vote.

Every employer governed by the Department of Labor and Industrial Relations must keep records of its employees and of the wages, hours, and other conditions and practices of employment.[54] Under the Workers' Compensation Law[55] every employer must keep a record of all injuries received by employees in the course of their employment.

IDAHO

Idaho Code § 41-3909 (1991) requires health maintenance organizations (HMOs) to establish and at all times maintain adequate records of their financial and business transactions, together with a medical record system adequate to provide accurate documentation of health maintenance care utilization by each enrollee. The HMO shall retain its general records with respect to a particular transaction for not less than six years after termination of the transaction.

---

52. Hawaii Revised Statute § 415-52, 415B-45 (1991).
53. *Id.* § 415B-45.
54. *Id.* § 371-11.
55. *Id.* § 386-95.

ILLINOIS

Hospitals must keep personnel records during the term of employment of hospital personnel and for the years thereafter required by state agency or federal requirements. Minimum contents include

- Application form or resume, or both, with current and background information sufficient to justify the initial and continuing employment of the individual

- Verification of license

- A record regarding the employee's specialized education, training, and experience

- Verification of identity

- Employment health examination and subsequent health services rendered to the employees to ensure that all are physically able to perform their duties

- Record of orientation to the job

- Continuing education

- Current information relative to periodic work performance evaluations (Illinois Administrative Code tit. 77, § 250.420 (1991))

Additional record requirements for hospitals include:

- Job descriptions. Under *id.* § 250.940, job descriptions shall be written for each position classification in the nursing services and shall delineate the functions, responsibilities, and qualifications for each classification. Copies of job descriptions shall be available to the nursing personnel.

- Nursing care plans (*id.* § 25.970). Each nursing care plan shall, at minimum, indicate

  - Patient's problems and what nursing care is needed

  - How it can best be accomplished

  - What methods and approaches are believed likely to be most successful

  - What modifications are necessary to ensure the best results

Each nursing care plan shall be initiated on the admission of the patient to the hospital and shall include a discharge plan.

- Unusual incidents. A procedure shall be established to investigate any unusual incidents that occur at any time on a patient care unit. The procedure shall include the making and disposition of incident reports.

Notation of incidents having a direct medical effect on a specific patient shall be entered in the medical record of that patient. Summarized reports shall be available to the Department of Public Health and shall be confidential in accordance with Section 9 of the Licensing Act (*id.* § 250.990).

- Nurses' meetings (*id.* § 250.1000), which shall be held on a regular basis, and proceedings of the meeting shall be recorded. Meetings may be organized consistent with the organizational plan of the nursing service.

- Education programs. *Id.* § 250.1010 requires documented evidence of attendance at each continuing education program, which must be planned, scheduled, documented by a written outline of its contents, and evaluated at least annually.

Section 250.2840 specifies that special care and special service units have available

- An updated list of resources to which clients may be referred

- A written policy requiring the review or revision, or both, and evaluations of the plan to assess the attainment of program goals

- Documentation of the date, results, and recommendations from the evaluation

Each alcoholism treatment program shall provide the Department with reports, and with such data or statistics, or both, as may be requested by the Department.

Section 300.1840 specifies that a skilled nursing facility shall also keep records regarding

- Any personal money, regardless of source, or valuables kept for a resident

- If purchases are made for a resident from these personal monies, proper receipts shall be kept and proper notations made in a separate bookkeeping system. These shall be available for review by the resident or his or her representatives.

- A record of any resident's belongings accepted by the facility for safekeeping. This shall be initiated at the time of admission. It shall be kept current and should be part of the resident's record.

- The Illinois Department of Public Health Resident Census and Movement Report

- A permanent chronological patient registry book showing date of admission, name of patient, and date of discharge or death. The Illinois Department of Public Health Census and Movement Report is acceptable as this registry.

- Records and daily time schedules on each employee as set forth in § 300.650.(C)

- Menu and food purchase records shall be maintained as set forth in 10.08(d) and § 300.2080(d) and (f).(C).

- Quarterly reports for all employees as needed for social security and unemployment compensation. These shall be made available to the Department on request.

The facility must file annual financial statements (*id.* § 300.210.(C)).

116 Illinois Statutes § 60 (Supp. 1991) states that unless a law requires a longer retention period, any business records may be destroyed after three years.

INDIANA

Other than medical records, the hospital must keep documents and records that show ownership and compliance with local, state, and federal laws and regulations and adherence to bylaws and regulations of the facility, as well as the general business records required of corporations, employers, and tax-payers.[56] Such records must be made available to representatives of the Hospital Licensing Council and the Board of Health. Such records include

- Certified copy of articles of incorporation (not required of governmental hospitals or individual ownership)

- Constitutions, bylaws, and regulations of the governing body and medical staff (signed and dated)

- Minutes of meetings of both the governing body and medical staffs, and their committees thereof. Such minutes shall be considered confidential.

- A current roster of members of the medical staff and their designated privileges

- A completed application for each member of the medical staff that includes the following data: date of application, professional education and training by school and year, date of licensure and number thereof in Indiana, Drug Enforcement Administration number, experience in the practice of medicine, type of medical staff appointment and delineation of privileges desired, Medicaid provider number, pledge to abide by rules and regulations of the hospital, and other items specified by the hospital and its medical staff

- The current Indiana licensure or certification number (and serial number if issued) issued by the applicable official agency for physicians, dentists, pharmacists, nurses, physical therapists, and others as required

---

56. Indiana Administrative Code tit. 410, r. 15-1-8 (1988).

- Personnel records for each employee of the facility, which include personal data, education and experience, evidence of participation in job-related educational activities, and records of employees that relate to pre-employment and subsequent physical examinations, immunizations, chest x rays, and tuberculin tests

  - Pharmacy permit when required by Indiana Board of Pharmacy

  - Transfer agreements with nursing homes and other hospitals where indicated[57]

As to tuberculosis hospitals, Indiana Code § 16-11-1-5 (Supp. 1991) specifies that the superintendent shall be the chief executive officer of the hospital and subject to the bylaws and rules of the hospital and to the powers of the board of managers.

- He or she shall cause proper accounts and records of the business and operations of the hospital to be kept regularly from day to day, in books and on the records provided for that purpose, and see that such accounts and records are correctly made up for the annual report to the board of managers, who shall incorporate them in their report to the said board of county commissioners.

- The superintendent shall keep proper accounts and records of the admission of all patients, their names, age, sex, color, race, nationality, marital condition, residence, occupation, and place of last employment.

Indiana Code § 16-11-1-13 specifies the duties of the business manager or purchasing agent. The business manager or purchasing agent shall keep proper accounts and records of the business and operations of the hospital, said accounts to be kept regularly from day to day in books and records provided for that purpose; see that such accounts and records are correctly made up for the annual report of the board of county commissioners; and present the same to the board of managers, who shall incorporate them in their report to said board of county commissioners.

For city hospitals in third-class cities, § 16-12.2-5-23 provides that hospital records and books are open for inspection by officials. The business records, books, papers, and physical property of the hospital shall be kept open at all reasonable times to the inspection and examination of

- The state board of accounts

- The mayor, the common council, and the board of public works and safety of the city

- The board of commissioners, the county council, and the judge of the circuit court of the county

---

57. *Id.* r. 15-1-8(1).

- Any other authorized local or state officer, board, or commission

As to tax records, Indiana Code § 6-2.1-7-2 provides that a taxpayer who fails to keep records of his gross income, and any other records that may be necessary to determine the amount of gross income tax he owes, for a period of three years, as required by § 6-8.1-5-4, commits a Class C infraction.

Under § 6-8.1-5-4, every person subject to a listed tax must keep books and records so that the department can determine the amount, if any, of the person's liability for that tax by reviewing those books and records. A person must retain such books and records and any state or federal tax return that the person has filed

- For an unlimited period, if the person fails to file a return or receives notice from the department that the person has filed a suspected fraudulent return, or an unsigned or substantially blank return

- In all other cases, for a period of at least three years after the date the final payment of the particular tax liability was due, unless after an audit, the department consents to earlier destruction

In addition, if the limitation on assessments provided in § 6-8.1-5-2 is extended beyond three years for a particular tax liability, the person must retain the books and records until the assessment period is over.

A person must allow inspection of the books and records and returns by the department or its authorized agents at all reasonable times.

For corporate records, § 23-1-53-1 spells out the requirements:

- A corporation shall keep as permanent records minutes of all meetings of its shareholders and board of directors, a record of all actions taken by the shareholders or board of directors without a meeting, and a record of all actions taken by a committee of the board of directors in place of the board of directors on behalf of the corporation.

- A corporation shall maintain appropriate accounting records.

- A corporation or its agent shall maintain a record of its shareholders, in a form that permits preparation of a list of the names and addresses of all shareholders in alphabetical order by class of shares showing the number and class of shares held by each.

- A corporation shall maintain its records in written form or in another form capable of conversion into written form within a reasonable time.

A corporation shall keep a copy of the following records at its principal office:

- Its articles or restated articles of incorporation and all amendments to them currently in effect

- Its bylaws or restated bylaws and all amendments to them currently in effect

- Resolutions adopted by its board of directors with respect to one or more classes or series of shares and fixing their relative rights, preferences, and limitations, if shares issued pursuant to those resolutions are outstanding

- The minutes of all shareholders' meetings, and records of all action taken by shareholders without a meeting for the past three years

- All written communications to shareholders generally within the past three years, including the financial statements furnished for the past three years

- A list of the names and business addresses of its current directors and officers

- Its most recent annual report delivered to the secretary of state (§ 23-1-53-3)

With regard to prepaid healthcare delivery plans, Indiana Code § 27-8-7-2 provides that a person may not establish or operate a prepaid healthcare delivery plan in Indiana without obtaining a certificate of authority. Any person may apply to the insurance commissioner for a certificate of authority to establish and operate a prepaid healthcare delivery plan that is in compliance with this chapter.

Each application for a certificate of authority is to be submitted to the commissioner on a form as prescribed, setting forth or accompanied by the following:

- The basic organizational documents, including the articles of incorporation, articles of association, partnership agreement, articles of admission, or other applicable documents in duplicate

- The bylaws or any similar documents of the organization in duplicate

- A statement describing the prepaid healthcare delivery plan's

  - Proposed method of marketing

  - Geographic area to be served, designated by county

  - Financial program

  - Sources of working capital and funding, including certified financial statements that show the assets, liabilities, and sources of financial support of the application as well as of any corporation, association, partnership, trust, or other organization owned or controlled by or affiliated with the applicant

  - Relationship to any parent or affiliate, and any proposed method of operation involving the parent or affiliate and the applicant

- Any proposed evidence of coverage to be issued by the applicant to enrollees

- A document appointing the commissioner as the applicant's attorney on whom legal process in any proceeding against it may be served, if the applicant is not domiciled in Indiana

- Any provider agreement forms, which must contain acceptable hold-harmless provisions applicable to enrollees

- A copy of any administrative or management agreements made between any persons and the applicant

- Any proposed charges or rates to be issued by the applicant to employers or enrollees

- A copy of the group contract, if any, that is to be issued to employers or enrollees

- A copy of reinsurance arrangements, agreements, or evidence of stop-loss coverage issued to the applicant

- Any other information required by the commissioner (*id.* § 27-8-7-4)

With regard to personnel records, Indiana Administrative Code tit. 410, r. 15-1-8 (1988), specifies that facilities must maintain

- Current roster of members of the medical staff and their designated privileges

- Completed application for each member of the medical staff, which includes the following data: date of application, professional education and training by school and year, date of licensure and number thereof in Indiana, Drug Enforcement Administration number, experience in the practice of medicine, type of medical staff appointment and delineation of privileges desired, Medicaid provider number, pledge to abide by rules and regulations of the hospital, and other items specified by the hospital and its medical staff

- The current Indiana licensure or certification number (and serial number if issued) issued by the applicable official agency for physicians, dentists, pharmacists, nurses, physical therapists, and others as required

- Personnel records for each employee of the facility, which include personal data, education and experience, evidence of participation in job-related educational activities, and records of employees that relate to pre-employment and subsequent physical examinations, immunizations, chest x rays, and tuberculin tests

For nursing home personnel records, Indiana Code § 16-1-46-10 (Supp. 1991) requires that a person who operates a nursing registry must maintain personnel records for employees. The records must include a record of the employee's

- License or certificate

- Education and training

- Health record, including a physician's statement that verifies that the employee is free of communicable diseases

- Orientation and experience in clinical work assignments

Under Indiana Code § 22-4-19-6 (Supp. 1991), labor and industrial safety records include true and accurate records containing such information as the Department of Labor and Industrial Services considers necessary. Such records shall be open to inspection and be subject to being copied by an authorized representative of the department at any reasonable time and as often as may be necessary. The director, the review board, or an administrative law judge may require from any employing unit any verified or unverified report, with respect to persons employed by it, that may be deemed to be necessary for the effective administration of this article.

Indiana State Board of Health Hospital Licensure Rules, Indiana Administrative Code tit. 410, r. 1-5-1-16 (1988), requires dietary services to maintain and periodically report a census of meals served and records of food and supplies used, including costs, to the hospital administration.

IOWA

Iowa Administrative Code r. 481-51.6(135B) (1990) requires hospitals to keep the following in addition to medical records: admission records, death records, birth records, and narcotic records.

All hospitals shall submit annually to the director of the Department of Public Health the Hospital Price Information Survey. All hospitals also must file annual reports with the Department within three months after termination of each fiscal year, including total number of admissions during year, bed capacity, average percentage of bed occupancy, total patient days, average length of stay, number of major operations, number of minor operations, number of autopsies, complete maternity statistics, and a report of any changes in the physical plant within the past year.

Under Rule 135C.23, healthcare facilities, defined as residential care facilities, nursing facilities, intermediate care facilities for the mentally ill, or intermediate care facilities for the mentally retarded, must keep contracts with residents for at least one year after their expiration.

Rule 481-59.19(4) requires skilled nursing facilities to keep incident records. Each skilled nursing facility shall maintain an incident record report and shall have available incident report forms. The report of incidents shall be in detail on a printed incident report form and cover all accidents where there is apparent injury or where hidden injury may have occurred and all accidents or unusual occurrences within the facility or on the premises affecting residents, visitors, or employees. A copy of the incident report shall be kept on file in the facility.

Under Rule 481-59.19(6), such facilities shall furnish statistical information concerning the operation of the facility to the department on request. Skilled nursing facilities shall keep employment records for each employee consisting of name and address of employee, social security number, date of birth, date of employment, experience and education, name and address of three references, position in the home, and date and reason for discharge or resignation (*id.*).

Residential care facilities shall maintain an incident record report under Rule 481-57.16(2) on file in the facility. Records shall be retained in the facility for five years following termination of services and retained in the facility upon change of ownership (Rule 481-57.16(3)).

Under Rule 481-57.16(4), residential care facilities must furnish statistical information to the department. Under Rule 481-57.16(5) such facilities must keep personnel records containing the following information: name and address of employee, social security number, date of birth, date of employment, experience and education, references, position in the home, and date and reason for discharge or resignation. Rule 481-58.15(4) requires each intermediate care facility to maintain an incident record report on file. Rule 481-58.15(5) specifies that records shall be retained within the facility for five years following termination of services and shall be retained within the facility on change of ownership.

Nursing homes under Iowa Administrative Code r. 441-81.4 (249A) (1990) must keep resident personal needs accounts with a separate ledger for each resident for crediting their money on hand with signed receipts for expenditures. Rule 441-81.6(1) specifies that failure to maintain fiscal records, including census records, medical charts, ledgers, journals, tax returns, canceled checks, source documents, invoices, and audit reports by or for a facility may result in penalties.

Nursing homes shall at a minimum maintain the following records for a minimum of three years or until an audit is performed, whichever is longer:

- All records required by the Department of Public Health and the Department of Inspections and Appeals

- Records of all treatments, drugs, and services for which vendors' payments have been made or are to be made under the medical assistance program, including the authority for and the date of administration of the treatment, drugs, or services

- Documentation in the patient's records that will enable the department to verify that each charge is due and proper prior to payment

- Financial records maintained in the standard, specified form including the facility's most recent audited cost report

- All other records as may be found necessary by the department in determining compliance with any federal or state law, rule, or regulation promulgated by the U.S. Department of Health and Human Services or by the department

- Census records to include the date, number of residents at the beginning of each day, names of residents admitted, and names of residents discharged

- Resident accounts

- In-service education program records

- Inspection reports pertaining to conformity with federal, state, and local laws

- Resident's personal records

- Resident's medical records

- Disaster preparedness reports

All records shall be retained within the facility on change of ownership.

Residential care facilities for the mentally handicapped must keep incident reports (Rule 481-62.18(135C)) and retain their records in the facility for five years following termination of services to the resident even when ownership changes. Personnel records must be current, accurate, complete, and confidential to the extent allowed by law. The record shall contain documentation of how the employee's or consultant's education and experience are relevant to the position for which hired. Such facilities must also keep health certificates for all employees available for review by the department.

Residential care facilities for the mentally retarded must furnish statistical information to the department on request (Rule 481-63.17(4)), and keep personnel records consisting of name and address of employee, social security number, date of birth, date of employment, experience and education, references, position in the home, and date and reason for discharge or resignation. These facilities must also keep incident reports on file (Rule 63.17(2)), and retain records in the facility for five years following termination of services and within the facility on change of ownership.

KANSAS

Kansas Administrative Regulations 28-34-2 (1990) gives some guidance as to required business records of hospitals when it details the information contained in annual reports to the licensing agency:

- Administration and ownership

- Classification

- Allocation of beds

- Special care services

- Patient statistics

- Surgical facilities, services, and procedures

- Outpatient and emergency room services

- Staff personnel

The Kansas Hospital Association *Record Retention Guide* suggests retention periods for administrative office records, business office records, personnel records, and others. Those guidelines include

- Permanent retention

  - Annual reports to board

  - Appraisal reports

  - Audit reports

  - Board minutes

  - Blueprints of buildings

  - Balance sheets (may be disposed of if general ledger is maintained)

  - Constitution with bylaws, together with all amendments

  - Construction contracts

  - Depreciation records

  - Education (continuing medical courses offered in hospital)

  - Endowments, trusts, bequests

  - Equipment operating instructions

  - Equipment records (by location)

  - Financial statements

  - Journals (general)

  - Ledgers (general)

  - Internal Revenue Service (IRS) exemption letters

  - Licenses, permits, contracts

  - Medical staff: personnel records, minutes of meetings, bylaws, rules and regulations, physician contracts

  - Policies and procedures

  - Property: deeds, title, and leases

- Reports (departmental)
- Statistics of hospital (annual)
- Vouchers (capital expenditures)

- Retention for 19 years
  - Patient accident and incident reports
  - Insurance policies (liability)
  - Nursing: minutes of meetings, policies and procedures, private duty name file, training

- Retention for 10 years
  - Cash receipts
  - Check vouchers
  - Equipment leases (10 years after expiration)
  - Purchase orders
  - Vouchers (cash)

- Retention for seven years
  - Check stubs (may be disposed of if other records of checks issued are maintained)
  - Credit and collection correspondence
  - Ledger cards (patient)
  - Posting audits

- Retention for six years
  - Check register
  - Purchase orders
  - Vouchers (welfare agency records)

- Retention for five years
  - Bank statements
  - Blue Cross income and expense summaries
  - Budgets
  - Cashier's tapes from bookkeeping machine
  - Census reports
  - Charge slips to patients

- Checks (payroll)

- Correspondence (routine)

- Deposits (bank)

- Equipment inspection reports

- Food costs

- Income, daily summary

- Medical care evaluation/audit

- Medicare cost reports (five years after final settlement)

- Medicaid cost reports (five years after final settlement)

- Meal counts

- Prospective rate review reports

- Utilization review

- Retention for four years

  - Correspondence, insurance

- Retention for three years

  - Communicable disease reports required by state and federal health departments

  - Survey and inspection reports (or until next inspection)

- Retention for two years

  - Menus

- Retention for one year

  - Inspection of grounds and buildings[58]

Under Kansas Administrative Regulations 28-34-5 (1990), a copy of the hospital's current bylaws must be available for review by the licensing agency.

Kansas Administrative Regulations 28-34-57 (1990) requires ambulatory surgical centers to maintain statistical and administrative records, as does Regulation 28-34-83 for recuperation hospitals. Both types of facilities must maintain attendance and minutes for medical staff meetings (Regulations 28-34-54 and 28-34-80), as must hospitals (Regulation 28-34-6).

Kansas Administrative Regulation § 28-4-373 (1990) provides some guidance as to maternity center business records. It requires records of the com-

---

58. Kansas Hospital Association Record Retention Guide, 2-5, 7-10.

munity advisory board to be kept on file in the maternity center. The regulation also requires the center to keep on file

- Separate written agreements with the practitioners responsible in the event of an emergency transfer of a patient to a hospital

- A written agreement with a hospital providing Level II or III care for admission of patients detailing how referrals will be made and to which units of the hospital patients will be admitted

- A written agreement with an ambulance service for emergency transfer of patients to the hospital, detailing how contacts will be made, the type of service to be provided, and the length of time required to complete the transfer

- Written personnel policies and operating practices that define the services of the facility and the duties and responsibilities of each staff member

- Health assessment record for every person living or working in the center

- Current license or certificate for each professional staff member

- Supplies and equipment inventory

- Record of submission of monthly reports on forms provided by the Kansas Department of Health and Environment

- Record of resterilization of sterile packs

- Record of evacuation drills

- Record of emergency light battery recharges

Kansas Statutes § 40-3211 (1990) requires health maintenance organizations (HMOs) to submit their books and records to examination by the commissioner of health.

KENTUCKY

902 Kentucky Administrative Regulations 20:016 § 3(3) (1991) requires a hospital to establish, maintain, and use administrative reports necessary to guide the operation, measure productivity and reflect the programs of the facility. Such reports shall include minutes of the governing authority and staff meetings, financial records and reports, personnel records, inspection reports, incident investigation reports, and other pertinent reports. A patient admission and discharge register, a birth register, and a surgical register must also be maintained. Finally, licensure inspection reports and plans of correction must be made available to the public on request.

Hospitals are also required to maintain detailed financial records in order to complete Medicaid cost reimbursement forms and supporting schedules (Supplemental Medicaid Schedules KMAP 1-8) and the Health Care Financing Administration Hospital and Health Care Cost Report Certification and Settlement Summary (HCFA Form 2552-89).

As to personnel records, Kentucky Revised Statutes Annotated § 337.320 (Baldwin 1992) requires employers to keep a record of the amount paid each pay period to each employee, the hours worked each day and each week by each employee, and such other information as the Secretary of Labor and Human Rights requires. Such records shall be kept on file for at least one year after entry. They shall be open for state inspection at any reasonable time, and every employer shall furnish a sworn statement of them to the secretary or a representative on demand.

902 Kentucky Administrative Regulations 20:016 § 3(9)(d) (1991) provides that the following information be included in each hospital employee's personnel record:

- Name, address, and social security number

- Health records

- Evidence of current registration, certification, or licensure of personnel

- Records of training and experience

- Records of performance evaluation

Personnel records on each employee must contain:

- Name, address, and social security number

- Health records (skin tests and chest x rays must be recorded as a permanent part of the personnel record)

- Evidence of current registration, certification, or licensure of personnel

- Records of training and experience

- Records of performance evaluation[59]

The dietary service's menus must be kept on file for 30 days. The hospital must also keep records of the pharmacy or drug room to maintain adequate control over the requisitioning and dispensing of all drugs and drug supplies, as well as charges to patients for drugs and pharmaceutical supplies, including a record of the stock on hand and of the dispensing of all controlled substances. Records shall also be kept indicating the receipt and disposition of all blood provided to patients. Reports of all laboratory services and tissue examinations will be filed with the patient's medical record, with duplicates kept in the department.

Kentucky Revised Statutes § 271B.16-010 (Baldwin 1992) requires that a corporation shall keep as permanent records minutes of all meetings of its

---

59. 902 Kentucky Administrative Regulations 20:016 § 3(9)(b) (1991).

shareholders and board of directors, and a record of all actions taken by shareholders, directors, or committees of the board of directors on behalf of the corporation.

Section 271B.16-010 also requires a corporation to maintain appropriate accounting records and a record of its shareholders. A corporation is also required to maintain at its principal office articles of incorporation, bylaws, and relevant amendments. Corporate records shall be maintained in writing or in other form capable of conversion to writing.

Charitable and educational corporations are required by § 273.233 to keep correct and complete books and records of account, corporate minutes, and a record of the names and addresses of their voting members.

LOUISIANA

For corporate records, Louisiana Revised Statutes § 12.103(A) (West 1990) provides some guidance to required records. Every corporation shall keep at its registered office, or at its principal place of business in or outside the state, books and accounts showing the amounts of its assets and liabilities, receipts and disbursements, and gains and losses; and records of the proceedings of the shareholders, of the directors, and of committees of the board.

Every corporation shall keep at its registered office, or at its principal place of business or at the office of a transfer agent in or outside the state, a share register, or a stock certificate record, giving the names of the share-holders and showing their respective addresses, as and if furnished by each shareholder, the number and classes of shares held by each, and the dates on which the certificates were issued (*id.* § 12.103(B)).

If such records are not kept at the registered office, information as to their location shall be made available at the registered office. Such records may be in written form or in any other form capable of being converted into written form within a reasonable time. On at least five days' written notice any shareholder, except a business competitor, who is and has been the holder of record of at least five percent of the outstanding shares of any class of a corporation for at least six months, shall have the right to examine, in person or by agent or attorney, at any reasonable time, for any proper and reasonable purpose, any and all of the records and accounts of the corporation and to make extracts therefrom (*id.* § 12.103(C)).[60]

Louisiana Revised Statutes § 12.223 (West 1990) specifies that every non-profit corporation shall keep at its registered office (1) records of the meetings of its members and directors, and of committees of the board; share and membership records giving the names and addresses of the members in alphabetical order by classes and series and the number of shares held by each; and records of its assets, liabilities, receipts, disbursements, gains, losses, capital, and surplus; and (2) separate records of all trust funds held by it.

---

60. *See* Louisiana Revised Statutes § 12.102 re corporate annual reports.

Whenever membership is terminated, this fact shall be recorded in the share or membership record together with the date on which the membership ceased, and transfers of shares shall similarly be recorded. These records may be in written form or in any other form capable of being converted into written form within a reasonable time. Every shareholder and voting member may examine in person, or by agent or attorney, at any reasonable time, the records of the corporation listed in subsection A of this section. If the articles or the trust agreement so provide, every corporation shall, within 90 days after the close of each fiscal year, mail an annual report, signed by the treasurer, to its members concerning any trust funds held by it, and the use made of such funds and the income thereof during such fiscal year.

Louisiana has no specific provisions governing mandatory personnel records.

MAINE

The regulations for the Licensure of General and Specialty Hospitals in the State of Maine require written minutes or reports of the executive committee, and records of medical staff committees verifying attendance by a majority of committee members. Medical staff committee meeting minutes must give evidence of

- A review of the clinical work done by the staff on at least a monthly basis

- Consideration of the hospital statistical report on admissions, discharge, clinical classifications of patients, autopsy rates, hospital infections, and other pertinent hospital statistics

- Short synopsis of each case discussed

- Name of discussants

- Duration of meeting

Personnel records of nursing must include application forms and verification of credentials. Nursing staff meetings must have minutes reflecting the purpose.[61]

MARYLAND

Maryland Regulations Code tit.10, § 07.02.07 (1991), requires hospitals (comprehensive care facilities and extended care facilities) to keep written employment applications containing the following on file:

- Employee's social security number

- Home address

- Educational background

---

61. State of Maine Regulations Governing the Licensure Functioning of General and Specialty Hospitals, ch. X, §§ (E)(94), (H)(1) (1972).

- Past employment with documentation that references have been considered by the facility. If the employee formerly worked in a nursing home, consideration shall be given to the record as it relates to abuse of patients, theft, and fires.

- The licensure of personnel employed as registered or licensed practical nurses shall be verified by the facility.

Title 10, § 07.01.25, requires hospitals to maintain a separate credentialing file for each physician, including documentation relating to the credentialing process.

Maryland Health–General Code Annotated § 19-717 (1990) specifies the requirements for annual reports by health maintenance organizations (HMOs), and § 19-718 permits the state insurance commissioner to examine the financial affairs of HMOs.

Home health agency personnel records shall include

- A certification that the employee is free from tuberculosis in a communicable form if the employee or volunteer

  - Will be involved in the direct care of tuberculosis patients, or

  - Is an immigrant from Africa, Asia, or Latin America

- Evidence of current licensure, certification, or registration, as appropriate

- Evidence of the individual's qualifications for the position

- Periodic performance evaluations

Maryland Annotated Code art. 15B § 2 (1991) specifies that unless a law requires a longer retention period, any business records may be destroyed after three years.

MASSACHUSETTS

Department of Public Health Regulations, Massachusetts Regulations Code tit. 105, § 130.120 (1990), requires hospitals to maintain the following records (under the responsibility of a trained medical record librarian or other responsible hospital employee):

- Daily census

- Register of admissions and discharges

- Register of outpatients

- Register of births

- Register of deaths

- Register of operations

- Narcotic register

- Emergency room admissions

Title 105 § 141.201 requires each hospice to maintain current, complete, and accurate administrative records, which shall include

- Updated articles of organization and bylaws

- Minutes of the meetings of the governing body

- An organizational chart

- Personnel records for each employee, including evidence of required license or registration number, and documentation of any specialty certification, education, and job experience

Cardiac rehabilitation programs shall maintain current, complete, and accurate administrative records in a safe location, including

- Updated articles of incorporation and bylaws, partnership agreement, or trust instrument, as appropriate. The documents shall specify the organizational structure of the governing body and the methods of the selection of its members.

- Minutes of the meetings of the governing body and of the members

- An organizational chart for the entire organization

- Written policies and procedures designed to safeguard the health and safety of patients and staff

- Personnel records for each employee, including evidence of any required license or registration number

- Documentation of any specialty certification, education, and job experience (*id.* tit. 105, § 143.007)

Title 105, § 142.503, provides for the same administrative records for freestanding birth centers as does Title 105, § 141.201, for hospices, and Title 105, § 140.301, for clinics (with minor additions).

As to long-term care facilities, Title 105, § 150.002, requires licensees to keep completed and signed application forms and employee records on the premises. Such records shall include

- Pertinent information regarding identification (including maiden name)

- Social security number, Massachusetts license or registration number (if applicable), and year of original licensure or registration

- Names and addresses of educational institutions attended, dates of graduation, degrees or certificates conferred, and name at the time of graduation

- All professional experience, on-the-job training, and previous employment in chronological order with name and location of employer, dates of employment, and reasons for terminating employment

Employee records shall also contain evidence of adequate health supervision, and the facility shall keep records of illnesses and incidents involving personnel while on duty.

Title 105, § 150.013, requires facilities to keep the following records on the premises:

- Daily census

- Employee records on all employees

- Patient care policies

- Incident, fire, epidemic, emergency, and other report forms

- Schedules of names, telephone numbers, dates, and alternates for all emergency or "on call" personnel

- A patient or resident roster approved by the Department of Public Health

- A doctor's order book with a stiff cover and indexed, looseleaf pages

- A bound narcotic and sedative book with a stiff cover and numbered pages

- A pharmacy record book with stiff cover and numbered pages

- A bound day and night report book with a stiff cover and numbered pages

- Individual patient or resident clinical records in stiff-covered folders

- Record forms for recording medical, nursing, social, and other service data

- Identifications and summary sheets on all patients or residents

- Record forms for listing patients' or residents' clothing, personal effects, and valuables

- In a skilled nursing care facility for children, an individual service plan for each resident

Title 105, § 360, requires hospitals to maintain manifests of infectious waste shipped offsite for disposal.

MICHIGAN

The Department of Public Health Rules and Minimum Standards for Hospitals requires hospitals to maintain the following administrative records at a minimum:

- Records of admissions and discharges

- Patients' records

- Daily census records

- Narcotic register

- Statistics regarding number of deaths

- Statistics regarding number of autopsies[62]

Rules for nursing homes and nursing care facilities specify that such facilities shall keep all of the following records in the home:

- A current patient register

- Contracts between the home and patients

- Patient clinical records

- Accident reports and incident work reports

- Employee records and work schedules[63]

Such records will include

- Name, address, telephone number, and social security number

- Licensure or registration number, if applicable

- Results of any preemployment or periodic physical examination

- Summary of experience and education

- Beginning date of employment, and position for which employed

- References, if obtained

- Results of annual chest x ray or intradermal skin test for tuberculosis

- For former employees, the date employment ceased and the reasons therefor

- A daily work schedule showing the number and type of personnel on duty in the home for the previous three months

---

62. Michigan Administrative Code r. 325.1028 (1987).
63. *Id.* r. 325.21101.

Nursing homes and nursing care facilities shall maintain a time record for each employee for not less than two years.[64]

Homes for the aged will keep a resident register, resident records, accident reports, incident reports, and employee records and work schedules in the home.[65] Employee records and the work schedules will contain the same information as for nursing homes immediately above.

Tuberculosis hospitals and other communicable disease units must maintain complete records of employee health programs.[66]

MINNESOTA

Minnesota Rules 9505.0205 (1991) requires providers receiving medical assistance payments to maintain medical, healthcare, and financial records, including appointment books and billing transmittal forms, for five years.

Rule 4640.1300 requires hospitals to maintain the following records:

- Record of admissions and discharges, total patient days, average length of stay, and number of autopsies performed. Separate data shall be maintained for adults and children excluding newborns, and newborn infants excluding stillbirths.

- Register of births

- Register of deaths

- Register of operations

- Register of outpatients

Rule 4675.0400, governing freestanding outpatient surgical centers, requires such facilities to maintain a record of each physician and dentist containing name, qualifications, experience, and present hospital affiliation, accompanied by a list of procedures and services he or she is authorized to perform.

Rule 4615.3000, governing maternal and infant health, requires grantees to maintain full and complete records concerning operation indefinitely unless state archives approve their destruction. Grantees shall keep contract records, financial records, food records, medical records, nutrition information and counseling records, and voucher records.

MISSISSIPPI

As to business records, Mississippi Code Annotated § 41-9-81 (1990) provides that the commissioners or board of trustees of hospitals owned and operated by counties, cities, towns, supervisory districts, or election districts have the

---

64. *Id.* r. 325.21105.
65. *Id.* r. 135.1851.
66. *Id.* r. 325.1060(6)(b).

authority to retire and destroy at their discretion any of the following business records at any time three years after they were prepared: intrahospital requisitions, inventory records of expendable supplies, temporary records pertaining to patients' charges, department reports, paid invoices, purchase orders, and similar documents of temporary use and value.

In addition, whenever such hospitals have retained business records that the law requires to be retained for indefinite periods or that are necessary on the basis of sound business practices and that shall have been so retained and preserved for a period of six years, the commissioners or board of trustees shall have the authority, in their discretion, to retire the same. However, this statute does not authorize the retirement, destruction, or disposal of any business records consisting of minutes or minute books; bylaws or rules and regulations; general ledgers; disbursement registers or journals; cash receipts registers; maintenance and investment accounts; inventory records; ledger cards; sheets or other records of unpaid accounts receivable; other evidence of unpaid indebtedness; budgets; audit reports; licenses or permits; abstracts or certificates of title; geological reports; engineering or architectural plans, specifications, or drawings; or any other business records that are required by law, court order, rules and regulations, or sound business practices to be retained permanently or for longer periods than six years.

Privately owned hospitals may retire any business records at such times as dictated by sound business practices and the reasonable accommodation of other interested parties except as otherwise provided by law, court order, or regulations (*id.*).

Any hospital may, at any time, microfilm or otherwise reproduce its business records. However, microfilming or use of other storage media does not permit destruction or retirement of any record that must be retained under this statute (*id.*).

Mississippi Code § 13-1-151 (1990) specifies that any business may dispose of original records after copying them, provided that every original record pertaining to any claim, tax, or report due the state shall be preserved for five years from the thirty-first day of December of the year in which such claim arose.

MISSOURI

Missouri's Rules of the Department of Health, Code of State Regulations, requires the following:

- Maintenance of records of meetings of the governing body

- Reporting to the Department of Health of the number of admissions and discharges during the year, number of births and deaths during the year, bed capacity, average percentage of bed occupancy, total patient days, average length of stay, number of surgical procedures, number of autopsies, and complete maternity statistics

- Maintenance of written minutes of meetings of the medical staff

- Records of biological spore assay tests if required by treatment methods, the approximate amount of waste sterilized or incinerated per hour measured by weight for load, and records of the proper operation of sterilization or incineration equipment

- Records of in-service training and continuing education in employees' personnel files

- Written accounts for residents' personal funds and property[67]

The Long-term Care Facility Regulations and Licensure Law of the Department of Social Services requires convalescent, nursing, and boarding homes to keep all financial information, data, and records relating to the operation and reimbursement of the facility for not less than seven years.[68] Intermediate care and skilled nursing facilities shall keep financial records related to facility operation for seven years following the end of the fiscal year.[69] Such facilities shall keep records of in-service training and individual personnel records including employee's name and address; social security number; date of birth; date of employment; experience and education; references, if available; position in the facility; record that the employee was instructed on residents' rights and received basic orientation; reason for termination, if applicable; a written statement signed by a licensed physician indicating that the employee is able to work in a long-term care facility; documentation of training received within the facility; and copies of licenses, transcripts, certificates, or statements evidencing competency for the position held. The facility shall retain personnel records for at least one year following termination of employment. The facility shall also keep written documentation on the premises showing actual hours worked by each employee.

Missouri Revised Statutes § 109.156 (1990) authorizes a business to destroy the original after it has microfilmed or otherwise reproduced a record.

MONTANA

Montana Administrative Rule 16.32.138 (1979) specifies the requirement for and contents of hospital annual reports, and Rule 16.32.139 does the same for annual financial reports. Annual reports by long-term care and personal care facilities are specified in Rule 16.32.140, by home health agencies in Rule 16.32.141, and by alcohol and drug treatment facilities in Rule 16.32.142. Obviously, these facilities must collect and maintain the information required to fulfill these reporting requirements.

---

67. Missouri Code Regulations tit. 19 §§ 30.20.011-20.050 (1990).
68. Missouri Revised Statutes § 198.052 (1990).
69. Missouri Code Regulations tit. 13, § 15-14.042 (1991).

Under Rule 16.32.138, every hospital shall submit an annual report to the Department of Health and Environmental Sciences no later than January 31 of each year on forms provided by the department. The annual reports must be signed by the hospital administrator and contain the following information:

- Whether the hospital has received Joint Commission on Accreditation of Healthcare Organizations (JCAHO) accreditation, and if so, for what period

- Beginning and ending dates of the hospital's reporting period, and whether the facility has been in operation for 12 full months at the end of the most recent reporting period

- A discussion of the organizational aspects of the project, including the following information:

  - The type of organization or entity responsible for the day-to-day operation of the hospital

  - Whether the controlling organization leases the physical plant from another organization. If so, the name and type of organization that owns the plant.

  - Any changes in the ownership, board of directors, or articles of incorporation during the past year

  - The name of the current chairman of the board of directors

  - If the controlling organization has placed responsibility for the administration of the hospital with another organization, the name and type of organization that manages the facility. A copy of the latest management agreement must be provided.

  - If the facility is operated as part of a multifacility system, the name and address of the parent organization

- Whether the hospital provides primarily general medical and surgical services, or specialty services (specify)

- Specific facilities and services provided by the hospital, bed capacities for each service (where applicable), and whether such services are provided full- or part-time, by hospital personnel or by contracting providers

- Newborn nursery statistics, including

  - Number of bassinets set up and staffed

  - Total number of births

  - Total newborn days

  - Neonatal intensive care admissions and inpatient days

- Surgery statistics, including

  - Number of inpatient and outpatient surgery suites

  - Number of inpatient and outpatient operations performed

  - Number of adult and pediatric open-heart surgical operations performed

  - Total adult and pediatric cardiac catheterization and intracardiac or coronary artery procedures

- Number of beds set up and staffed, and total inpatient days (excluding newborns) in each basic inpatient service category

- Inpatient statistics including

  - Number of licensed hospital beds (excluding bassinets and long-term care beds)

  - Number of admissions (excluding newborns)

  - Number of discharges (including deaths)

  - Number of deaths (excluding fetal deaths)

  - Census on last day of reporting period (excluding newborns)

- Information on other services, including number of rooms or units, number of inpatient and outpatient procedures, and number of outpatient visits in at least the following areas:

  - Emergency room

  - Organized outpatient department

  - X-ray, ultrasound, nuclear medicine, cobalt therapy, CT scans

  - Physical therapy

  - Respiratory therapy

  - Renal dialysis

  - Other ancillary services

- Information on changes in total number of beds during the reporting period

- Whether there is a separate long-term care unit, and if so, how many beds

- Patient origin data, including every town of origin and number of discharges

- Total Medicare and Medicaid admissions and inpatient days

- Size of medical and nonmedical staff, including number of active and consulting physicians, medical residents, and trainees, registered and licensed professional or vocational nurses, and all other personnel

- Name of person to contact in the event the department has questions about the information provided in the annual report

According to Rule 16.32.139, every hospital shall submit an annual financial report to the department no later than January 31 of each year on forms provided by the department. The annual financial report must be signed by the hospital administrator and include the following information:

- Hospital revenues for both acute and long-term care units, including

  - Gross revenue from inpatient and outpatient service

  - Deductions for contractual adjustments, bad debts, charity, and so forth

  - Other operating revenue

  - Nonoperating revenue (such as government appropriations, mill levies, contributions, grants, and so forth)

- Hospital expenses for both acute and long-term care units, including

  - Payroll expenses for all categories of personnel

  - Nonpayroll expenses, including employee benefits, professional fees, depreciation expense, interest expense, others

- Detail of deductions for both acute and long-term care units, including

  - Bad debts

  - Contractual adjustments (specifying Medicare, Medicaid, Blue Cross, or other)

  - Charity/Hill-Burton

  - Other

- Medicaid and Medicare program revenue for both acute and long-term care units

- Unrestricted fund assets, including dollar amounts of

  - Current cash and short-term investments

  - Long-term debts

  - Gross plant and equipment assets deductions for accumulated depreciation

  - Long-term investments

- Other
- Unrestricted fund liabilities, including dollar amounts of
  - Current liabilities
  - Long-term debts
  - Other liabilities
  - Unrestricted fund balance
- Restricted fund balances, with identification of specific purposes for which funds are reserved, including plant replacement and expansion, and endowment funds
- Capital expenditures made during the reporting period, including expenditures, disposals, and retirements for land, building, and improvements; fixed and movable equipment; and construction in progress
- Whether a permanent change in bed complement or in the number of hospital services offered will result from any capital acquisition projects begun during the reporting period (specify)
- Whether a certificate of need or Section 1122 approval was received for any projects during the reporting period, and if so, the total capital authorization included in such approvals

Rule 16.32.140 governs annual reports by long-term care and personal care facilities. Every long-term care and personal care facility shall submit an annual report to the department no later than January 31 of each year on forms provided by the department. The annual report must be signed by the facility administrator and must include the following information:

- The facility's reporting period and whether the facility was in operation for a full 12 months at the end of the reporting period
- A discussion of the organization aspects of the project, including the following information
  - The type of organization or entity responsible for the day-to-day operation of the facility
  - Whether the controlling organization leases the physical plant from another organization. If so, the name and type of organization that owns the plant
  - Any changes in the ownership, board of directors or articles of incorporation during the past year
  - The name of the current chairman of the board of directors

- If the controlling organization has placed responsibility for the administration of the hospital with another organization, the name and type of organization that manages the facility. A copy of the latest management agreement must be provided.

- If the facility is operated as part of a multifacility system, the name and address of the parent organization

- Utilization information, including

  - Licensed bed capacity (skilled and intermediate)

  - Whether the facility is certified for Medicare or Medicaid

  - Number of beds currently set up and staffed

  - Total patient census on first day of reporting period; total admissions, discharges, patient deaths, and patient-days of service during the reporting period

  - Patient census on last day of reporting period, broken down by sex and age categories

- Financial data, including

  - Total annual operating expenses (payroll and nonpayroll)

  - Closing date of financial statement

  - Sources of operating revenue, indicating percent received from Medicare, Medicaid, private pay, insurance, grants, contributions, and other

- Staff information, including number of full- and part-time registered and licensed professional nurses

- Patient origin data, including patients' counties of residence, and number of admissions from state institutions and from out of state

- Name of person to contact should the department have any questions regarding the information on the report (R. 16.32.141)

According to Rule 16.32.141, every home health agency shall submit an annual report to the department no later than January 31 of each year on forms provided by the department. The report must be signed by the administrator of the agency and must include the following information:

- Whether the agency has Medicare certification, and if so, the term of such certification

- The agency's reporting period, and whether the agency was in operation for a full 12 months at the end of the reporting period

- A discussion of the organizational aspects of the project, including the following information:

- The type of organization or entity responsible for the day-to-day operation of the agency

- Whether the home health agency is owned by the same organization that controls it. If not, the name and type of organization that owns the agency

- Any changes in the ownership, board of directors, or articles of incorporation of the agency during the past year

- The name of the current chairman of the board of directors of the agency

- If the controlling organization has placed responsibility for the administration of the agency with another organization, the name and type of organization that manages the facility. A copy of the latest management agreement must be provided.

- If the agency is operated as a part of a multifacility system, the name and address of the parent organization

- A listing of specific services provided by the agency, and the number of people served and number of visits made for each service

- A description of the geographic area served by the agency

- The number of persons served by the agency and the number of new cases acquired by the agency during the reporting period

- Financial data, including

  - Payroll and nonpayroll expenses

  - Closing date of financial statement

  - Sources of operating revenue, indicating percentage received from Medicare, Medicaid, private pay, insurance, grants, contributions, or other

- Staff information, including number of full-time, part-time and con-tracted registered and licensed professional nurses, home health aides, student nurses, and others

- The name of the person to contact should the department have ques-tions regarding the information on the report

Every alcohol and drug treatment facility shall submit an annual report to the department no later than January 31 of each year on forms provided by the department. The report must be signed by the facility administrator and must include the following information:

- The facility's reporting period, and the number of days the facility was open during the period

- Type of licensure (hospital, long-term care facility, other)

- Duration of inpatient treatment program

- The type of organization or entity responsible for the day-to-day operation of the facility

- Utilization information, including number of inpatient beds, admissions, and patient-days, and number of outpatient clients and service contacts

- Total inpatient and outpatient alcohol unit revenues

- Number of first admissions, listed by age, race, sex, and education

- Percent of revenue received from Medicare, Medicaid, insurance, private pay, CHAMPUS, Indian health service, and other sources

- Number of clients who have received previous treatment

- Discharge data, including number of clients who completed treatment or were referred elsewhere

- Patient origin data, indicating number of patients from each county or out of state (*id.* r. 16.32.142)

Montana Code Annotated § 39-51-603 (1990), governing unemployment insurance, requires each employer to keep true and accurate work records containing such information as the department may prescribe.

NEBRASKA

Nebraska Administrative Rules and Regulations 175-9-002.01A (1979), Regulations and Standards for Hospitals, requires each hospital to keep written minutes of meetings and actions of the governing body. The chief executive officer shall maintain a written record of all business transactions and patient services rendered in the hospital (*id.* 175-9-002.02A). Summaries of meetings of the nursing staff shall be retained and available to all staff members for one year (*id.* 175-9-003.01A6). Records of radiation exposure shall be maintained for not less than two years (*id.* 175-9-003.03B6). The pharmacy must maintain an accurate inventory of stock supply every two years and have monthly documented inspections. Dietary services must have a written orientation plan and a record of each person's orientation, a record of in-service educational programs, job descriptions, minutes of monthly meetings, staff schedules, and weekly duty schedules on file (*id.* 175-9-003.03G1e). The dietary service must also maintain a list of patients, identified by name, location, and diet order (*id.* 175-9-003.03G2). Hospitals must maintain records of social services provided patients, which need not be part of the medical record (*id.* 175-9-003.03H). Rule 175-9-003.03J3 requires anesthesia equipment maintenance records to reflect regular inspection and approval for use prior to the administration of anesthesia.

Intermediate care facilities shall keep findings of any inspection or investigation regarding a nursing home's compliance with the Nebraska Nursing Home Act or rules and regulations adopted thereunder, together with the nursing home response, so they are available to the public not later than 21 departmental working days after the findings are available to the nursing home (Nebraska Administrative Rules and Regulations 175-8-002.02). Rule 175-8-002.09 requires the facility to keep all records required by these regulations on the licensed premises and available to inspection by the Department of Health. Statistical reports giving information on previous years' operation shall be kept available for review by the Department (*id*. 175-8-002.11). The administrator is responsible for establishing and implementing facility policies for administrative, personnel, and preservation and maintenance of resident and facility records (*id*. 175-8-003.01). He or she shall make certain that records of care and reports of paid employees are available for inspection by the Department. Daily staff schedules of employees shall be kept in writing and they and individual time records shall be retained for not less than three years (*id*. 175-8-003.02). The facility must maintain a written account of resident funds with receipts and itemized accounting (*id*. 175-8-003.02F6).

In addition to medical records, the facility must maintain admissions and discharge cards (*id*. 175-8-003.04B1), a chronological admission register (*id*. 175-8-003.04B2), and the following records pertaining to residents:

- Records of leaves, absences, and returns of residents, which shall include at least the time left and the time returned, destination or purpose, and in whose charge the resident was placed

- Accident and incident reports, which include the date, time, and action taken

- Records pertaining to resident financial matters, resident possessions, and statements of resident rights and responsibilities (*id*. 175-8-003.04C)

The facility must also maintain:

- Daily census record

- Records to substantiate its retention of residents whose economic status changes so that they become eligible for Medicaid if such residents have resided in the facility for at least one year, unless 10 percent of the facility's residents are receiving or are eligible for Medicaid

- Written policies and procedures that govern all services provided by the facility

- A written disaster plan

- Records of each orientation and in-service or other training program including names of staff attending, subject matter of the training, names and qualifications of instructors, dates of training, length of training sessions, and any written materials provided

- Contracts with outside resources to furnish required facility services not provided directly by the facility

- Personnel records

- Records pertaining to construction, maintenance, sanitation, equipment, and supplies for the facility

- Records pertaining to any waivers of these regulations (*id.* 175-8-003.04C)

Nebraska Administrative Rules and Regulations 175-12-002.02 (1987) governs skilled nursing facilities. Such facilities must keep findings of any inspection or investigation regarding a nursing home's compliance with the Nebraska Nursing Home Act or rules and regulations adopted thereunder, together with the nursing home response, so they are available to the public not later than 21 departmental working days after the findings are available to the nursing home (*id.*). Under 175-12-002.09, all required records must be kept on the premises and be available for inspection by the Department. The administrator is responsible for establishing and implementing policies pertaining to administration, personnel, and preservation and maintenance of resident and facility records (*id.* 175-12-003.01L), and ensuring that reports demonstrating competent supervision and direction of personnel are maintained. He or she shall make certain that records of care and reports of paid employees are available for inspection by the Department. Daily staff schedules of employees shall be kept in writing, and they and individual time records shall be retained for not less than three years (*id.* 175-12-003.02D). Such facilities must keep written accounts of all resident funds, including an accounting, and have a facility employee designated to be responsible for resident accounts (*id.* 175-12-003.02F6). These facilities must keep records virtually identical to those specified above for intermediate care facilities (*see* 175-12-003.04C and 175-12-003.04D).

Residential care facilities under the Rules and Regulations for Residential Care Facilities must keep records of menus as served for not less than 14 days (Nebraska Administrative Rules and Regulations 175-11-006.09B3 (1984)). Employee files on each employee must contain

- Copy of pre-employment physical

- Copy of results of annual tuberculosis skin test and date of the test

- If the employee cannot have a skin test because of a known reaction, then a copy of the results of a chest x ray including date must be on file.

- A record shall be maintained of all orientation and in-service training, including a notation of type of training, length of training, name of employee or employees, date, and signature of person providing the training (*id.* 175-11-007.03).

Such facilities must also maintain an incident record and report (id. 175-11-008.01).

Personnel records for home health agencies must include

- The title of each individual's position and a description of the duties and functions assigned to that position

- The qualifications for the position

- Evidence of licensure, certification, or approval, if required

- Performance evaluations made within six months of employment and annually thereafter

- Pre-employment health assessment or physical exam, given in accordance with agency policies, which shows evidence of good general health[70]

Other than clinical records, home health agencies must maintain the following records:

- Written policies and procedures governing services provided by the agency

- Policies and procedures governing admission to ensure only individuals whose needs can be met by the agency or by providers of services under contract to the agency will be admitted as patients

- Policies and procedures governing discharge

- Policies and procedures describing the method used to receive complaints and recommendations from the patients and to ensure agency response

- Records of each orientation and in-service or other training program, including the signature of staff attending, subject matter of the training, the names and qualifications of instructors, dates of training, length of training sessions, and any written materials provided

- Contracts with outside resources to furnish agency services not provided directly by the home health agency

- Personnel records

- Quality assurance records[71]

Regulations and Standards Governing Treatment Centers for Persons with Alcohol Problems or the Chemically Dependent indicate that such centers must keep operational statistics including

- Number of residents accepted, separately identifying new admissions and readmissions

---

70. Nebraska Administrative Rules and Regulations 175-14-004.03 (1988).
71. *Id.* 175-14-006.02.

- Number of beds or treatment slots available

- Number of applications for admission rejected and reasons for such actions

- Number and reasons for terminations or discharges, separately identifying terminations against advice

- Length of stay

- Plans of resident at time of leaving the center[72]

Statistics on the operation of the center (halfway house) must be kept up to date monthly and reported to the Department of Health and Division on Alcoholism, and must include the same statistics as above.[73]

Rules and Regulations Governing Drug Treatment Centers require such facilities to provide statistical reports giving information on previous years' operation on or before March 1 of each year.[74] Its personnel files must include a job description for each member of the center staff, as well as memoranda relevant to job performance including a yearly evaluation.

Regulations and Standards for Domiciliary Facilities require them to maintain personnel records including a copy of pre-employment physical (food service personnel only), copy of skin test results, and job description.[75]

Regulations and Standards for Health Clinics require statistical reports giving information on the previous year's operation including, but not limited to, caseload, admissions, terminations, and services rendered.[76] Each health clinic shall maintain accurate, current, and complete administrative records of its operations that extend over a period of time of not less than five years unless the facility has not been in operation that long, in which case the records shall cover the period for which the clinic has been in operation.[77] Employment records must be retained at least five years after termination of employment and include information on the employee's length of service, performance, training, and previous work experience.

NEVADA

Facilities that treat patients, including hospitals, convalescent care facilities, nursing care facilities, detoxification centers, and specialized medical healthcare facilities must file with the Department of Human Resources the following financial statements and reports: a balance sheet detailing the assets, liabilities, and net worth of the institution for its fiscal year, and a statement of income and expenses for the fiscal year. Such reports are public records.[78]

---

72. *Id.* 175-1-005.14 (1974).
73. *Id.* 175-1-007.15.
74. *Id.* 175-1-002.06.
75. *Id.* 175-1-003.05.
76. *Id.* 175-1-002.06.
77. *Id.* 175-7-004.01 (1975).
78. Nevada Administrative Code ch. 449, § 490 (1986).

Records need not be kept permanently. Nevada Revised Statutes § 51.135 (1991) provides that business records are admissible in any form, so long as they are made at or recorded near the time of the transaction. The information in the records must be transmitted by a person having knowledge of the transaction, as shown by testimony of the record custodian or some other qualified witness.[79]

As to general business records, Nevada Administrative Code ch. 449, § 310(4) (1991), requires all healthcare institutions to submit annual reports to the health division as prescribed by the state health officer on forms provided by the division.

Section 449.313 requires hospital governing bodies to keep minutes of meetings held to carry on the necessary business of the hospital. Minutes must reflect the pertinent business conducted.

With regard to financial and tax records, Nevada Revised Statutes § 372.735 (1991) requires sellers, retailers, and persons consuming tangible personal property purchased from a retailer to keep records, receipts, invoices, and other pertinent papers as required by the Revenue and Taxation Department for four years.

Section 372.740 allows the Revenue and Taxation Department to examine books, papers, records, and equipment of any person selling tangible personal property or any person liable for use tax.

Section 449.490 requires facilities for the diagnosis, care, and treatment of illness, including hospitals, convalescent care facilities, nursing care facilities, detoxification centers, and all specialized medical healthcare facilities, to file with the Health Department the following financial statements or reports annually:

- Balance sheet detailing the assets, liabilities, and net worth of the institution for the fiscal year

- Statement of income and expenses for the fiscal year

- Proposed operating budget at least 30 days before the start of the following fiscal year

Corporate records are governed by Nevada Revised Statutes, ch. 449, § 490 (1989), which provides exhaustive statutory requirements for private corporations and lists the following documents that every corporation must keep at its principal office in Nevada:

- Certified copy of certificate or articles of incorporation, and all amendments

- Certified copy of bylaws and all amendments

- Stock ledger or duplicate stock ledger, revised annually, containing the names and addresses of all stockholders and number of shares owned in lieu of the stock ledger. Corporations may substitute a statement naming the custodian of the ledger and the address where the custodian keeps the ledger.[80]

---

79. *Theriault v. State,* 92 Nev. 185, 547 P.2d 668 (1976).
80. Nevada Administrative Code ch. 449, § 78.105 (1989).

Nevada Revised Statutes § 78.105 (1991) lists the following documents that every corporation must keep at its principal office in Nevada:

- Certified copy of its certificate or articles of incorporation, and all amendments

- Certified copy of bylaws and all amendments

- Stock ledger or duplicate stock ledger, revised annually. The ledger must contain the names and addresses of all stockholders and number of shares owned.

- In lieu of the stock ledger, a statement naming the custodian of the ledger, and address where the custodian keeps the ledger

A professional corporation must file a statement with the secretary of state, each year on its anniversary, showing the names and addresses of all stockholders, directors, officers, and employees of the corporation. The statement must certify that all stockholders, directors, officers, and employees of the corporation are licensed or legally authorized to render professional service in Nevada. The statement must not contain any fiscal information, and is in lieu of any regular annual report of corporations required by Nevada Revised Statutes § 89.090 (1989).

A professional association must file a statement with the secretary of state, on or before July 1 of each year, showing the names and addresses of all members and employees of the association. The statement must certify that all members and employees of the association are licensed or legally authorized to render professional service in Nevada (*id.* § 89.250).

NEW HAMPSHIRE

New Hampshire's Licensure Rules and Regulations for Hospitals do not contain any specific requirements for maintenance of business records (New Hampshire Code Administrative Rules for Hospitals, Department of Health and Human Services Regulations 802 (1986)). *Id.* 803.11 requires nursing homes to maintain personnel records, which include qualifications, licensure if indicated, health examination by a physician (which shall be pre-employment or up to three months post-employment), and results of annual tuberculosis tests, with results of follow-up of reactors to tuberculosis testing.

Home healthcare provider business records must contain

- Documentation of services provided

- Annual report

- Current financial report

- Current service contracts or agreements including

  - Description of service provided

- Delineation of responsibility of each agency

- Fiscal arrangements

Id. 808.12 contains detailed requirements on records required of clinical laboratories. All test records and reports must be kept for not less than two years. Such facilities must also keep current personnel records, including the employee's training, qualifications, and experience with verified dates of previous and current employment.

Unless a law designates a specific period, business records may be destroyed three years after they were made.[81]

NEW JERSEY

New Jersey Standards for Hospital Facilities, New Jersey Administrative Code tit. 8, § 43B-5.1 (1985), requires hospitals to maintain appropriate personnel records, including employment and health records and documentation of required tuberculin and other tests. *Id.* § 43B-6.3 requires records of attendance and adequate minutes of medical staff meetings.

Hospitals must maintain the following records, along with such additional records as shall be required to document the overall operation and to provide statistical data to the Department of Health:

- Record of admissions and discharges

- Case and clinical records

- Daily census

- Register of births

- Register of operative procedures

- Narcotic register

- Death records

- Autopsy records

- Consultations

- Record of emergency and clinic services (*id.*)

NEW MEXICO

New Mexico Statutes § 30-44-5 (1991) notes that any person who fails to retain medical and business records relating to the Medicaid reimbursement for five years commits the crime of failure to retain records.

---

81. New Hampshire Statutes Annotated § 337-A: 2 (1990).

NEW YORK

Department of Health Memorandum, Health Facilities Series H-40, specifies that the chief executive officer must develop and implement personnel policies that cover, among other items, the maintenance of an accurate, current, and complete personnel record for each hospital employee and the recorded medical history for all personnel, along with their other medical records (New York Compilation Codes Rules and Regulations tit. 10, §405.3(b) (1988)).

Section 405.3(d) requires that the hospital maintain and, on request, immediately furnish to the Department of Health copies of all documents including, but not limited to

- All records related to patient care and services

- The certificate of incorporation or the partnership agreement and the certificate of conducting business under an assumed name as required by General Business Law, § 130

- The reports of hospital inspections and surveys of outside agencies, with statements attached specifying the steps taken to correct any hazards or deficiencies or to carry out the recommendations contained therein

- All contracts, leases, and other agreements entered into by the governing authority pertaining to the ownership of the land, building, fixtures, and equipment used in connection with the operation of the hospital

- All licenses, permits, and certificates required by law for the operation of the hospital and also for those departments and staff members, where required

- Operating procedure manuals for all services or units of the hospital organization. These manuals shall be reviewed at least biennially by the hospital or more frequently as determined appropriate by each service or unit and be made available to all services and units of the hospital.

- All bylaws, rules, and regulations of the hospital and all amendments thereto, listing the names and addresses and titles of offices held for all members of the governing authority and revisions thereof. Also, a copy of the bylaws, rules, and regulations of the medical staff and all amendments of the medical staff and revisions thereof, a copy of the current annual report, and financial statements of the hospital

- Copies of all complaints received regarding patient care and documentation of the follow-up actions taken as a result of the investigation of these complaints

- Copies of all incident reports

- A listing of the names and titles of the members of each committee of the hospital

- Written minutes of each committee's proceedings. These minutes shall include at least the following

  - Attendance

  - Date and duration of the meeting

  - Synopsis of issues discussed and actions or recommendations made

- Any record required to be kept by law (*id.* § 405.3(d))

The hospital shall report in writing to the Office of Professional Medical Conduct with a copy to the appropriate area administrator of the Department's Office of Health Systems Management within 30 days of the occurrence of denial, suspension, restriction, termination or curtailment of training, employment, association, or professional privileges or the denial of certification of the completion of training of any physician, registered physician's assistant, or registered specialist's assistant licensed or registered by the New York State Department of Education for reasons related in any way to any of the following:

- Alleged mental or physical impairment, incompetence, malpractice, misconduct, or endangerment of patient safety or welfare

- Voluntary or involuntary resignation or withdrawal of association or of privileges with the hospital to avoid the imposition of disciplinary measures

- The receipt of information concerning a conviction of a misdemeanor or a felony

These reports must contain the name and address of the individual, the profession and license number, the date of the hospital's action, a description of the action taken, and the reason for the action or the nature of the action or conduct that led to the resignation or withdrawal and the date thereof (*id.* § 405.3(e)(1)). Section 405.3(e)(2) establishes a similar requirement for health profession students serving in a clinical clerkship, an unlicensed health professional serving in a clinical fellowship or residency, or an unlicensed health professional practicing under a limited permit or a state license.

The infection control officer of the hospital must maintain a log of occurrences of infections and communicable diseases (*id.* § 405.11(b)(4)).

Records of radiologic services including interpretations, consultations, and therapy shall be filed with the patient's record, and duplicate copies kept in the radiology department (*id.* § 405.15(a)(5)).

The hospital will ensure that all tests, examinations, and procedures of its laboratory services are properly recorded and reported, including filing reports with the patient's medical record and keeping duplicate copies in a manner that permits ready identification and accessibility (*id.* § 405.16(c)(2)(ii)). In addition, the facility must keep records on file indicating the receipt and disposition of all blood and blood products acquired by the hospital (*id.* §405.16(e)(5)).

The director of the pharmacy will ensure that his or her personnel keep current and accurate records of the transactions of the pharmacy including

- A system of record keeping and bookkeeping in accordance with the policies of the hospital for

    - Maintaining adequate control over the requisitioning and dispensing of all drugs and pharmaceutical supplies

    - Charging patients for drugs and pharmaceutical supplies

- A record of inventory and dispensing of all controlled substances maintained

- The labeling of all inpatient and outpatient medications

All abuses and losses of controlled substances must be reported to the director and the medical staff, as appropriate (*id.* §§ 405.17(a)(7) and 405.17(c)(3)).

The admission and discharge register of the emergency service must include the following information for every individual seeking care:

- Date, name, age, gender, zip code

- Expected source of payment

- Time and means of arrival, including name of ambulance service for patients arriving by ambulance

- Complaint and disposition of the case

- Time and means of departure, including name of ambulance service for patients transferred by ambulance

The emergency service must develop a medical record for every patient seen in the service, and integrate or cross-reference these records with the inpatient and outpatient medical record system to ensure the timely availability of previous patient care information and shall contain the prehospital care report or equivalent report for patients who arrive by ambulance (*id.* §§ 405.19(c)(6) and 405.19(c)(7)).

The hospital must also maintain, in the maternity and newborn service, a register of births containing the name of each patient admitted; date of admission; date and time of birth; type of delivery; names of physicians, nurse midwives, assistant, and anesthetists; sex, weight and gestational age of infant; location of delivery; and fetal outcome of delivery. Any delivery for which the institution must file a birth certificate shall be listed in this register (*id.* §§ 405.21(c)(2)–(4)).

Section 405.8 requires hospitals to report immediately to the Department of Health's Office of Health Systems Management any of the following incidents, followed up by written notification within seven days. Reportable incidents include

- Patients' deaths in circumstances other than those related to the natural course of illness, disease, or proper treatment in accordance with generally accepted medical standards. Injuries and impairments of bodily functions, in circumstances other than those related to the natural course of illness, disease, or proper treatment in accordance with generally accepted medical standards, that necessitate additional or more complicated treatment regimens or that result in a significant change in patient status, are also reportable.

- Fires or internal disasters in the facility that disrupt the provision of patient care services or cause harm to patients or personnel

- Equipment malfunction or equipment user error during treatment or diagnosis of a patient, which did or could have adversely affected a patient or personnel

- Poisoning occurring within the facility

- Reportable infection outbreaks

- Patient elopements and kidnappings

- Strikes by personnel

- Disasters and other emergency situations external to the hospital environment that adversely affect facility operations

- Unscheduled termination of any services vital to the continued safe operation of the facility or to the health and safety of its patients and personnel, including but not limited to the termination of telephone, electric, gas, fuel, water, heat, air conditioning, rodent or pest control, laundry services, food, or contract services

The hospital will provide a copy of its investigative report to the area administrator within 24 hours of its completion, documenting all hospital efforts to identify and analyze the circumstances surrounding the incident and to develop and implement appropriate measures to improve the overall quality of patient care. The report shall include

- An explanation of the circumstances surrounding the incident

- An updated assessment of the effect of the incident on the patient(s)

- A summary of current patient status, including follow-up care provided and postincident diagnosis

- A chronology of steps taken to investigate the incident that identifies the date(s) and person(s) or committee(s) involved in each review activity

- The identification of all findings and conclusions associated with review of the incident

- Summaries of any committee findings, and recommendations associated with review of the incident

- A summary of all actions taken to correct identified problems, to prevent recurrence of the incident or to improve overall patient care, or both, and to comply with other requirements of this regulation (*id.* § 405.11(d))

The New York State Statewide Planning and Research Cooperative System (SPARCS) is a statewide centralized healthcare system that incorporates data from the uniform bill and uniform discharge abstract. This law requires hospitals to submit to the Department the patient review instrument data required of residential healthcare facilities as well as ambulatory surgery data submitted by hospitals and freestanding centers. Among other requirements, this law requires hospitals to maintain their accounts and records in accordance with the *American Hospital Association Manual,* Chart of Accounts for Hospitals, on an accrual basis except where an alternate system is mandated by law. Hospitals must submit a certified uniform financial report and a uniform statistical report of hospitals within 120 days after the close of the fiscal year.[82]

New York Public Health Law § 2803-b (McKinney 1992) requires every organization that operates, conducts, or maintains a hospital, and the officers thereof, to furnish to the Department of Health with respect to each licensed hospital, within 120 days after the close of the fiscal year, all of the following reports:

- A balance sheet detailing the assets, liabilities, and net worth of the hospital at the end of its fiscal year

- A statement of income, expenses, and operating surplus or deficit for the annual period ending on the balance sheet date

- A statement detailing the source of application of all funds expended by the hospital for the period encompassed by the income

- A report of hospital expenditures that allocates the costs of non–revenue-producing departments of a hospital to the other non–revenue- and revenue-producing centers that they serve. This cost center data must be accompanied by a sufficiently detailed statistical report containing data describing the hospital's basic services and patient statistics, which identifies costs related to categories of hospital services delivered to patients by each department of the hospital.

Public Health Law § 2805-g (McKinney 1992) requires every hospital to maintain, as public information for public inspection, records containing copies of all inspection reports pertaining to the agency that have been filed or issued by any government agency for 10 years from the date the reports were issued or filed.

---

82. New York Compilation Codes Rules and Regulations tit. 10, Ch. V, subch. A, art. 1, Pt. 400, § 400.18 (1988).

Section 2805 notes that no state, county, or municipal hospital qualifies for an operating certificate unless it maintains a record of all charges and collections made by any person, partnership, organization, or other entity whatsoever for services rendered to patients in the hospital including the person making the charge, the amount, and the purpose for which the charge was made.

Section 2805-a requires every general hospital to file with the commissioner of health within 120 days after the end of the fiscal year a certified report showing its financial condition and all of its financial transactions, including receipts and expenditures during the fiscal year. The report must include

- The facility's operations and accomplishments

- Its receipts and disbursements, or revenues and expenses, during such fiscal year in accordance with generally accepted accounting principles by categories, clinical services, and departments as set forth under the bylaws of the institution and including but not limited to salaries and other benefits, personnel expenses, operating expenses, equipment and supplies, and all other direct and indirect disbursements allocated to each department and clinical service

- Assets and liabilities at the end of its fiscal year including the status of reserves, depreciation, special or other funds, and including the receipts and payments of these funds

- Loans and investments, interest, rents, and profits from investments of the hospital

- The location of any real property owned by the hospital

Every general hospital shall also submit

- A report of hospital expenses incurred in providing services during the period covered by the reports issued under this section for which payment was not received and is not anticipated, which identifies as bad debts or charity care the cost of services provided to emergency inpatients, nonemergency inpatients, emergency ambulatory patients, clinic patients, and referred or private ambulatory patients for which the hospital did not receive and does not anticipate payment

- A statement of anticipated capital-related expenses as defined in subdivision 8 of § 2807-c for the forthcoming calendar year at least 120 days, or such shorter period as the commissioner shall determine, prior to the commencement of such year

Every general hospital shall submit a monthly report of gross inpatient revenue received and within 120 days after the end of the calendar year a certified annual report of gross inpatient revenue received for hospital inpatient service.

Under New York Public Health Law § 2803-l (McKinney 1992), voluntary nonprofit general hospitals must prepare and make available to the public a statement showing on a combined basis the financial resources of the hospital and related corporations and the allocation of available resources to hospital purposes including the provision of free or reduced service charges.

NORTH CAROLINA

North Carolina Administrative Code tit. 10, r. 03.0200 (1991), requires hospitals to keep the following essential documents on file in their administrative offices

- Certificate of incorporation (if incorporated)

- Bylaws of the governing authority (if applicable)

- Bylaws of the medical staff

- Minutes of the governing authority (if applicable)

- Minutes of the medical staff and staff committees

- Applications of all current members of the medical staff and professional and technical personnel containing qualifications and supporting documentation documenting conformity with requisite professional licensing laws, action by staff committees, and the governing authority

- Insurance policies, mortgages, deeds and other contracts (or true copies) to which the hospital is a party

- Rules and recommendations of the division of facility services regulating the operation of hospitals

- Report of the most recent inspection by the Joint Commission on Accreditation of Healthcare Organizations (JCAHO) (if applicable)

- Necessary licenses, permits, and certificates for the hospital and for certain staff personnel, as required (*id.* tit. 10 r. 03C.0306)

Title 10, r. 03C.0707, requires the blood bank to keep records indicating the receipt and disposition of all blood handled. Rules 03C.0803 and 03C.0804 require the x-ray department to keep permanent records of personnel exposures to ionizing radiation. Rule 03C.1303 requires that if narcotics administered from the hospital stock are procured under a federal permit, each dose shall be recorded on a permanent narcotic record, which must provide the date, hour, name of patient, kind of narcotic, dose, and by whom administered. The pharmacy must keep records of its transactions (*id.* r. 03C.1303).

Nursing home administrators must maintain records relative to operating costs and statistical records of the operation of the facility that provide a viable audit trail for at least two years. These records shall include, but not be limited to, detailed information indicating the time worked by and salary paid to all employees, food invoices, and daily census information, including admissions and discharges (*id.* r. 03H.0309).

Under Title 10, r. 03T.0303, hospices must maintain records of operating costs, annual budgets, and statistical records for not less than five years. Records shall include, as a minimum: hours worked by staff, including volunteers; patient census information including number of referrals, admissions, and discharges; patient diagnoses; service location (home or inpatient); and other appropriate statistical data required for the operation of the hospice or by the state's Medical Facilities Plan. Hospices must maintain personnel records, which include education, training, previous experience, verification of license when applicable, and other qualifications (*id.* r. 03T.0401). Hospices must also maintain records of the content of volunteer training sessions and on the subject of in-service, with attendance records for both (*id.* tit. 10 r.r. 03T.0401, 03T.0402 (Feb. 1976)).

NORTH DAKOTA

North Dakota Century Code §26.1-18-27 (1991) requires every health maintenance organization (HMO) to file annual reports, on or before March 1, verified by at least two principal officers, with the commissioner covering the preceding calendar year. These reports should include

- A financial statement of the organization, including its balance sheet and receipts and disbursements for the preceding year certified by an independent public accountant

- Any material changes in the information submitted pursuant to § 26.1-18-03 (required information for a certificate of authority)

- The number of persons enrolled during the year, the number of enrollees terminated during the year, and the number of enrollees as of the end of the year

- A summary of information pertaining to review of applications for certificates of authority, including procedures for developing, compiling, evaluating, and reporting statistics relating to the cost of its operations, the pattern of utilization of its services, the availability and accessibility of its services, and any other matters reasonably required by the commissioner

- Any other information relating to the performance of the HMO necessary to enable the commissioner to carry out his or her duties under this chapter

North Dakota Century Code § 23-17.3-05 (1991), standards of licensure for home health agencies, requires that they maintain personnel folders on all agency employees, indicating that qualified personnel are available to render designated services. Where hospital or long-term care personnel are utilized by the hospital or long-term care facility to treat agency patients during the normal working hours, the hospital's or facility's personnel folder meets this requirement for that facility's employees. Home health agencies that contract for staff to provide services shall maintain in the personnel folders a current written agreement with personnel serving under that contract. The agency will also maintain full information in its files relating to ownership of the agency. In those situations where the agency is incorporated for profit, the files must contain names and addresses of the corporate officers and of each person having a 10 percent or greater interest in the ownership of the agency. If services are provided by arrangement with other agencies or organizations, the home health agency shall ensure that the other agencies or organizations furnish qualified and trained personnel.

Under § 23-17.3-09, home health agencies shall submit annually to the Department of Health a complete description of their operations, including name, address, location, or principal place of business; ownership; identification of administrative personnel responsible for home health services; and the nature and extent of the programs.

OHIO

Ohio has some record-keeping requirements scattered within its administrative code. For example, Ohio Administrative Code § 5101:3-3-26 (1990) requires long-term care facility cost report filing, record retention, and disclosure as a condition for participation in the medical assistance program. Long-term care facilities other than state-operated facilities must submit cost reports containing an itemized listing of incurred costs and services for the cost-reporting year or for the period of participation in the Medicaid program if less than a year. Such facilities must maintain financial, statistical, and medical records supporting the cost reports or claim for services rendered to residents for the longer of seven years, or six years after the fiscal audit has been adjudicated.

Under § 5101:3-26-07, health maintenance organizations (HMOs) must submit reports to the Department of Human Services as follows:

- Annual audited financial statements no later than 120 days after the close of the HMO's fiscal year

- Annual disclosure statements

- Quarterly financial, service utilization, and statistical reports, no later than 45 days after the end of each calendar quarter

- A copy of the HMO's annual certificate of authority from the Ohio Department of Insurance

- Financial or utilization and statistical reports on a monthly basis when the Department determines that a concern exists regarding the quality or the delivery of services, or the fiscal operations or solvency of the HMO

OKLAHOMA

According to the Oklahoma Department of Health and Department of Libraries, records of public health care facilities must be retained as specified in the Records Management Act, Oklahoma Statutes tit. 67, § 201 and following. Private facilities should maintain their records in accordance with the Uniform Preservation of Private Records Act, tit. 67, § 251 and following. § 252 states that unless another law specifies a different retention period, business records may be destroyed after the expiration of three years from the making of such records. This section does not apply to minute books of corporations or to records of sales or other transactions involving weapons, poisons, or other dangerous articles or substances capable of use in the commission of crimes.

Title 63, § 1-1910, requires nursing homes to keep the following for public inspection:

- A complete copy of every inspection report of the facility received from the Department during the past three years

- A copy of every order pertaining to the facility issued by the Department or a court during the past three years

- A description of the services provided by the facility and the rates charged for those services as well as items for which a resident may be separately charged

- A copy of the statement of ownership

- A record of licensed, certified, or registered personnel who are employed or retained by the facility and responsible for resident care

- A complete copy of the most recent inspection report of the facility received from the Department

Title 63, § 1-818.19, requires group homes for developmentally disabled or physically handicapped persons to retain the following for public inspection:

- A complete copy of every inspection report of the group home received from the Department during the past three years

- A copy of every order pertaining to the group home issued by the Department or a court during the past three years

- A description of the services provided by the group home and the rates charged for those services as well as items for which a resident may be separately charged

- A copy of the statement of ownership

- A record of licensed, certified, or registered personnel who are employed or retained by the group home and responsible for resident care

- A complete copy of the most recent inspection report of the group home received from the Department

- A complete copy of any current contract or agreement between the group home and the Department of Human Services for the care, treatment, training, habilitation, or rehabilitation of residents of the group home

OREGON

Publicly and privately held health care facilities must file prospective budgets and service rate information annually with the state agency responsible for their regulation.[83] This requirement does not apply to physicians in private practice.[84]

Oregon Administrative Rules § 333-86-055(9) (1986) exempts general records of long-term care facilities from specific medical records retention requirements, allowing such a facility to establish its own practices for record retention.

State agencies responsible for healthcare facilities may specify required accounting and financial reporting systems, and the facilities must then adopt the systems specified within the next fiscal year. Such systems include records and reports of revenues, income, expenses and other outlays, and assets and liabilities.[85] The state agency may authorize groups of healthcare facilities to submit consolidated balance sheets, and income and expense statements.[86]

State agencies may further examine a healthcare facility's records and accounts, by full or partial audit as necessary, using either their own staff or any qualified independent third party.[87]

A corporation must keep the following permanent records:

- Minutes of all meetings of its shareholders and boards of directors

- Records of all actions taken by committees, the shareholders, or board of directors without a meeting

- Appropriate accounting records

- Record of shareholders, including names and addresses and number of shares

A corporation shall keep copies of the following records at its principal or registered office:

- Articles of incorporation and bylaws

- Resolutions by board of directors creating shares of stock

- Minutes of all shareholders' meetings and records of actions taken by shareholders for the past three years

---

83. Oregon Revised Statutes § 442.210 (1989).
84. *Id.* § 442.450.
85. *Id.* § 442.425 (1989).
86. *Id.* § 442.425(4).
87. *Id.* § 442.430.

- All written communications to shareholders within the past three years

- A list of names and business addresses of current directors and officers

- A copy of the most recent annual report[88]

All domestic corporations, and foreign corporations transacting business within Oregon, must deliver an annual report to the secretary of state by the corporation's anniversary date. The annual report shall include

- Name of the corporation and the state or country under whose law it is incorporated

- Address of the registered office and name of registered agent

- Address of principal office, if different

- Names and addresses of officers

- Classification of category of primary business activity

- Federal employer identification number

- Any other information required by the secretary of state[89]

Oregon Administrative Rules include rules detailing nonmedical record-keeping requirements for various departments in healthcare facilities. Examples of nonmedical records include the following:

- Joint Commission on Accreditation of Healthcare Organizations (JCAHO) certificates, surveys, and inspection reports, which must be submitted with license renewal applications[90]

- Written evidence of corrective actions under way or completed in response to JCAHO recommendations, including progress reports[91]

- Written definitions of facility and department organization, authority, responsibility, and relationships; written patient care policies and procedures; and written provisions for systematic evaluation of programs and services[92]

- Written personnel policies and procedures, which shall be made available to personnel; job descriptions for each position delineating qualifications, duties, authority, and responsibilities for each position, as well as an annual work performance evaluation for each employee with appropriate records maintained[93]

---

88. *Id.* § 60.771.
89. *Id.* § 60.787.
90. Oregon Administrative Rules 333-500-100(2)(A) (1991).
91. *Id.* at 333-500-100(2)(B).
92. *Id.* at 333-505-030(2).
93. *Id.* at 333-505-040.

- Documentation of any actions taken regarding tuberculin testing and results for each employee[94]

- Written facility-wide quality assurance program, with quarterly documentation of quality assurance activities[95]

- Written patient care policies, with documentation of annual evaluation[96]

- Nursing documentation of patient admission assessment and written plan of care documentation

- Certification of nurses and nurse assistants

- Documentation of qualifications of nurse assistants whose functions include administration of noninjectable medications[97]

- Written nursing service philosophy, objectives, standards of practice, policy and procedure manuals, and nursing job descriptions, as well as nursing personnel policies and procedures for staff capacity; and written quality assurance program for nursing service[98]

- Written isolation procedures in accordance with universal precautions[99]

- Written admission, transfer, and discharge policies and procedures[100]

- Written policies for a facility-wide infection control program with annual review of such policies[101]

PENNSYLVANIA

55 Pennsylvania Code § 1101.51 (1991) requires providers to retain for at least four years all medical and fiscal records that fully disclose the nature and extent of services rendered to medical assistance recipients. *Id.* § 1163.475 requires hospitals to maintain utilization review records for a minimum of four years from the date of submission of the year-end cost report. Hospitals participating in the medical assistance program must keep patient statistics and fiscal records on the cost of, and charges for, services provided to medical assistance recipients in a distinct-part psychiatric unit, a distinct-part drug and alcohol rehabilitation unit, a hospital-based nursing facility, and other inpatient settings. Such hospitals must retain complete, accurate, and auditable medical and fiscal records for four years for medical assistance patients (*id.* §§ 1101.51 and 1163.43), as must hospitals and hospital units under cost reim-

---

94. *Id.* at 333-505-040(7)(b)(9).
95. *Id.* at 333-505-060.
96. *Id.* at 333-510-000.
97. *Id.* at 333-510-020.
98. *Id.* at 333-510-040.
99. *Id.* at 333-510-060(14).
100. Including at least the items listed in Rule 333-510-070(1)(a) through (g).
101. Including at least the items listed in Rule 333-515-010(1)(a) to (d).

bursement principles under *id.* § 1163.443. Hospitals being reimbursed for distinct-part unit services shall keep separate patient statistics and fiscal records on the cost of, and charges for, services provided to medical assistance patients in each distinct-part unit being reimbursed (*id.*).

Providers enrolled in pharmaceutical assistance contracts for the elderly under 6 Pennsylvania Code § 22.62 (1991) shall retain for at least four years all fiscal records and other records necessary to disclose the full nature and extent of prescription drugs both covered and not covered by such contracts.

Primary health centers under the Health Care Services Malpractice Act must keep board meeting minutes in accordance with generally accepted accounting and business procedures.[102]

Nursing facilities must maintain adequate financial records and statistical data for the proper determination of costs payable under the medical assistance program. Such records shall include all ledgers, books, records, and original evidence of cost (purchase requisitions, purchase orders, vouchers, vendor invoices, requisitions for supplies, inventories, time cards, payrolls, bases for apportioning costs, and the like) that pertain to the determination of reasonable costs and are auditable. The facility shall maintain such records for not less than four years from the date the facility submits the cost report to the department.[103]

Shared health facilities operators shall maintain proper records of medical assistance recipients for a minimum of four years, including

- The full name, address, and medical assistance record number of each recipient

- The dates of visits by a recipient to providers in the share health facility, a statement as to whether the recipient is instructed to return for further treatment, and the dates of return visits

- The major complaint and diagnostic impressions for each visit to a provider in the shared health facility

- Pertinent history and physical examinations rendered by each provider in the shared health facility

- A listing of medications prescribed by a provider in the shared health facility

- The precise dosage and prescription regimens for each medication prescribed by a provider in the shared health facility

- Orders for x rays, laboratory work, and diagnostic tests written by or under the direction of a provider at the shared health facility

- The results of tests ordered

---

102. 28 Pennsylvania Code § 7.2 (1991).
103. 55 Pennsylvania Code § 1181.213 (1991).

- The medical documentation justifying the necessity of diagnostic procedures ordered by a practitioner in a shared health facility, regardless of whether the procedure is performed directly by the onlining practitioner or by someone under the direct supervision of the practitioner, or is referred to another practitioner or purveyor

- Referrals by practitioners in the shared health facility to other providers and the reasons for the referrals.[104]

Adult day care centers records shall include

- Statement of service provider objectives for the adult day care program

- Personnel policies, including job descriptions, salary, and benefits for paid staff, assignments for volunteers, and affirmative action policies

- Record of employee pre-employment and annual medical evaluations

- Daily menus for meals and nutritional snacks for the preceding three months

- Emergency evacuation plans, drill procedures, and staff responsibilities

- Plan for emergency medical care, including provider agreements with ambulance service, emergency room care, and the county MH/MR Crisis Intervention Unit

- Current certificate from state or local authorities relating to fire and panic regulations

- Insurance policies[105]

34 Pennsylvania Code § 315.2 (1991) requires employers to keep records of employees' exposure to specific chemical substances as required by the federal Occupational Safety and Health Administration (OSHA).

RHODE ISLAND

1990 Acts and Resolves R23-17-HOSP § 8 details the records that the governing body of a healthcare facility is required to maintain. These include written bylaws, rules and regulations, and amendments to them. The bylaws and rules should include specifications for the publication of an annual report and a certified financial statement (*id.* § 8.5(k)).

The hospital is also required by *id.* § 11.2 to maintain clearly written definitions of its organization, authority, responsibility, and relationships.

Hospitals must also maintain written admission, transfer, and discharge policies and procedures.

---

104. *Id.* § 1102.34 (1991).
105. *Id.* § 2380.93.

Section 15.0-15.5.2 requires hospitals to establish and maintain records in a uniform manner to facilitate periodic uniform reporting to the state. Each hospital shall report detailed financial and statistical data pertaining to its operations, services, and facilities. This information shall include

- Utilization of hospital facility and services

- Unit cost of hospital services

- Charges for rooms and services

- Financial condition of the hospital

- Quality of hospital care

Concerning personnel records, *id.* § 12 spells out a hospital's personnel record-keeping requirements. Hospital personnel records must include

- Written personnel policies and procedures

- A job description for each position

- Work performance evaluation programs with appropriate records

Effective October 1, 1989, licensed hospitals in the state are required to report financial and statistical data as required by *id.* Appendix B. To ensure anonymity of the reported data, it should be identified by only the medical record number or the hospital assigned number.

Appendix B requires quarterly reporting of data on discharges taking place during the periods ending March 31, June 30, September 30, and December 31. Data relating to discharges after January 1, 1990, must be submitted no later than 90 days after the end of the three-month period covered in the report. Corrected data must be submitted within 30 days of a request for such correction by the Office of Health Statistics.

Hospitals shall retain copies of all data and corrections submitted for no less than one year after the end of the three-month period covered.

For specific provisions regarding data to be reported and methods of transmission of data, see sections II and III of Appendix B.

SOUTH CAROLINA

South Carolina Minimum Standards for Licensing of Hospitals and Institutional General Infirmaries contain some record-keeping requirements.[106] Such facilities must maintain

- A personnel record folder for each employee[107]

---

106. South Carolina Code Regulations 61-16 (1982).
107. *Id.* § 204.

- A record of each accident or incident occurring in the facility, including medication errors and adverse drug reactions[108]

- Written minutes of medical staff meetings[109]

- Written minutes of nursing staff meetings[110]

- Records indicating the receipt and disposition of all blood handled[111]

- Duplicate written, signed reports on each x ray and therapy treatments in the x-ray department[112]

- A record of the stock and distribution of all controlled substances in Schedule II[113]

- Written reports of checks of sterilizer performance[114]

- Records of menus as served for at least 30 days[115]

- Records of all foods and supplies purchased by the dietary service[116]

The Minimum Standards for Licensing of Intermediate Care Facilities in South Carolina require

- Written documentation of in-service programs to include program content and persons attending[117]

- Monthly statistical records containing name, case number, age, sex, dates of admission, discharge, or death, and days of care rendered during the month[118]

- Fire reports for every fire regardless of size or damage that occurs in the facility[119]

- A record of each accident or incident occurring in the facility, including medication errors and drug reactions[120]

- Written transfer agreements that provide reasonable assurance that transfer of residents will be made between the hospital and the intermediate care facility whenever the attending physician deems that such

---

108. *Id.* § 206.2.
109. *Id.* § 303.
110. *Id.* § 403.
111. *Id.* § 602.2.
112. *Id.* § 603.2.
113. *Id.* § 604.3.
114. *Id.* § 605.3.
115. *Id.* § 806.
116. *Id.*
117. South Carolina Code Regulations 61-14 § 204 (1980).
118. *Id.* § 207.
119. *Id.*
120. *Id.*

transfer is medically appropriate. If such an agreement cannot be established, documented evidence that the facility in good faith to effect a transfer agreement[121]

- Personnel changes of administrators or licensed nursing personnel[122]

- Disaster plan[123]

- Records that the facility conducted planned in-service programs at regular intervals for all ancillary personnel[124]

- Documentation of destroyed medications[125]

- Separate control sheets on Schedule II drugs containing date, time administered, name of resident, dose, signature of individual administering, name of physician ordering drug, and balances as verified by drug inventory[126]

- Records of menus as served, maintained for at least 30 days[127]

- Records of tests of firefighting and related equipment[128]

- Documentation of fire drills, including date and time, how conducted, results of drill, and names of individuals attending[129]

Minimum Standards for Licensing Intermediate Care Facilities–Mental Retardation Providing Sleeping Accommodations for 15 Residents or Less require such facilities to keep

- A current roster of all management personnel and all employees[130]

- Monthly statistical reports containing name, case number, age, sex, date of admission, and date of discharge for each resident in the facility during all or any part of the month. This report must also provide the total number admissions, discharges, deaths, and days of care rendered during the month.[131]

- Fire reports[132]

- Incident reports, including medication errors, drug reactions, and resident accidents[133]

---

121. *Id.*
122. *Id.*
123. *Id.*
124. *Id.* § 604.
125. *Id.* § 1005.
126. *Id.*
127. *Id.* § 1107.
128. *Id.* § 1202.
129. *Id.*
130. South Carolina Code Regulations § 203 (1980).
131. *Id.* § 206.
132. *Id.*
133. *Id.* § 1203.

- Separate records shall be maintained for narcotics, depressants, stimulants, psychotherapeutic, and other controlled drugs containing the following information: date, time administered, name of resident, dose, signature of individual administering dose, and balance as can be verified by drug inventory.[134]

Regulation No. 61-17, Minimum Standards for Licensing Nursing Care Facilities and Institutional Nursing Infirmaries in South Carolina, requires such facilities to keep

- A written employment application containing information as to age, education, training, experience, health, and personal background of each employee[135]

- Documentation of in-service training programs including program content and attendance[136]

- Accident or incident reports, including medication errors and drug reactions[137]

- Monthly statistical record including name; case number; age; sex; dates of admission, discharge, or death; and days of care rendered during the month[138]

- Any changes of administrators or licensed nursing personnel[139]

- Fire reports[140]

- Transfer agreements as noted above[141]

- Records of receipt, administration, and disposition of all drugs[142]

- Records of destruction of medications[143]

- Separate control sheets on Schedule II drugs containing date, time administered, name of patient, dose, signature of person administering, name of physician ordering drugs, and balances as verified by drug inventory[144]

- Records of menus as served for at least 30 days[145]

- Records of fire equipment and other inspections[146]

---

134. *Id.* § 1205.
135. *Id.* § 204 (1980).
136. *Id.*
137. *Id.* § 207.
138. *Id.*
139. *Id.*
140. *Id.*
141. *Id.*
142. *Id.* § 605.
143. *Id.*
144. *Id.*
145. *Id.* § 1107.
146. *Id.* § 1202.

SOUTH DAKOTA

Administrative Rules of South Dakota, R. 44:04 (1991), requires ambulatory surgery centers to maintain personnel records on each employee, including job application, professional licensing information, and health information (*id*. R. 44:04:16:06), and keep records and attendance of medical staff meetings (*id*. R. 44:04:16:07). The pharmaceutical service must keep records of stock supplies of all drugs and an accounting for all items purchased and dispensed (*id*. R. 44:04:16:13).

Rule 44:14:25:02 requires drug and alcohol abuse agencies to present fiscal reports to the board of directors or its delegate at least quarterly showing the variances between the projected revenues and expenditures and the actual revenues and expenditures for each specific income source and each specific expense category in the agency budget. The report shall also break down revenues and expenditures by program (R. 44:14:25:02). Their personnel files shall include

- Copies of the employee's certificate, license, or other credentials

- Documentation of pre-employment education, training, and experience completed by the employee

- Copies of the employee's performance reviews

- Any employee health clearances, including the tuberculin test results

- Documentation of any disciplinary actions taken against the employee

- Documentation of any commendations

- Documentation of in-service training and continuing education (R. 44:14:27:10)

Residential programs shall keep a separate record of the receipt and disposition of Schedule II drugs (R. 44:14:35:03).

Health maintenance organizations (HMOs) shall submit the following statistics to the secretary of health by March 1 of each year:

- Average income per enrollee per month and expense per enrollee per month

- Cost statistics reflecting the cost required to provide services by the 20 most frequently occurring primary diagnoses

- Gross utilization totals, including use by the 20 most frequently occurring primary diagnoses, hospital discharges, surgical hospital discharges, hospital bed days, outpatient visits, laboratory tests and x rays, physician encounters, and nonmedical encounters

- Service area demographic characteristics, including the age, sex, and geographic residence of enrollees who use HMO services

- Statistics indicating the number of total enrollees whose source of premium payment is by Medicare, Medicaid, employer paid, and private pay

- A list of personnel and office hours revealing the availability of services

- Enrollee disease-specific and age-specific mortality rates

TENNESSEE

With regard to hospital business records, except as otherwise provided by law, order or decree of a court, or applicable rules and regulations, any hospital may retire any business records, as defined in Chapter 15, at such times as in its judgment may conform to sound business practices and the reasonable accommodation of other interested parties. Any hospital may, in its discretion, and at any time, cause any part of its business records to be reproduced in the same manner as hospital records.[147]

Tennessee's nursing home regulations specify that nursing homes will keep a copy of current inspection reports and fire safety reports on file. They will also keep legible copies of the following records and reports concerning the facility for the 36 months following their issuance

- Local fire safety inspections

- Local building code violations

- Fire marshal reports

- Department licensure and fire safety inspections and surveys

- Department quality assurance surveys, including follow-up visits, and certification inspections, if the facility has entered into an agreement to provide services to the Medicaid or Medicare medical assistance program

- Federal Health Care Financing Administration surveys and inspections, if any

- Orders of the commissioner or board, if any

- Comptroller of the State Treasury's audit reports and findings, if any[148]

Facilities shall maintain such records and reports at a single file at a location convenient to the public and during normal business hours, they shall be promptly produced for the inspection of any person who requests to view them. The facility must notify each resident and each person assuming any financial responsibility for a resident of the availability of these reports to the public, of their location within the nursing home, and each resident or responsible person must be given an opportunity to inspect the file before entering into any monetary agreement with the facility. Nursing homes shall

---

147. Tennessee Code Annotated § 24-7-110 (1990).
148. Tennessee Compiled Rules and Regulations tit. 1200, ch. 8-6-.01(3) (1990).

also maintain a duplicate of records pertaining to the money agreement between the nursing home and the patient.[149]

Nursing home employee health records shall contain a verification of a physical examination by a physician for employment and an annual health evaluation. Nursing homes shall keep employee personnel records on all employees, including verification of the credentials of licensed employees and verifying references. These records shall show the name, position assignment, qualification, professional experience, date hired, and date the person left or was dismissed, as well as a verification of physical examination by a physician for employment in a nursing home, showing that the employee is free of infectious disease. Nursing homes will maintain accurate narcotic records and incident reports.[150]

TEXAS

Texas Business and Commerce Code § 35.48 (1991) specifies that unless a state agency specifies a different retention period, business records must be retained for three years.

Texas Department of Health, Hospital Licensing Standards ch. 12, § 3.1.3.7 (1991), specifies special care facilities' personnel records must contain sufficient information to support placement in the assigned position (including a resume of training and experience). Where applicable, a current copy of the person's license or permit shall be in the file.

Texas Revised Civil Statutes art. 71-4438e(3) (West 1991) requires each hospital to submit to the Department of Health financial and utilization data, based on its latest audited financial records, including data relating to that hospital's

- Total gross revenue, including
  - Medicare gross revenue
  - Medicaid gross revenue
  - Other revenue from state programs
  - Revenue from local government programs
  - Local tax support
  - Charitable contributions
  - Other third-party payments
  - Gross inpatient revenue
  - Gross outpatient revenue
- Total deductions from gross revenue including
  - Charity care

---

149. *Id.*
150. *Id.* tit. 1200, ch. 8-6-.06(4).

- Bad debt
- Contractual allowance
- Any other deductions
- Total admissions, including
  - Medicare admissions
  - Medicaid admissions
  - Admissions under a local government program
  - Charity care admissions
  - Any other type of admission
- Total discharges
- Total patient days
- Average length of stay
- Total outpatient visits
- Total assets
- Total liabilities
- Total cost of reimbursed and unreimbursed care for indigent patients
- Total cost of reimbursed and unreimbursed medical education

Any portion of this data that relates to a specific patient or any financial data that refers to a provider or facility is confidential. Disclosure of such information is a misdemeanor.

The Hospital Licensing Standards of the Texas Department of Health require hospitals to keep written records of board meetings and of executive committee meetings (ch. 12, § 1-6.1.3). The hospital must keep individual files for each physician including applications for the medical staff, recommendations, type of privileges, and other applicable data. Chapter 12, § 1-8.1-7, requires the facility to keep minutes of meetings of the nursing staff.

The commissioners court may authorize hospital district boards in counties of at least 190,000 to transfer, destroy, or otherwise dispose of district records, other than medical records, that are more than five years old and are of no further use to the district as official records.[151] Similarly, municipal hospital authorities' governing bodies may authorize their boards to transfer, destroy, or otherwise dispose of authority records, other than medical records, that are more than five years old and are of no further use to the authority as official records.[152]

---

151. Texas Health and Safety Code § 281.073 (West 1991).
152. *Id.* § 262.030.

UTAH

Utah's Health Facility Licensure Rules specify certain record-keeping requirements other than medical records. Utah Administrative Rules 432-100-4.103 (1990) requires each licensed hospital to keep written records of board meetings. Under Rule 432-100-4.201, the hospital administrator must maintain a current record of all business transactions and patient services rendered in the hospital. Rule 432-100-7.412 requires hospitals to keep a record of admissions, discharges, and number of autopsies performed and vital statistics including registers of births, deaths, operations, and narcotics administered.

Nursing care facility administrators must complete, submit, and file all reports required by the Department of Health (Rule 432-150-4.201). The licensee must maintain written transfer agreements with one or more hospitals or nearby health facilities to facilitate the transfer of patients and essential patient information (Rule 432-150-4.502). The facility must maintain accurate records of patients' monies and valuables entrusted to its care, including a copy of the receipt furnished to the patient or the person responsible for the patient (Rule 432-4.802). Facilities must keep attendance records of recreational activities (Rule 432-5.602).

Small healthcare facility administrators must complete, submit, and file all reports required by the Department of Health (Rule 432-200-4.202). The administrator will document periodic employee performance evaluations (*id.*). Under Rule 432-200-4.501, the facility shall secure and update contracts for required professional and other services not directly provided by the facility including

- The effective and expiration dates of the contract

- A description of the goods or services provided by the contractor to the facility

- A statement that the contractor will conform to the standards required by Utah law or rules

The facility shall also maintain written transfer agreements under Rule 432-200-4.502. Each licensee shall also keep accurate records of patients' monies and valuables, including a copy of the receipt furnished to the patient or person responsible for the patient (Rule 232-4.802). Mental retardation facilities have similar requirements for the administrator to complete, submit, and file records under Rule 432-201-4.402, and to account for client funds under Rule 432-201-4.602.

Residential care facilities shall maintain complete and accurate records as required by the Department of Health to determine compliance with licensure rules, and shall make provision for the filing, safe storage, and easy accessibility of records. Records shall be protected against access by unauthorized individuals. Each facility shall maintain the following records:

- General policies and procedures including but not limited to

- Personnel

- Acceptance, retention, and discharge

- Residents' rights

- Disaster and emergency

- Medication assistance

- Housekeeping, laundry, and maintenance schedules (facilities licensed for nine or more only)

- A copy of any variance requests granted by the Department

- A statement signed by the licensee delegating responsibility to the administrator

- Agreements

- Personnel records (see below)

- Resident records

- A three-month record of daily work schedules indicating staff assignments and hours of duty (facilities licensed for nine or more)

- A three-month record of menus including substitutions

- A three-month record of logs indicating significant events or changes in any resident's condition and the facility's action

- One-year record of incident or accident reports (Rule 432-250-4.501)

Residential care facilities must maintain personnel records for at least three years following termination of employment. The record shall include at least the following:

- Employment application including

  - Employee's full name, social security number, birth date, and date of application

  - Home address and telephone number

  - Educational background and experience

- Position, date of employment, termination date, and reason for leaving (Rule 432-250-4.502)

Residential care facilities shall also keep accurate records of patients' monies and valuables, including a copy of the receipt furnished to the patient or person responsible for the patient (Rule 432-250-4.701).

Freestanding ambulatory surgical centers shall secure and update contracts for services not provided directly by the facility, which shall include a statement that the contractor will conform to the standards required by the licensure rules (Rule 423-500-4.601). The licensee shall also maintain transfer agreements (Rules 423-500-4.601 and 423-500-4.602).

Under Rule 432-550-4.203, the administrator of a birthing facility shall complete, submit, and file records and reports required by the Department. Rule 432-550-4.501 requires the facility to maintain personnel records for employees and to retain them for terminated employees for a minimum of one year following termination of employment. Birthing facilities shall secure and update contracts for services not provided directly by the facility, which shall include a statement that the contractor will conform to the standards required by the licensure rules (Rules 432-550-4.601 and 432-550-4.602). The licensee shall also maintain transfer agreements (*id.*).

Home health agency administrators have the responsibility to complete, submit, and file all records and reports required by the Department (Rule 432-700-3).

VERMONT

Vermont Statutes Annotated tit. 18, § 1955 (1991), requires hospitals to file the following information at the time and place and in the manner established by the Health Data Council:

- Budget for the forthcoming fiscal year

- Financial information, including but not limited to costs of operation, revenues, assets, liabilities, fund balances, other income, rates, charges, units of services, and wage and salary data

- Scope-of-service and volume-of-service information, including but not limited to inpatient services, outpatient services, and ancillary services by type of service provided

- Utilization information

- New hospital services and programs proposed for the forthcoming fiscal year

- Projected three-year capital expenditure budget

- Such other information as the council may require

Hospitals shall adopt a fiscal year that shall begin on October 1 (*id.*).

Vermont Statutes Annotated tit. 33, § 7114 (1991), requires nursing homes to file annually and on request such information, data, statistics, or schedules as the licensing agency may require. The agency shall have the power to examine the books and accounts of any facility operated by any licensee if it is the opinion of the secretary that the examination is necessary to carry out the purposes of this chapter.

As to corporate records, Vermont Statutes Annotated tit. 11, § 1896(a) (1991), requires each corporation to keep correct and complete books and records of account and minutes of the proceedings of its shareholders and board of directors. Each corporation also must keep at its registered office or principal place of business, or at the office of its transfer agent or registrar, a record of its shareholders, giving the names and addresses of all shareholders and the number and class of the shares held by each.

Under *id.* § 2372, each corporation shall keep correct and complete books and records of account and shall keep minutes of the proceedings of its members, board of directors and committees having any of the authority of the board of directors; the corporation also shall keep at its registered office or principal office in the state a record of the names and addresses of its members entitled to vote.

VIRGINIA

Virginia's Rules and Regulations for the Licensure of General and Special Hospitals provide little guidance for maintenance of hospital business records. Part III does require such facilities to keep a complete set of legible drawings showing construction, fixed equipment, and mechanical and electrical systems installed or built along with a complete set of installation, operation, and maintenance manuals for the installed equipment. They shall also maintain complete design data for their building(s) including structural design loadings, summary of heat loss assumptions and calculations, estimated water consumption, and electric power requirements of installed equipment.[153]

Rules and Regulations for the Licensure of Nursing Homes require individual personnel records comprising employee qualifications; evidence of current professional licensure or certification, where applicable; employee health record; and incident and accident reports (Virginia Regulations pt. III, § 7.0 (1982)). Section 25.5 requires maintenance of a record of fire drills to include date, time required to carry out appropriate emergency procedures, number of patients involved, and number of personnel participating. Section 41.0 requires maintenance of drawings and manuals similar to those detailed above for hospital construction or equipment installation.

WASHINGTON

Hospital personnel records must include a record of tuberculin skin tests, reports of x-ray findings, or exemptions.[154] Hospitals shall also keep a record of the orientation, on-the-job training, and continuing education provided to an employee.[155] Other hospital records required by this regulation include

---

153. Virginia Regulations pt. III, § 606.0 (1982).
154. Washington Administrative Code § 248-18-070 (1986).
155. *Id.* § 284-18-229.

equipment maintenance and inspection records,[156] laundry inspections,[157] and record of planned menus (kept for one month).[158] Census reports are required, including a daily inpatient census report on admissions to inpatient services, births, and discharges including deaths and transfer to another healthcare facility, as well as periodic (at least monthly) reports on admissions to outpatient services, the number of emergency care patients, and analyses of hospital services.[159] Reports on referred outpatient diagnostic services shall be retained for at least two years. The master patient index card shall be retained for at least the same period as the medical records to which it pertains. Data in inpatient and outpatient registers shall be retained at least three years. Data in an emergency service register shall be retained for the same period as medical records. However, retention of emergency service registers beyond three years after the last entry therein is optional if the facility includes all outpatient emergency care patients in the master patient index. Data in the operation register, the disease and operation indexes, the physicians' index, and annual reports on analyses of hospital services shall be retained at least three years. In the event of transfer of ownership, not only patient records but registers, indexes, and analyses of hospital services shall remain with the hospital and shall be retained by the new owner in accordance with state law. If the hospital ceases operation, it shall make arrangements for preservation of reports on patient care data along with medical records and get approval by the department.

Washington Administrative Code 388-87-007 (1986) requires providers to keep all records necessary to disclose the extent of services the provider furnishes to recipients of medical assistance.

In the event of a transfer of ownership of a hospital, patients' medical records, registers, indexes, and analyses of hospital services shall remain with the hospital and shall be retained and preserved by the new owner (*id.* § 248-18-440).

WEST VIRGINIA

West Virginia Legislature tit. 64 W. Va. Legislative Rules Department of Health: Hospital Licensure, series 12, § 7.2.1.b (1987), requires hospitals to keep permanent, signed minutes of all meetings of the governing authority and of its committees, including a record of attendance.

Hospitals must include in their annual license applications information concerning the voting members of their boards of directors whom they have designated as consumer representatives as well as women, minority, or handicapped representatives (*id.* § 7.2.3). Each hospital shall maintain a file con-

---

156. *Id.* § 248-18-150.
157. *Id.* § 248-18-170.
158. *Id.* § 248-18-180.
159. *Id.* § 248-18-440.

taining affidavits by its consumer representatives as to their consumer category (*id.* § 7.2.6). Each hospital shall maintain a file that shall contain the procedure established by the board of directors to ensure the consideration of women, racial minorities, and the handicapped in the selection of consumer representative board members and documentation that such procedure has been followed.

The dietary department shall maintain records on the number of persons, by job descriptions, employed full-time or part-time in the dietary department, the number of hours each employee works weekly, and a job description of each type of dietary department position with verification that each employee has been familiarized with his or her duties and responsibilities. The department shall keep menus for at least four weeks (*id.* § 10.4.2).

The facility should delineate clinical privileges of the medical staff in writing, and all members shall sign a document specifying that the bylaws, rules, and regulations have been read (*id.* § 14.1.1).

The following records shall be available in the nursing department:

- A list of all licensed nursing personnel, including private duty and per diem nurses, with each individual's current West Virginia license number

- Personnel records including application forms and verification of credentials and character references for each department employee

- The current nursing care policy and procedure manuals

- Minutes and records of attendance at all meetings

- A list of the nursing department committees and other committees on which nursing is represented

- A master staffing plan for the current year (*id.* § 14.2.3)

The hospital shall maintain records of planned continuing educational activities for nursing personnel, which include the methods used and an evaluation of their effectiveness.

Nursing homes shall keep the following records on file in their administrative offices:

- Documentation of the facility's professional and administrative staff meetings

- Documentation of visits by professional consultants employed by the facility

- A current copy of the licensure regulations

- A copy of the facility's current policy and procedures manual, containing copies of all policies and procedures required by the provisions of these regulations

- Reports of all inspections by government agencies, together with summaries of corrective action taken in response to each report during the previous five years

- Reports of any other inspections required by these regulations

- Copies of contracts and agreements, including agreement for the provision of professional services by outside agencies or contractors, to which the facility is a party

- Documents demonstrating control and ownership of the facility

- Bylaws of the governing body, if applicable

- Reports of accidents or incidents involving patients

- Records of all transactions conducted by the facility involving personal funds of patients in the facility during the previous five years

- All menus prepared by the facility

- Records of food purchases

- A copy of the facility's emergency evacuation plan

- A chronological record of all patients admitted to the facility with an identifying number, date of admission, and where appropriate, date of discharge

- All other records required by state or federal laws or regulations (West Virginia Legislature, tit. 64 W. Va. Legislative Rules Department of Health: Nursing Home Licensure, series 13, § 7.9 (1987))

Such facilities shall maintain a confidential personnel record for each employee containing sufficient information to support the employee's assignment. The records shall contain at least the following information:

- A dated application for employment that includes a resume of the applicant's training and experience and verification by references

- An employee health record containing the results of pre-employment and annual physical examination, including tuberculosis

- Evaluations of work performance signed by employee and supervisor

- Subsequent change of status forms including change of address, salary adjustments, merit increases, or promotions

- Current licensure, registration, or certification status demonstrating appropriate licensure, registration, or certification, and periodic verification

- A summary record of each employee's in-service training

Section 7.5, governing nursing homes, requires an admission contract, governing the relationship of the patient to the facility, to be kept on file for five years from the date it is terminated. Nursing homes must also keep all such records in their administrative offices. Such records may be photocopied.

WISCONSIN

Wisconsin Administrative Code, § HSS 124.05 (Feb. 1988), requires hospitals to keep written minutes or reports reflecting business conducted by the executive committee and other committees, including the finance, joint conference, and plant and safety management committees. Under § HSS 124.06, the chief executive officer is responsible for maintaining an accurate, current, and complete personnel record for each employee and for providing any required information to the Department of Health and Social Services and for providing reasonable means for the department to examine records and gather information. Section HSS 124.07 requires records of employee health assessments.

Both the chief executive officer and the chief of the medical staff are responsible for documenting the monitoring and evaluation activities performed under the hospital's quality assurance program (*id.* § HSS 124.10). The facility must keep written records of the hospital utilization review activities and findings (*id.* § HSS 124.11).

Section HSS 124.12 requires the hospital to keep adequate minutes of medical staff meetings sufficient to document for those members who did not attend the general nature of the business conducted, the decisions reached, and the findings and recommendations of the medical staff.

Records shall be kept of the transactions of the pharmacy or drug room, and the managing or consulting pharmacist shall maintain, in cooperation with the business office, a satisfactory system of records and bookkeeping for maintaining adequate control over the requisitioning and dispensing of all drugs and pharmaceutical supplies and charging patients for drugs and pharmaceutical supplies (*id.* § HSS 124.15).

The dietary service shall maintain a systematic record of all diets (*id.* § HSS 124.16).

Laboratories shall keep duplicate records of the authenticated laboratory report filed in the patient's medical record for at least two years (*id.* § HSS 124.17). The pathologist shall keep duplicate records of examination reports in the laboratory (*id.*). Radiological services shall keep copies of reports, printouts, films, scans, and other image records for at least five years. Copies of nuclear medicine interpretations, consultations, and therapy shall be retained by the services as must records of cumulative radiation exposure for staff, records of the receipt and disposition of radiopharmaceuticals, documentation of instrument performance, and records of inspection (*id.* § HSS 1224.18).

Wisconsin Administrative Code § HSS 132 (Mar. 1989), governing nursing homes, provides that nursing homes shall keep current, separate records of each employee that contain sufficient information to support assignment to the employee's current position and duties (*id.* § HSS 132.45). Section HSS 132.62, governing nursing services, requires weekly time schedules indicating the names and classifications of nursing personnel and relief personnel assigned on each nursing unit for each tour of duty. Section HSS 132.65, pharmaceutical services, requires the facility to keep records of all medication returned for credit and proof-of-use records for Schedule II drugs.

Section HSS 134, Facilities for the Developmentally Disabled Rules, requires such facilities to keep all records not directly related to resident care for at least two years, including

- A separate record for each employee kept current and containing sufficient information to support assignment to the employee's position and duties, and records of staff work schedules and time worked

- All menus and records of modified diets, including the average portion size of items

- A financial record for each resident, which shows all personal funds held by the facility and all receipts, deposits and disbursements made by the facility

- Any reports that document compliance with applicable sanitation, health, and environmental safety rules and local ordinances, and written reports of inspections and actions taken to enforce these rules and local ordinances

- Records of inspections by local fire inspectors or departments, records of fire and disaster evacuation drills, and records of tests of fire detection, alarm, and extinguishing equipment

- Documentation of professional consultation by registered dietitians, registered nurses, social workers and special professional services providers, and other persons used by the facility as consultants

- Medical transfer service agreements and agreements with outside agency service providers

- A description of subject matter, a summary of contents, and a list of instructors and attendance records for all employee orientation and in-service programs (HSS 134.47)

Wisconsin Administrative Code § HSS 3.12 (July 1988) requires community-based residential facilities to maintain separate personnel records on each employee containing

- Name and address of employee

- Social security number

- Date of birth

- Date of employment

- Job-related experience and orientation

- Educational qualifications

- Date of discharge or resignation

WYOMING

Information provided by the Wyoming Records Management Archives, Records Management and Micrographics Services, gives guidance for county publicly funded hospitals that should suffice for other facilities as well. Retention periods include

- Permanent in office or transfer to state archives

  - Board of trustees—minutes of meetings and supportive documents

  - Legal notices

  - Capital improvement projects records

  - Delineation of hospital privileges

  - Lease agreements

  - Licenses and permits—permanent

  - Master organizational chart (destroy duplicates at discretion)

- Permanent in hospital

  - Nuclear Regulatory Commission license

  - Radioisotopes records (receipts, transfer, use, storage, delivery, and disposal)

Other retention periods

- Administrative

  - Board of trustees—correspondence. Retain five years, then transfer to state archives for evaluation

  - Analysis of daily census. Summary information—retain seven years, then destroy at discretion. Detailed analysis—retain three years, then destroy at discretion

  - Budget files. Retain five years, then destroy at discretion

  - Contracts and agreements with other agencies. Retain five years, then transfer to state archives after review by hospital administrator for continued legal or administrative value

- Correspondence—administrator. After five years, administrator will review for transfer to state archives or microfilm and destroy

- Deeds, abstracts of title, and other property records. Permanent in office as long as property held, then transfer to state archives

- Equipment records. Retain for life of equipment plus five years, then destroy

- Fire drill records. Retain three years, then destroy

- Incident reports. Retain three years, then destroy unless litigation pending

- Inspection records. Retain five years, then destroy at discretion (insurance policies may recommend longer retention)

- Inventory records. Retain five years, then destroy at discretion

- Licenses and permits—periodically renewable. Retain five years after expiration, then destroy

- Minutes of meetings—committees. Retain five years, then destroy at discretion of administrator

- State and Local Government Information Report (EEO-4 Form) (if required to file with the Equal Employment Opportunity Commission). Retain three years, then destroy at discretion

- Patient registration forms—duplicates. Destroy at discretion

- Accounting

  - Accounts receivable adjustments. Retain two years, then destroy

  - Accounts receivable payments. Retain two years, then destroy; or microfilm at discretion, then destroy

  - Audits. Permanent or retain four years, then microfilm and destroy

  - Bank reconciliation statement. Retain two years, then destroy

  - Bank statements, canceled checks, checkbook stubs, check copies, and deposit slips. Retain five years, then destroy

  - Cash flow report. Retain five years, then destroy

  - Financial reports—daily and monthly. Retain two years, then destroy

  - Financial reports—year end. Retain five years, then destroy

  - Ledger sheets. Permanent in office or retain five years, then microfilm and destroy

- Petty cash reconciliation and request for reimbursement. Retain two years, then destroy

- Rates and charges. Retain ten years, then transfer to state archives; or microfilm at discretion and destroy

- Receipts and transmittals records. Retain five years, then destroy

- Receiving report. Retain two years, then destroy

- Reconciling items. Retain two years, then destroy

- Requisition and charges—patient services. Retain two years, then destroy

- Uncollectible debt records and certification statements. Retain two years after the governing body has directed that the debt be discharged and extinguished, then destroy

- Uniform billing form. Retain three years, then destroy

- Blood bank

  - Blood bank laboratory reports. Retain five years, then destroy

  - Blood donor records—information and release. Retain 10 years, then destroy

  - Blood transfusion record book. Retain 10 years, then destroy

- Central supply

  - Inventory control sheet or record. Retain five years, then destroy

- Insurance

  - Insurance claims paid. Retain five years, then destroy

  - Outpatient and inpatient insurance information forms. Retain one year after account is paid in full, then destroy

  - Provider billing for medical and other health services, medical insurance benefits, or physician's medical insurance benefits. Retain one year after account is paid in full, then destroy

  - Services or supplies provided by CHAMPUS. Retain two years after account paid in full, then destroy

- Laboratory

  - Autopsy reports and worksheets. Retain five years, then destroy

  - Laboratory quality control records. Retain three years, then destroy

  - Laboratory reports and worksheets. Retain three years, then destroy (original in medical records)

- Log books. Retain three years, then destroy

- Maintenance records. Retain three years, then destroy

- Specimens

  - Wet tissue. Retain one week after reported, then destroy

  - Paraffin blocks. Retain ten years if cancer case; five years if not, then destroy

  - Slides. Retain five years, then destroy

  - Blood smears. Retain one week, then destroy

  - Serum and cell samples. Retain three days, then destroy

- Statistical reports—lab. Retain five years, then destroy

- Maintenance

  - Inspection logs. Retain for life of equipment plus five years, then destroy at discretion

  - Preventative maintenance card. Retain for life of equipment plus five years, then destroy

- Nursing

  - Nursing history, nursing care plan, or healthcare plan and discharge records. If copies are maintained, retain three years, then destroy. Transfer originals to medical records

  - Private duty nurse records. Retain two years, then destroy

  - Shift schedules. Retain two years, then destroy

  - Ward personnel assignment shifts. Retain one year, then destroy

- Personnel and payroll

  - Collective bargaining agreements. Retain three years after superseded, then destroy at discretion

  - Earning record. Retain four years, then destroy

  - Employee contracts. Retain three years after termination, then destroy at discretion

  - Employee performance appraisal or evaluation records. If not periodically updated, destroy by shredding or burning because of confidential nature

  - Time cards or time sheets. Retain four years, then destroy

- Group enrollment card—health or life. Retain four years after inactive, then destroy
- Insurance claims (personnel only). Retain one year after settlement and if no litigation is pending, then destroy by shredding or burning because of confidential nature
- Job descriptions. One copy permanent in office. Destroy duplicates at discretion
- Payroll deduction authorization card—credit unions. Retain four years after no longer in force, then destroy by shredding or burning
- Payroll garnishment records. Retain four years after inactive, then destroy by shredding or burning
- Personnel file (master file) (employee physical examinations and medical history; termination records; chronological record and salary history; personnel information request forms; new employee registration sheet, applications, and hiring records). Permanent in office or retain four years after separation, then transfer to state archives or microfilm and destroy at discretion by shredding or burning. Other personnel records may be destroyed by shredding or burning four years after separation.
- Personnel hiring records. Retain two years after position filled, then destroy by shredding or burning
- W-2 wage and tax statement. Retain year-end forms four years, then destroy
- W-4 form (employees withholding exemption certificate). Retain four years after separation from employment or superseded, then destroy
- Worker's compensation records. Retain six years, then destroy
- Social security (F.I.C.A.) report—quarterly. Retain four years or until audited by Social Security, then destroy
- Pharmacy
  - Controlled substances—purchase orders. Retain five years, then destroy
  - Daily record of narcotics administered and narcotic disposition record. Retain five years, then destroy
  - Narcotics inventory control register. Retain five years, then destroy
  - Narcotic requisition. Retain five years, then destroy
  - Official order form for Schedule I and II controlled substances. Retain five years, then destroy

- Patient prescription log. Retain seven years, then destroy

- Perpetual inventory of controlled substances. Retain five years, then destroy

- Prescriptions. Retain seven years, then destroy

- Quality assurance

  - Infection control worksheets. Retain three years, then destroy

  - Quality assurance studies. Retain three years, then destroy

  - Quality control forms. Retain five years, then destroy

  - Quality control strips. Destroy at discretion

  - Room dismissal record. Retain three years, then destroy

  - Sterilization monitors. Retain five years, then destroy

- Surgery

  - Operating room register. Retain three years, then destroy

- X ray

  - Calibration reports—equipment. Retain 10 years, then transfer to state archives or microfilm at discretion and destroy

  - Diagnostic ultrasound report. Retain five years, then destroy (original in medical records)

  - Index file card. Retain five years, then destroy

  - Radiation reports. Retain five years, then transfer to state archives or microfilm at discretion and destroy

  - Records of radioisotopes—receipts, transfer, use, storage, delivery, and disposal. Retain five years, then transfer to state archives or microfilm at discretion and destroy

  - Requests for X-rays. Retain two weeks, then destroy

  - X-ray register of tests. Retain five years, then destroy

  - X-ray report forms. Retain department copy with x-ray film five years, then destroy (original in medical records)

  - X rays (film)—original. Retain five years, then destroy at discretion. Destroy copies at discretion[160]

---

160. Wyoming State Archives, Museum, and Historical Department, *Records Disposal Manual for Wyoming County Hospitals* (Feb. 20, 1987).

CHAPTER 17

What Media Can You Use for Business Records?

Media Generally

The dynamic nature of today's information technology applies to business records as well as to medical records. Healthcare providers must weigh the costs of retaining this critical information in original form versus other media. *See* Chapter 4 for a discussion of the considerations inherent in the selection of storage media.

Microfilming is permitted by almost all states and by the U.S. government.[1] However, providers must be certain that their staffs conduct microfilming during the regular course of business and "in good faith," that is, not only for records that are involved in an investigation or litigation. The provider should also be sure that it can produce a readable copy of the microfilmed records. Microfilm is most appropriate for bulky records of the same size that do not require frequent access.

Optical storage media has aspects of both microfilm and computer stored data. Like microfilm, optically stored data is hard to alter, but, like magnetic computer data, optically stored data cannot be read without being translated into visually readable form. Consequently, the evidentiary advantage microfilm has over computer-generated data, its unalterability, should result in unalterable optical storage data's admissibility. State statutes or evidence codes that talk about "any other information storage device" or use similar language should encompass optical storage systems. The Federal Rules of Evidence definition of "duplicate" as including "other equivalent techniques which accurately reproduce the original" would seem to authorize the use of optical storage systems (Rule 1001(4)). A recent amendment to the Uniform Photographic Copies of Business and Public Records Act would add optical imaging to the list of authorized reproductive techniques.

Information, such as Medicare payment data, recorded on a computer or other electronic device, and its output, such as a hard-copy printout, become the original physical records of that data and thereby become part of the provider's business records, subject to the same retention requirements.

Output, such as the printout, that is visually intelligible may be retained in that form in the regular course of business. The situation is more compli-

---

1. 28 U.S.C. § 1732 (1992).

cated when the output is not visually intelligible, such as a magnetic tape. In such cases, any future use of the data, as in a court case, would require turning the data into a written or visually understandable form.

Should the provider retain the unintelligible "original" or reproduce the output in an intelligible form and store it? The answer depends, in part, on state law. Under federal and many state laws, data can be reproduced from an unintelligible form and used as evidence. The law calls such evidence "duplicate originals."[2] However, providers must create and store the data in conformance with their established procedures in the normal course of their business. Facility personnel must, of course, properly operate the recording devices for such information to be admissible in court.

Federal Laws

28 U.S.C. § 1732 (1992) governs business and public records. The statute provides that if any business, institution, member of a profession or calling, or any department or agency of government, in the regular course of business, keeps any memorandum, writing, entry, print, or representation of any act, transaction, occurrence, or event, and in the regular course of business records, copies, or reproduces the original by any photographic, photostatic, microfilm, microcard, miniature photographic, or other process that accurately reproduces the original, the entity may destroy the original unless its preservation is required by law. Such reproduction is admissible in evidence to the same extent as the original was.

When a statute requires indefinite retention of a record, the retention of a photographic, microphotographic, or other reproduction suffices.[3] Photographs or microphotographs made in compliance with federal regulations have the same effect as the originals and are originals for the purposes of admissibility in evidence.[4]

The Public Health Service permits microfilming or other adequate copies of records required of grantees.[5] The Internal Revenue Service also permits the use of microfilm.[6]

The Food and Drug Administration,[7] the Occupational Safety and Health Administration (OSHA),[8] and the Veterans Administration also permit microfilming of records.[9]

Under federal law, no one may reproduce, by microfilm or otherwise, certain documents, such as naturalization records (i.e., certificates of citizen-

---

2. Federal Rule of Evidence § 1001(4).
3. 42 U.S.C. § 2112(a).
4. 44 U.S.C. § 3312.
5. *See* 45 C.F.R. § 74.20 (1991).
6. Revenue Procedure 81-46 1981-2 CB 621; Revenue Ruling 75-265, 1975 CB 460.
7. 21 C.F.R. § 58.195(g) (1991).
8. 29 C.F.R. § 1910.20 (1991).
9. 38 C.F.R. § 17 (1991).

ship), military identification cards, obligations or securities of the United States, currency, stamps, social security cards, copyrighted material without permission of the copyright holder, and licenses.[10]

State Laws

Although not all states specify what media are permissible for medical and other healthcare records, all states have laws governing business records. Some states may only specify whether business records reproduced by a particular medium are admissible in evidence, but such a law is sufficient to tell the healthcare provider what media it should consider, because records that are not admissible in evidence are not much help. If, for example, a business record shows that the facility complied with some state regulation, but the record is inadmissible, it will not help the facility avoid liability if it is taken to trial.

Many states have adopted rules based on the federal rules of evidence or Rule 803(6) of the Uniform Rules of Evidence. Others have adopted the Uniform Photographic Copies of Business and Public Records Act and the Uniform Business Records as Evidence Act.

ALABAMA

The Alabama Code § 12-21-44(a) (1991) covers business records generally and permits them to be photostated, photographed, or microphotographed on plate or film. Such copies are admissible in evidence (*Id.* § 12-21-43).

ALASKA

Alaska permits business records to be copied by photostatic, microfilm, microcard, or miniature photographic means, or reproduction in the regular course of business.[11]

ARIZONA

Arizona permits microfilming of records that may be used in court, regardless of whether the hard copy is extant. Business records may be copied by photostatic, microfilm, microcard, miniature photographic, or other reproduction in the regular course of business.[12]

ARKANSAS

Rule 1003 of the Arkansas Rules of Evidence states that a copy is admissible to the same extent as an original unless a genuine question exists as to the

---

10. E.g., 18 U.S.C. § 474 (1992) (treasury notes); 50 U.S.C. § 462 (1992) (Selective Service registration certificates).
11. Alaska Rule of Civil Procedure 44(c).
12. Arizona Revised Statutes Annotated § 12-2262 (1991).

authenticity of the original. Rule 1001 (4) defines "duplicates" as counterparts of the original made by photography, including enlargements or miniatures, mechanical or electronic rerecording, chemical reproduction, or other equivalent techniques that accurately reproduce the original. Business records may be reproduced by photograph, photostat, microfilm, microcard, miniature photographic, or other process that accurately reproduces the original,[13] and such records are admissible in evidence (*Id.* § 25-18-101).[14]

CALIFORNIA

The California Evidence Code § 1550 (West 1992) permits photostatic, microfilm, microcard, miniature photographic, or other photographic copy or reproduction to be admitted into evidence if made and preserved as a business record in the regular course of business. Business records are admissible in evidence (*Id.* §§ 1270–1272).

COLORADO

Colorado Revised Statutes §§ 13-26-102 (1991) permits copies by photographic, photostatic, microfilm, microcard, or other process that accurately reproduces or forms a durable medium for reproducing the original. Such reproductions are admissible in evidence.

CONNECTICUT

Connecticut General Statutes § 52-180 (1990) permits copying of business and public records by any photographic, photostatic, microfilm, microcard, miniature photographic, or other process that accurately reproduces or forms a durable medium for reproducing the original. Business records are admissible in evidence.

DELAWARE

Under Delaware's Uniform Rules of Evidence, a "duplicate" is a counterpart produced by the same impression as the original, or from the same matrix, or by means of photography, including enlargements and miniatures; mechanical or electronic rerecording; chemical reproduction; or other equivalent techniques that accurately reproduce the original (Rule 1001). Duplicates are admissible to the same extent as the original unless a genuine question is raised as to the authenticity of the original or unless it would be unfair to admit the duplicate instead of the original (Rule 1003). Records of regularly conducted activities are admissible if kept in the regular course of business (Rule 803(6)).

---

13. Arkansas Code Annotated § 16-46-101 (1991).
14. *Id.* § 25-18-101.

DISTRICT OF COLUMBIA

The District of Columbia follows the federal rules.

FLORIDA

The Florida Evidence Code specifies that duplicates are admissible to the same extent as the original unless the document is a negotiable instrument, a security, or any other writing that evidences a right to the payment of money, is not itself a security agreement or lease, and is of a type that is transferred by delivery in the ordinary course of business with any necessary endorsement or assignment. Such documents are admissible unless a genuine question is raised as to the authenticity of the original, or unless it would be unfair to admit the duplicate instead of the original.[15] A "duplicate" is a counterpart produced by the same impression as the original, or from the same matrix, or by means of photography, including enlargements and miniatures; mechanical or electronic rerecording; chemical reproduction; or other equivalent techniques that accurately reproduce the original or an executed carbon copy not intended by the parties to be an original.[16]

GEORGIA

The Georgia Code Annotated § 24-5-26 (Michie 1991) provides that a photostatic, microphotographic, or photographic reproduction of any original writing made in the regular course of business is admissible in evidence regardless of whether the original is available. Corporations may maintain their records "in written form or in another form capable of conversion into written form within a reasonable time" (*id.* § 14-2-1601). That statute recently added nonerasable optical images to the list of approved media.

HAWAII

Rule 803 of Hawaii's Uniform Rules of Evidence, governing hearsay exceptions, states that records including memoranda, reports, and data compilations of acts, events, conditions, opinions, or diagnoses, in any form, made in the course of a regularly conducted activity, in a timely manner, are not excluded by the hearsay rule.

Hawaii adds that a "duplicate" is a counterpart produced by the same impression as the original, or from the same matrix, or by means of photography, including enlargements and miniatures; mechanical or electronic rerecording; chemical reproduction; or other equivalent techniques that accurately reproduce the original (Rule 1001).

---

15. Florida Statutes Annotated § 90.953 (West 1990).
16. *Id.* § 90.951.

IDAHO

Idaho provides that if any business, institution, member of a profession or calling, or any department or agency of government, in the regular course of business, keeps any memorandum, writing, entry, print, or representation of any act, transaction, occurrence, or event, and in the regular course of business records, copies, or reproduces the original by any photographic, photostatic, microfilm, microcard, miniature photographic, or other process that accurately reproduces the original, the entity may destroy the original unless its preservation is required by law.[17] Such reproduction is admissible in evidence to the same extent as the original.

ILLINOIS

Illinois statutes define a copy as a "reproduction or durable medium for making a reproduction obtained by any photographic, photostatic, microfilm, microcard, miniature photographic or other process which accurately reproduces or forms a durable medium for reproducing the original."[18] If made in the regular course of business, such reproductions are admissible in evidence.[19]

The preservation of reproductions is equivalent to the preservation of originals.[20]

INDIANA

Indiana authorizes businesses to reproduce their records by any "photographic, photostatic or miniature photographic process which correctly, accurately, and permanently copies . . . the original."[21] A corporation may maintain its records in written form or in another form capable of conversion into written form within a reasonable time.[22]

IOWA

Iowa provides that if any business, institution, member of a profession or calling, or any department or agency of government, in the regular course of business, keeps any memorandum, writing, entry, print, or representation of any act, transaction, occurrence, or event, and in the regular course of business records, copies, or reproduces the original by any photographic, photostatic, microfilm, microcard, miniature photographic, or other process that accurately reproduces the original, the entity may destroy the original unless

---

17. Idaho Code § 9-417 (1991).
18. Illinois Revised Statutes ch. 116, ¶ 59 (1991).
19. *Id.* ch. 110, ¶ 236.
20. *Id.* ch. 116, ¶ 61.
21. Indiana Code § 34-3-15-1 (1991).
22. *Id.* § 32-1-52-1.

its preservation is required by law.[23] Such reproduction is admissible in evidence to the same extent as the original was. A 1991 act added electronic imaging and electronic data processing to the list of authorized media and also required that the reproduction be legible.[24]

KANSAS

Kansas statutes state that a corporation may, in the regular course of business, microfilm or reproduce business records by any other information storage device if the reports can be converted into clearly legible form within a reasonable period.[25] Photostatic, microfilm, microcard, miniature photographic, or other photographic copies made in the regular course of business are admissible in evidence.[26]

KENTUCKY

Kentucky provides that if any business, institution, member of a profession or calling, or any department or agency of government, in the regular course of business, keeps any memorandum, writing, entry, print, or representation of any act, transaction, occurrence, or event, and in the regular course of business records, copies, or reproduces the original by any photographic, photostatic, microfilm, microcard, miniature photographic, or other process that accurately reproduces the original, the entity may destroy the original unless its preservation is required by law.[27] Such reproduction is admissible in evidence to the same extent as the original.

LOUISIANA

Louisiana statutes allow any business to record, copy, or reproduce its records by any photographic, photostatic, or miniature photographic process that correctly, accurately, and permanently copies, reproduces, or forms a medium for copying and reproducing on a film or other durable material, if the reproduction is done in the regular course of business.[28]

MAINE

Business records are governed by Maine Revised Statutes Annotated tit. 16, § 456 (West 1991), which provides that if in the regular course of business a company keeps any memorandum, writing, entry, print, or representation of any act, transaction, occurrence, or event, and records, copies, or reproduces

---

23. Iowa Code § 622.30.2 (1991).
24. *Id.*
25. Kansas Statutes Annotated § 17-6514 (1990).
26. *Id.* § 60-469.
27. Kentucky Revised Statutes Annotated § 422.105 (Baldwin 1990).
28. Louisiana Revised Statutes Annotated § 3733 (West 1991).

the original by any photographic, photostatic, microfilm, microcard, miniature photographic, or other process that accurately reproduces the original, such reproduction is admissible in evidence to the same extent that the original was.

MARYLAND

The Maryland Courts and Judicial Proceedings Code Annotated art. 15B, § 1 (1990), defines a copy as a "reproduction or durable medium for making a reproduction obtained by any photographic, photostatic, microfilm, microcard, miniature photographic or other process which accurately reproduces or forms a durable medium for so reproducing the original." Such reproductions are admissible in evidence if made in the regular course of business (*id.* §§ 10-101 and 102).

MASSACHUSETTS

Massachusetts specifies that if any business, institution, member of a profession or calling, or any department or agency of government, in the regular course of business, keeps any memorandum, writing, entry, print, or representation of any act, transaction, occurrence, or event, and records, copies, or reproduces the original by any photographic, photostatic, microfilm, microcard, miniature photographic, or other process that accurately reproduces the original, the entity may destroy the original unless its preservation is required by law.[29] Such reproduction is admissible in evidence to the same extent as the original.

MICHIGAN

A business may record, copy, or reproduce its records by any photographic, photostatic, microfilm, microcard, or miniature photographic process that correctly reproduces the original, and may thereafter dispose of the original. Such copies made in the usual course of business are admissible under Michigan laws.[30]

MINNESOTA

Minnesota provides that if any business or similar organization, in the regular course of business, keeps or records a writing and causes it to be recorded, copied, or reproduced by any photographic, photostatic, microfilm, microcard, miniature photographic, optical disk imaging, or other process that accurately reproduces the original, it may be destroyed unless preservation is required by law.[31] Duplicates are admissible to the same extent as originals.[32]

---

29. Massachusetts General Laws ch. 233, § 79e (1992).
30. Michigan Compiled Laws §§ 600.2146–48 (1990).
31. Minnesota Statutes § 600.135 (1991).
32. Minnesota Rule of Evidence 1003.

MISSISSIPPI

Mississippi permits businesses to reproduce their records by any photographic, photostatic, or miniature photographic process that correctly, accurately, and permanently reproduces the original on a film or other durable material. Such reproductions are admissible in evidence.[33]

MISSOURI

Missouri provides that reproductions of original records shall be deemed to be originals for all purposes, provided the reproductions are equal in resolution to microfilm. Such reproductions are admissible in evidence in all courts or administrative agencies.[34] Business records are admissible in evidence if made during the regular course of business.[35]

MONTANA

Montana Rules of Evidence provide that a duplicate—a counterpart of the original produced by means of photography, mechanical or electric rerecording, chemical reproduction, or other equivalent techniques that accurately reproduce the original—is admissible to the same extent as the original unless someone raises a genuine question as to the original's authenticity.[36]

NEBRASKA

Nebraska statutes provide that a duplicate is admissible to the same extent as an original unless a genuine question exists as to the authenticity of the original or unless it would be unfair to admit the duplicate.[37] A duplicate is defined as a counterpart produced by the same impression as the original, or from the same matrix, or by means of photography, mechanical or electronic recording, chemical reproduction, or other equivalent techniques that accurately reproduce the original.[38]

NEVADA

Nevada defines a "duplicate" as a counterpart produced by a number of methods, such as photography, including enlargements and miniatures; mechanical or electronic rerecording; chemical reproduction; or other equivalent techniques.[39] A duplicate is admissible to the same extent as an original unless a genuine question exists as to the authenticity of the original, unless

---

33. Mississippi Code Annotated § 13-1-151 (1991).
34. Missouri Revised Statutes § 109.130 (1990).
35. *Id.* § 536.070.
36. Montana Rules of Evidence 1001 and 1003.
37. Nebraska Revised Statutes § 27-1003 (1990).
38. *Id.* § 27-1001.
39. Nevada Revised Statutes § 52.195 (1989).

it would be unfair to admit the duplicate, or if the custodian was authorized to destroy the original after duplicating it and did so.[40]

NEW HAMPSHIRE

For business records in general, New Hampshire defines a duplicate as a "reproduction or durable medium for making a reproduction obtained by any photographic, photostatic, microfilm, microcard, miniature photographic or other process which accurately reproduces or forms a durable medium for so reproducing the original."[41] Keeping such reproductions complies with all state laws requiring preservation of business records.[42] Records made in the regular course of business, including reproductions, are admissible in evidence.[43]

NEW JERSEY

New Jersey statutes provide that if any business, institution, member of a profession or calling, or any department or agency of government, in the regular course of business, keeps any memorandum, writing, entry, print, or representation of any act, transaction, occurrence, or event, and records, copies, or reproduces the original by any photographic, photostatic, microfilm, microcard, miniature photographic, or other process that accurately reproduces the original, the entity may destroy the original unless its preservation is required by law.[44] Such reproduction is admissible in evidence to the same extent that the original was.

NEW MEXICO

The New Mexico Rules of Evidence define a duplicate as "a counterpart produced by the same impression as the original, or from the same matrix, or by means of photography, including enlargements or miniatures, or by mechanical or electronic re-recording, or by chemical reproduction, or by other equivalent technique which accurately reproduces the original" (Rule 1001). A duplicate is admissible to the same extent as an original, unless a genuine question is raised as to the authenticity of the original or unless it would be unfair to admit the duplicate into evidence (Rule 1003).

NEW YORK

In New York, any business records made in the regular course of business are admissible in evidence.[45] If any business, or similar entity, in the regular

---

40. *Id.* § 52.245.
41. New Hampshire Revised Statutes Annotated §§ 337-A:1 to A:6 (1991).
42. *Id.*
43. *Id.* §§ 520:1–520:3.
44. New Jersey Revised Statutes § 2A:82-38 (1991).
45. New York Civil Practice Laws and Rules 4518 (McKinney 1992).

course of business, keeps or records a writing and causes it to be recorded, copied, or reproduced by any photographic, photostatic, microfilm, microcard, miniature photographic, optical disk imaging, or other process that accurately reproduces the original, the original may be destroyed unless preservation is required by law.[46]

NORTH CAROLINA

North Carolina statutes allow corporations,[47] and nonprofit organizations[48] to reproduce records or keep them on any information storage device, provided that they can be converted to legible form within a reasonable time. Such duplicates are admissible in evidence. If any business or member of a profession in the regular course of business keeps or records a memorandum, writing, entry, print, or representation, and records, copies, or reproduces it by any photographic, photostatic, microfilm, microcard, miniature photographic, or other process that accurately reproduces or forms a durable medium for reproducing the original, the entity may destroy the original unless it holds the record in a custodial or fiduciary capacity or unless its preservation is required by law.[49] Such reproductions are admissible in evidence.

NORTH DAKOTA

A memorandum, report, record, or data compilation, in any form, of acts, events, conditions, opinions, or diagnoses, made at or near the time, by or from information transmitted by a person with knowledge, is an exception to the hearsay rule, if kept in the regular course of business, unless the source of the information or method or circumstances indicate lack of trustworthiness.[50] A "duplicate" is a "counterpart produced by the same impression as the original, or from the same matrix, or by means of photography, including enlargements and miniatures; mechanical or electronic re-recording; chemical reproduction; or other equivalent techniques that accurately reproduce the original" (Rule 1001). A duplicate is admissible unless a genuine question is raised as to the authenticity of the original or it would be unfair to admit the duplicate instead of the original (Rule 1003).

OHIO

Ohio code specifies that a "photograph" includes a microphotograph, a roll or strip of film, a strip of microfilm, or a photostatic copy. Such a photograph is admissible in evidence if made in the regular course of business.[51] Similarly,

---

46. *Id.* 4539.
47. North Carolina General Statutes § 55-37.1 (1991).
48. *Id.* § 55A-27.1.
49. *Id.* § 8-45.1.
50. North Dakota Rule of Evidence 803(6).
51. Ohio Revised Code Annotated § 2317.41 (Baldwin 1991).

the Ohio Uniform Rules of Evidence define a "duplicate" as a counterpart produced by the same impression as the original, or from the same matrix, or by means of photography, including enlargements and miniatures; mechanical or electronic re-recording; chemical reproduction; or other equivalent techniques that accurately reproduce the original (Rule 1001). A duplicate is admissible unless a genuine question is raised as to the authenticity of the original or it would be unfair to admit the duplicate instead of the original (Rule 1003).

OKLAHOMA

Under Oklahoma Statutes, a duplicate means a reproduction or durable medium for making a reproduction obtained by any photographic, photostatic, microfilm, microcard, miniature photographic, or other process that accurately reproduces or forms a durable medium for so reproducing the original.[52] If in the regular course of business a person makes reproductions of original business records, the preservation of such reproductions constitutes compliance with any state law requiring that business records be kept or preserved.[53]

OREGON

Oregon permits photographic, microphotographic, or photographic reproduction of records. The Oregon Evidence Code provides that a duplicate is admissible in evidence to the same extent as an original unless a genuine question is raised as to the authenticity of the original or, unless in the circumstances, it would be unfair to admit the original.[54]

PENNSYLVANIA

Pennsylvania Statutes provide that if any business or member of a profession, in the regular course of business, keeps or records a memorandum, writing, entry, print, or representation, and records, copies, or reproduces it by any photographic, photostatic, microfilm, microcard, miniature photographic, or other process that accurately reproduces or forms a durable medium for reproducing the original, the entity may destroy the original unless its preservation is required by law.[55] Such reproductions are admissible in evidence,[56] as are records kept in the regular course of business.[57]

---

52. Oklahoma Statutes tit. 67, § 251 (1991).
53. *Id.* § 253.
54. Oregon Revised Statutes § 40.560 (1989).
55. Pennsylvania Statutes Annotated tit. 42, § 6109 (1991).
56. *Id.*
57. *Id.* § 6108.

RHODE ISLAND

The Rhode Island Rules of Evidence provide that records of regularly conducted activity, kept in the regular course of business, are admissible (Rule 803(6)). A duplicate is defined as a counterpart produced by the same impression as the original, or from the same matrix, or by means of photography, mechanical or electronic rerecording, chemical reproduction, or by ar.y other equivalent technology that accurately reproduces the original (Rule 1101(4)). Such duplicates are admissible unless a genuine question exists as to their authenticity or, unless under the circumstances, it would be unfair to admit the duplicate (Rule 1003).

SOUTH CAROLINA

The South Carolina Code Annotated § 19-5-610 (Law. Co-op. 1990) states that if any business, or member of a profession, in the regular course of business keeps or records a memorandum, writing, entry, print, or representation, and records, copies, or reproduces it by any photographic, photostatic, microfilm, microcard, miniature photographic, or other process that accurately reproduces or forms a durable medium for reproducing the original, the entity may destroy the original in the regular course of business unless it holds the record in a custodial or fiduciary capacity or unless its preservation is required by law. Such reproductions are admissible in evidence (*id.*). Photographic copies of business records and disposal of the originals are authorized (*id.* § 39-1-40).

SOUTH DAKOTA

South Dakota Rules of Evidence define a "duplicate" as a "counterpart produced by the same impression as the original, or from the same matrix, or by means of photography, including enlargements and miniatures, or by mechanical or electronic rerecording, or by chemical reproduction, or by other equivalent techniques which accurately reproduce the original."[58] Such duplicates are admissible unless a genuine question is raised as to the authenticity of the original or it would be unfair to admit the duplicate instead of the original.[59] If any business or member of a profession during the regular course of business reproduces a record by a photographic, photostatic, microfilm, microcard, miniature photographic, or other process that accurately reproduces or forms a durable medium for reproducing the original, the original may be destroyed in the regular course of business unless held in a custodial or fiduciary capacity or unless its preservation is required by law. Such reproduction is admissible in evidence.[60]

---

58. South Dakota Codified Laws Annotated § 19-18-1(4) (1991).
59. *Id.* § 19-18-3.
60. *Id.* § 19-7-12.

TENNESSEE

A memorandum, report, record, or data compilation, in any form, of acts, events, conditions, opinions, or diagnoses, made at or near the time, by or from information transmitted by a person with knowledge, is an exception to the hearsay rule, if kept in the regular course of business, unless the source of the information or method or circumstances indicate lack of trustworthiness.[61] A "duplicate" is a "counterpart produced by the same impression as the original, or from the same matrix, or by means of photography, including enlargements and miniatures, or by mechanical or electronic rerecording, or by chemical reproduction, or by other equivalent techniques which accurately reproduce the original" (Rule 1001). Such duplicates are admissible unless a genuine question is raised as to the authenticity of the original (Rule 1003).

TEXAS

The Texas Rules of Evidence provide that records of a regularly conducted activity, kept in the regular course of business, are admissible (Rule 803(6)). A duplicate is defined as a counterpart produced by the same impression as the original, or from the same matrix, or by means of photography, mechanical or electronic rerecording, chemical reproduction, or by any other equivalent technology that accurately reproduces the original (Rule 1101(4)). Such duplicates are admissible unless a genuine question exists as to their authenticity or unless, under the circumstances, it would be unfair to admit the duplicate (Rule 1003).

The Texas Business and Commerce Code governs retention of business records and defines them as including letters, words, sounds, or numbers, or their equivalent, recorded by handwriting, typewriting, printing, photostat, photograph, magnetic impulse, mechanical or electronic recording, or another form of data compilation.[62]

UTAH

The Utah Code provides that if any business or member of a profession during the regular course of business reproduces a record by a photographic, photostatic, microfilm, microcard, miniature photographic, or other process that accurately reproduces or forms a durable medium for reproducing the original, the original may be destroyed in the regular course of business unless held in a custodial or fiduciary capacity or unless its preservation is required by law. Such reproductions are admissible in evidence.[63]

---

61. Tennessee Rule of Evidence 803(6).
62. Texas Business and Commerce Code Annotated § 35.48 (West 1991).
63. Utah Code Annotated § 78-25-16 (1992).

VERMONT

Vermont Statutes Annotated tit. 12, § 1701 (1991), specify that if any business or member of a profession during the regular course of business reproduces a record by a photographic, photostatic, microfilm, microcard, miniature photographic, or other process that accurately reproduces or forms a durable medium for reproducing the original, the original may be destroyed unless held in a custodial or fiduciary capacity or unless its preservation is required by law. Such reproductions are admissible in evidence (*id.*)

VIRGINIA

Concerning business records, Virginia defines copies to include photographs, microphotographs, photostats, microfilm, microcard, printouts or other reproductions of electronically stored data, or any other reproduction of an original from a process that forms a durable medium for its recording, storing, and reproducing. Such copies made in the regular course of business are admissible in evidence.[64]

WASHINGTON

Business records are governed by the Washington Revised Code § 5.46.010 (1991), which specifies that if any business or member of a profession during the regular course of business reproduces a record by a photographic, photostatic, microfilm, microcard, miniature photographic, or other process that accurately reproduces or forms a durable medium for reproducing the original, the original may be destroyed in the regular course of business unless held in a custodial or fiduciary capacity or unless its preservation is required by law. Such reproductions are admissible in evidence (*id.*).

WEST VIRGINIA

The West Virginia Rules of Evidence provide that records of regularly conducted activity, kept in the regular course of business, are admissible (Rule 803(6)). A duplicate is defined as a counterpart produced by the same impression as the original, or from the same matrix, or by means of photography, or by a mechanical or electronic rerecording, or by chemical reproduction, or by any other equivalent technology that accurately reproduces the original (Rule 1101(4)). Such duplicates are admissible unless a genuine question exists as to their authenticity or, unless under the circumstances, it would be unfair to admit the duplicate (Rule 1003).

---

64. Virginia Code Annotated § 8.01-391 (Michie 1991).

WISCONSIN

For records generally, Wisconsin's Rules of Evidence define a "duplicate" as a counterpart produced by the same impression as the original, or from the same matrix, or by means of photography, including enlargements and miniatures, mechanical or electronic rerecording, chemical reproduction, or by any other equivalent technique that accurately reproduces the original.[65] A duplicate is admissible to the same extent as the original, unless a genuine question is raised as to the authenticity of the original or unless it would be unfair to admit the duplicate in lieu of the original.[66] Businesses and professions are permitted to destroy originals if they have made a copy by a photographic, photostatic, microfilm, microcard, miniature photographic, or other process that accurately reproduces the originals. Such copies are admissible.[67] Records made in the regular course of business are admissible as against a hearsay objection.[68]

WYOMING

The Wyoming Rules of Evidence provide that records of regularly conducted activity, kept in the regular course of business, are admissible (Rule 803(6)). A duplicate is defined as a counterpart produced by the same impression as the original, or from the same matrix, or by means of photography, mechanical or electronic rerecording, chemical reproduction, or by any other equivalent technology that accurately reproduces the original (Rule 1101(4)). Such duplicates are admissible unless a genuine question exists as to their authenticity or, unless under the circumstances, it would be unfair to admit the duplicate (Rule 1003).

---

65. Wisconsin Statutes § 910.1 (1989-1990).
66. *Id.* § 910.03.
67. *Id.* § 889.29.
68. *Id.* § 908.03(6).

Condition of Participation: Medical Record Services, Health Care Financing Administration, 42 C.F.R., Chapter 4, § 482.24

The hospital must have a medical record service that has administrative responsibility for medical records. A medical record must be maintained for every individual evaluated or treated in the hospital.

(a) Standard: Organization and staffing: The organization of the medical record service must be appropriate to the scope and complexity of the services performed. The hospital must employ adequate personnel to ensure prompt completion, filing, and retrieval of records.

(b) Standard: Form and retention of record. The hospital must maintain a medical record for each inpatient and outpatient. Medical records must be accurately written, promptly completed, properly filed and retained, and accessible. The hospital must use a system of author identification and record maintenance that ensures the integrity of the authentication and protects the security of all record entries.

  (1) Medical records must be retained in their original or legally reproduced form for a period of at least five years.

  (2) The hospital must have a system of coding and indexing medical records. The system must allow for timely retrieval by diagnosis and procedure, in order to support medical care evaluation studies.

  (3) The hospital must have a procedure for ensuring the confidentiality of patient records. Information forms or copies of records may be released only to authorized individuals, and the hospital must ensure that unauthorized individuals cannot gain access to or alter patient records. Original medical records must be released by the hospital only in accordance with Federal or State laws, court orders, or subpoenas.

(c) Standard: Content of record. The medical record must contain information to justify admission and continued hospitalization, support for the diagnosis, and describe the patient's progress and response to medications and services.

  (1) All entries must be legible and complete, and must be authenticated and dated promptly by the person (identified by name and disci-

pline) who is responsible for ordering, providing, or evaluating the service furnished.

(i)   The author of each entry must be identified and must authenticate his or her entry.

(ii)   Authentication may include signatures, written initials, or computer entry.

(2)   All records must document the following, as appropriate:

(i)   Evidence of a physical examination, including a health history, performed no more than seven days prior to admission or within 48 hours after admission.

(ii)   Admitting diagnosis.

(iii)   Results of all consultative evaluations of the patient and appropriate findings by clinical and other staff involved in the care of the patient.

(iv)   Documentation of complications, hospital acquired infections, and unfavorable reaction to drugs and anesthesia.

(v)   Properly executed informed consent forms for procedures and treatments specified by the medical staff, or by Federal or State law if applicable, to acquire written patient consent.

(vi)   All practitioner's orders, nursing notes, reports of treatment, medication records, radiology, and laboratory reports, and vital signs and other information necessary to monitor the patient's condition.

(vii)   Discharge summary with outcome of hospitalization, disposition of care, and provisions for follow-up care.

(viii) Final diagnosis with completion of medical records within 30 days following discharge.

Recommended Retention Period for Hospital Records

To be used when your state or the federal government does not specify a retention period.

Record	Suggested Period of Retention	Remarks
Administrative Offices		
Accident (or incident reports)	6 years	
Annual reports	Permanent	
Appraisal reports	Permanent	
Audit reports	Permanent	
Birth records to local government	Permanent	
Census (daily)	5 years	
Communicable disease reports	3 years	
Constitution and bylaws	Permanent	
Construction projects	Permanent	
Correspondence	5 years	Retain only that of continuing interest. Review annually.
Death records to local government	Permanent	
Endowments, trusts, bequests	Permanent	
Insurance policies, expired	6 years	
Licenses, permits, contracts	Permanent	
Minutes of meetings of board of directors, executive committees, and medical staff	Permanent	
Permits (alcohol & narcotics)	Life of permit plus 6 years	

Record	Suggested Period of Retention	Remarks
Physician's personnel records	Permanent	
Policies and procedure manuals	Life of manual plus 6 years	
Property records		
deeds, titles	Permanent	
leases	Term of lease plus 6 years	
Reports (departmental)	Many daily and nonannual reports can be destroyed after year-end statistics are compiled	
Statistics on admissions, services, discharges	Permanent	

Admissions and Discharges

Listings	6 years	
Register	Permanent	

Business Office

Alien—statement of income paid	So long as contents may be material in the administration of an Internal Revenue law (26 C.F.R. 1.6001-1)	
Bank statements	6 years	
Budgets	5 years	
Cash receipts	6 years	
Cashier's tapes from bookkeeping machine	5 years	
Charge (slips) to patients	5 years	
Checks (canceled)		
Payroll	7 years	

Record	Suggested Period of Retention	Remarks
Voucher	10 years	
Check registers	6 years	
Correspondence		
Credit and collections	7 years	
General	6 years	
Insurance	4 years	
Deposits (bank)	2 years	
Equipment (depreciation records)	Permanent	
Income (daily summary)	5 years	
Income tax returns	Permanent	
Invoices		
Fixed assets	Permanent/life of Asset plus 6 years	
Accounts receivable	6 years	
Accounts payable	6 years	
Journals (general)	Permanent	
Ledgers (general)	Permanent	
Ledger cards (patients')	7 years	
Payroll		
Bonds	10 years	
Insurance	8 years	
Individual earnings	Term of employment plus 6 years	
Journals	25 years	
Rate schedules	6 years	
Social security reports	4 years	
Time cards	5 years	
Withholding tax exemption (W-4 forms)	4 years	
Withholding tax statements (W-2 forms)	4 years after taxes paid	
Posting audits	7 years	
Unemployment tax records	4 years	
Vouchers		
Capital expenditures	Permanent/life of item plus 6 years	
Cash	10 years	
Welfare agency records	7 years	

Record	Suggested Period of Retention	Remarks
Clinic		
Appointment books	3 years	
Encounter statistics	1 year	Daily and monthly reports
Medical records	10 years from date of last visit	
Patients' name index	Permanent	
Social service confidential case Histories	5 years	
Welfare agency records	7 years	
Dietary		
Food costs	5 years	
Meal counts	5 years	
Menus	2 years	
Engineering		
Blueprints of buildings	Permanent	
Calibration records	6 years	
Equipment records by location	Life of equipment plus 6 years	
Equipment records in inspection and maintenance	5 years including meter charts	
Equipment operating instructions	Life of equipment plus 6 years	
Inspection of grounds and buildings	1 year	
Maintenance log	6 years	
Purchase orders	10 years	
Temperature charts	2 years	
Watchman clock dials	2 years	
Work orders	2 years	
Laboratory, Therapy and X ray		
Appointment books	3 years	

Record	Suggested Period of Retention	Remarks
Blood banks		
Adverse reactions to transfusions	5 years	
Blood donor histories, examination, consent, reactions, and results of required tests performed on plasmapheresis and cytapheresis donors	5 years	
ABO and Rh types	5 years	
Blood test results, interpretations, and release (issue) data for compatibility testing	5 years	
Final disposition of blood and components	5 years	
Refrigeration and blood inspection records	5 years	
Transfusion request records	5 years	
Electrocardiogram tracings	10 years—unusual cases permanent	
Electroencephalogram tracings	Until litigation is settled. Uncut tracings to be retained in medical-legal disputes. 5 years for normal cut-outs (reduced approximately five-sixths), 10 years for abnormal cut-outs	
Fetal monitoring	Permanent/10 years	
Index to patient's records	10 years; unusual cases Permanent	
Psychiatric reports to state health departments	Permanent	
Radioisotopes (receipt, transfer use, storage, delivery, disposal, and reports of overexposure	Permanent (10 C.F.R. 30.51)	

Record	Suggested Period of Retention	Remarks
Registers (chronological of tests)	5 years or until hospital statistics are compiled	
Requests for tests	2 weeks	
Research papers published	Permanent	
Test results (clinical laboratory)	3 months except for cases of unusual interest	
Therapy treatment records (inpatient and outpatient)	5 years where not duplicated in medical records	

Medical Records

Record	Suggested Period of Retention	Remarks
Annual reports to government agencies	Permanent	
Birth registration copy	Permanent	
Death registration copy	Permanent	
Delivery room log	Permanent	
Disease index	10 years to permanent	
Emergency room reports	10 years	
Fetal heart rate monitoring	10 years	
Operation index	10 years to permanent	
Indexes to patients' medical records	Permanent	
Patient index	Permanent	
Patients' medical records	10 years after most recent care usage	
Physician index	10 years	
Surgery log	Permanent	
Tumor registry files	Permanent	

Miscellaneous Departments

Record	Suggested Period of Retention	Remarks
Housekeeping room record	5 years	
Return goods memoranda	1 year if records are duplicated in business office	

Record	Suggested Period of Retention	Remarks
Nursing		
Application (nonemployees)	2 years	
Attendance and time records	2 years. Copy in business office	
Minutes of meetings	Permanent	
Personnel records	6 years after termination	
Policies and procedures	6 years after revision	
Private duty name file	6 years after last use	
Staffing records	6 years	
Training (course outlines and examinations)	Permanent	
Personnel		
Absence reports	5 years	
Application (nonemployees)	4 years	
Employee health records	5 years after termination of employment	
Employee history	5 years in full. After 5 years, reduce to payroll card rate	
Garnishment records	7 years	
Job classifications	Permanent	
Overtime reports	5 years	
Payroll and time records	5 years	
Pension records	Permanent	
Vacation lists	2 years	
Volunteer service (certification of hospital workers)	2 years after termination	
Pharmacy		
Controlled substances (inventory and orders)	2 years	

Record	Suggested Period of Retention	Remarks
Controlled substances (dispensed and administered)	2 years. In a separate file keep daily records showing kind and quantity of narcotics dispensed or administered, the names and addresses of persons on whose authority and the purpose for which dispensed or administered (21 C.F.R. 304.04).	
Methadone	3 years. Maintain clinical record for each patient showing dates, quantity, and batch or code mark (21 C.F.R. 310.505).	
Other prescriptions	2 years	

Public Relations

Record	Suggested Period of Retention	Remarks
Clipping (historical)	Permanent	
Contributor records	Permanent	
Photographs (institutional)	Permanent	
Publications (house organs)	Permanent	

Purchasing and Receiving

Record	Suggested Period of Retention	Remarks
Packing slips	3 months	
Purchase orders	2 years. Copy on record on voucher in business office	
Purchase requisitions	3 years	
Receiving report	5 years. Copy on record on voucher in business office	
Returned goods credit	2 years. Copy on record on voucher in business office	

American Medical Association's Confidentiality Statement

The information disclosed to a physician during the course of the relationship between physician and patient is confidential to the greatest possible degree. The patient should feel free to make a full disclosure of information to the physician in order that the physician may most effectively provide needed services. The patient should be able to make this disclosure with the knowledge that the physician will respect the confidential nature of the communication. The physician should not reveal confidential communications or information without the express consent of the patient, unless required to do so by law.

The obligation to safeguard patient confidences is subject to certain exceptions which are ethically and legally justified because of overriding social considerations. Where a patient threatens to inflict serious bodily harm to another person and there is a reasonable probability that the patient may carry out the threat, the physician should take reasonable precautions for the protection of the intended victim, including notification of law enforcement authorities. Also, communicable diseases, gun shot and knife wounds should be reported as required by applicable statutes or ordinances.

Section 5.05, *Current Opinions of the Council on Ethical and Judicial Affairs of the American Medical Association,* 1989. Reprinted with permission.

Uniform Photographic Copies of Business and Public Records Act

Photographic copies of business and public records as evidence.

(a) This section may be cited as the Uniform Photographic Copies of Business and Public Records as Evidence Act.

(b) (1) If any business, institution, member of a profession or calling, or any department or agency of government, in the regular course of business or activity has kept or recorded any memorandum, writing, entry, print, representation or combination thereof, of any act, transaction, occurrence or event, and in the regular course of business has caused any or all of the same to be recorded, copied or reproduced by any photographic, photostatic, microfilm, microcard, miniature photographic, or other process which accurately reproduces or forms a durable medium for so reproducing the original, the original may be destroyed in the regular course of business unless its preservation is required by law.

(2) Such reproduction, when satisfactorily identified, is as admissible in evidence as the original itself in any judicial or administrative proceeding whether the original is in existence or not and an enlargement or facsimile of such reproduction is likewise admissible in evidence if the original reproduction is in existence and available for inspection under direction of court.

(3) The introduction of a reproduced record, enlargement or facsimile does not preclude admission of the original.

(c) This section shall be so interpreted and construed as to effectuate its general purpose of making uniform the law of those states which enact it.

Uniform Business Records as Evidence Act

(a) This section may be cited as the "Uniform Business Records as Evidence Act."

(b) The term "business" shall include every kind of business, profession, occupation, calling or operation of institutions, whether carried on for profit or not.

(c) A record of an act, condition or event, shall, insofar as relevant, be competent evidence if the custodian or other qualified witness, testifies to its identity and the mode of its preparation, and if it was made in the regular course of business, at or near the time of the act, condition or event, and if, in the opinion of the court, the sources of information, method and time of preparation were such as to justify its admission.

(d) This section shall be so interpreted and construed as to effectuate its general purpose to make uniform the law of those states which enact it.

AHA Statement on Preservation of Medical Records

Since a hospital or other health care institution is seldom requested to produce medical records older than ten (10) years for clinical, scientific, legal, or audit purposes, it is ordinarily sufficient to retain the medical records of cases ten (10) years after the most recent patient care usage in the absence of legal considerations. Accordingly, it is recommended that complete patient medical records in health care institutions usually be retained either in the original or reproduced form, for a period of ten (10) years after the most recent patient care usage. After this period, such records may be destroyed unless destruction is specifically prohibited by statute, ordinance, regulation, or law, provided that the institution:

1. retains basic information such as dates of admission and discharge, names of responsible physicians, record of diagnoses and operations, operative reports, pathology reports, and discharge resumes for all records so destroyed;

2. retains complete medical records of minors for the period of minority plus the applicable statute of limitations as prescribed by statute in the state in which the health care institution is located;

3. retains complete medical records of patients under mental disability in like manner as those of patients under disability of minority; and

4. retains complete patient medical records for longer periods of time when requested in writing by one of the following:

   a. an attending or consultant physician of the patient,

   b. the patient or someone acting legally in his behalf, or

   c. legal counsel for a party having an interest affected by the patient medical records.

Glossary

Abstract. A condensation of a record.

Accredited record technician (ART). A person who is certified as an expert, although not on as high a level as a registered record administrator, by the American Medical Record Association.

Acquisition. The takeover of another business by a purchaser.

Admission. An acknowledgment that an allegation of the opposing party in a lawsuit is true.

Authentication. An attestation that something, such as a record, is genuine.

Consent. Voluntary agreement. Consent may be express (oral or written) or implied (demonstrated by silence or actions).

Defendant. The party against whom a plaintiff brings a lawsuit seeking some relief from a harm that the defendant allegedly caused him or her.

Deposition. A written record of oral testimony, in the form of questions and answers, made before a notary or other public officer, to discover evidence for a lawsuit or to be read into evidence at trial.

Discovery. Pretrial proceedings in which the opposing parties get factual information concerning the matter in controversy. The tools of discovery are depositions, interrogatories, requests for admissions, inspections of documents, physical and mental examinations, and inspections.

Duplicate. One of two documents that are the same. Many state and federal laws provide that certain copies, such as microfilm copies, are duplicate originals.

Felony. A serious offense usually punishable by death or imprisonment in the state penitentiary for one year or more.

Informed consent. Agreement based upon complete understanding of the nature of the undertaking including the risks thereof.

Interrogatories. Written questions asked by one side to a lawsuit of another party. The person queried must answer in writing, under oath. Used in discovery proceedings.

Media. The materials upon which information is stored, such as microfilm or diskette.

Medical record. A record that identifies the patient and specifies the care he or she received.

Merger. The union of two or more businesses or organizations into a single new one.

Microfilm. A photographic medium on which documents can be greatly reduced in size.

Minor. A person who has not yet reached the age of majority so as to be considered an adult by law.

Misdemeanor. Any crime that is not a felony. A minor offense usually punishable by a lesser penalty than imprisonment in the state penitentiary for one year.

Negligence. A failure to use due care.

Original document. An authentic writing as opposed to a copy.

Plaintiff. The party who brings a lawsuit complaining of some harm done him or her by the defendant.

Punitive damages. Sometimes called exemplary damages. Damages in excess of the amount that would compensate the plaintiff for injury suffered awarded to punish the defendant for misconduct.

Record. As a noun, the preservation of information or data on some medium so that it may be read at some future time.

Records management. The supervision of records so that they are properly created, processed, stored and retrieved, and disposed of.

Records retention program. The plan that specifies how long a facility keeps its records.

Regular course of business. Doing business activities in accordance with your usual habit or custom.

Registered record administrator (RRA). A person who is registered as such an expert by the American Medical Record Association.

Regulation. A rule issued by a governmental agency other than the legislature. Unless a regulation conflicts with the constitution or a statute, it has the force of law.

Statute of limitations. A period of time, fixed by federal or state law, during which a plaintiff may bring a lawsuit and after which, his or her claim is barred.

Subpoena. A subpoena commands a person to appear at a trial or other hearing and give testimony.

Subpoena *duces tecum.* A subpoena *duces tecum* commands the person to bring with him or her certain records or documents in his or her custody or possession.

Index

About the Author

Jonathan P. Tomes is Visiting Associate Professor at IIT Chicago—Kent College of Law, where he teaches hospital law and other subjects. As a retired army officer, he adjudicated and defended medical malpractice claims against government healthcare providers. He is the author of a number of books in healthcare legal issues, including *The Trustee's Guide to Understanding Medical Staff Privileges* (HFMA, 1992) *Antitrust Law: A Guide for the Healthcare Professional* (HFMA, 1993). *Healthcare Fraud, Waste, Abuse and Safe Harbors: The Complete Legal Guide* (Probus/HFMA, 1993).